Handbook of
Medical Device
Design

Handbook of
Medical Device
Design

edited by
Richard C. Fries
Datex-Ohmeda, Inc.
Madison, Wisconsin

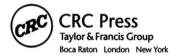

CRC Press
Taylor & Francis Group
Boca Raton   London   New York

CRC Press is an imprint of the
Taylor & Francis Group, an informa business

ISBN: 0-8247-0399-5

This book is printed on acid-free paper.

Headquarters
Marcel Dekker
270 Madison Avenue, New York, NY 10016
tel: 212-696-9000; fax: 212-685-4540

The publisher offers discounts on this book when ordered in bulk quantities. For more information, write to Special Sales/Professional Marketing at the headquarters address above.

Current printing (last digit):
10 9 8 7 6 5 4 3 2

PRINTED IN THE UNITED STATES OF AMERICA

To

Alexa Bayley Fries

whose smile, laughter,

and enthusiasm for life

make you a very special young lady

Preface

The medical device field is one of rapid technological innovation. The process of designing and producing medical devices has become an increasingly more difficult one, as the number of standards and regulations constantly increases, the functionality of devices becomes more complex, and the expectations of the customer regarding price, reliability, and life cycle costs becomes more demanding.

This handbook has been written to give those professionals working in the development and use of medical devices practical knowledge about biomedical technology, regulations, and their relationship to quality health care. This handbook includes practical techniques which a developer and manufacturer of medical devices may incorporate in their processes to improve the methodology of designing and manufacturing medical devices, but to improve the functionality and reliability of the device as well.

The layout of the handbook follows a typical product development process. Section 1 addresses the determination and documentation of device requirements. The first action is determining customer needs. Once these have been determined, product and then design specifications must be developed and documented, including designing for manufacturing and designing for service. This is also the time to establish certain reliability and quality metrics that can be monitored throughout the product development cycle.

Section 2 addresses the current regulatory and standards issues. Of special interest to medical device manufacturers are FDA regulations, the ISO 9000 series, the Medical Device Directives. In addition, the section discusses current standards and regulations from countries such as Canada, Japan, and Australia. The section also address intellectual property considerations, such as patents, copyrights, and trademarks.

Section 3 discusses actual design issues, by specialty, as well as corollary issues pertinent to completing a well conceived, well controlled design. Current design topics are discussed in the areas of electrical, mechanical, software, industrial design, and human factors. Preparing and maintaining the necessary project files is discussed with examples of what is included in each. Other important issues that are addressed in this section include biocompatibility, safety/risk analysis, reliability, third party certification, technical documentation, translations, and life cycle costs.

Section 4 addresses the important topics of verification and validation. Once the design is completed, it must be verified that its functionality meets the requirements that were originally documented. In addition, the design must be proven to be robust and reliable over time. An overview of verification and validation is provided followed by a detailed investigation of electrical, mechanical, and software verification and validation.

Section 5 examines the manufacturing process, because even if the product is designed to meet appropriate standards and to be very reliable, unless the product is manufactured to the same high standards, the product will be a failure. This section discusses the various aspects of the manufacturing process, the validation of the manufacturing process, the particular requirements of the Quality System Regulation that apply to manufacturing, and finally, how to prepare for a quality system audit.

Knowledge of essential design, product development, quality assurance, and regulatory requirements and techniques is an essential part of every medical device development process. It is hoped that this handbook will be an invaluable resource in helping medical device manufacturers develop a safe, effective, and reliable product development process.

I am indebted to the authors, not only for their contributions, but for advice and suggestions that helped shape this text.

Richard C. Fries

Contents

Preface...*v*
Contributors..*xvii*

Section 1   Standards and Regulations.....................................1

Chapter 1   FDA Regulations...3
                Richard C. Fries
1.1   History of Device Regulation..4
1.2   Device Classification..5
1.3   Registration and Listing..9
1.4   Good Laboratory Practices (GLP)...............................10
1.5   Good Manufacturing Practices (GMP)........................10
1.6   Human Factors...11
1.7   Design Control..11
1.8   Software..12
1.9   The FDA Inspection...14
1.10   Dealing with the FDA..15
                References..16

Chapter 2   Preparing an FDA Submission....................................21
                Richard C. Fries
2.1   Device Classification..22
2.2   The Traditional 510(k)..26

2.3   Special 510(k)..34
2.4   Abbreviated 510(k)..36
2.5   Declaration of Conformity to a Recognized Standard..........37
2.6   PMA Application...38
2.7   Investigational Device Exemptions............................40
2.8   Software Classification..43
           References..44

Chapter 3 European Standards and Regulations............................49
           Richard C. Fries
3.1   The European Regulatory Scene................................51
3.2   European Directives..52
3.3   European Standardization Bodies..............................53
3.4   European Standards Development Process....................55
3.5   Other European Standards Considerations....................58
3.6   Conformity Assessment and Testing...........................60
3.7   European Organization for Testing and Certification..........62
3.8   Examples of European Directives and Regulations............64
3.9   Medical Informatics..67
3.10   The Global Harmonization Task Force........................69
           References..72

Chapter 4 The Medical Device Directives.................................75
           Richard C. Fries
4.1   Definition of a Medical Device.................................76
4.2   The Medical Device Directives Process........................77
4.3   Choosing the Appropriate Directive............................77
4.4   Identifying the Applicable Essential Requirements............78
4.5   Identification of Corresponding Harmonized Standards.......81
4.6   Assurance that the Device Meets the Essential
           Requirements and Harmonized Standards....................82
4.7   Classification of the Device.....................................91
4.8   Decision on the Appropriate Conformity
           Assessment Procedure...94
4.9   Type Testing...97
4.10   Identification and Choice of a Notified Body.................98
4.11   Establishing a Declaration of Conformity....................102
4.12   Application of the CE Mark....................................103
4.13   Conclusion..103
           References..105

Chapter 5 The Basics of ISO 9001......................................107
           Tina Juneau
5.1   Historical Perspective...108

Contents

5.2	ISO 9001 Revision Year 2000	108
5.3	Requirement Synopses	110
	References	132

Chapter 6	Design of Medical Devices for the Canadian Market	133
	Paul Fabry	
6.1	Fundamental Safety and Effectiveness Principles	134
6.2	Device Classification	137
6.3	Labeling	137
6.4	Standards and the Design Process	139
6.5	Implant Registration	141
6.6	*In Vitro* Diagnostic Devices (IVDDs)	142
6.7	Electrically Operated Medical Devices	142
6.8	Medical Devices Incorporating Plumbing Features	146
6.9	Summary	146
	References	147

Chapter 7	Pacific Rim Standards and Regulations	149
	Richard C. Fries	
7.1	Australia	150
7.2	Japan	158
7.3	Russia	162
7.4	China	163
	References	164

Chapter 8	Overview of Software Standards	167
	Nancy George	
8.1	History	169
8.2	Major Standards Organizations	171
8.3	The FDA's Interest in Standards	171
8.4	ISO/IEC 12207 Information Technology – Software Life Cycle Process	172
8.5	The FDA Recognizes ISO/IEC 12207	174
8.6	Tailoring ISO/IEC 12207 for the Medical Device Business Sector	181
8.7	Summary	200
	References	200

Section 2	**Determining and Documenting Requirements**	**203**

Chapter 9	Defining the Device	205
	Richard C. Fries	
9.1	The Product Definition Process	207

Contents

9.2	Overview of Quality Function Deployment	210
9.3	The QFD Process	210
9.4	Summary of QFD	218
9.5	The Business Proposal	219
	References	226
Chapter 10	Documenting Product Requirements	227
	Richard C. Fries	
10.1	Requirements, Design, Verification, and Validation	227
10.2	The Product Specification	232
10.3	Specification Review	234
10.4	The Design Specification	234
10.5	The Software Quality Assurance Plan (SQAP)	236
10.6	Software Requirements Specification (SRS)	240
10.7	The Software Design Description (SDS)	243
	References	246
Chapter 11	Medical Device Records	249
	Richard C. Fries	
11.1	The Design History File (DHF)	250
11.2	The Device Master Record (DMR)	252
11.3	The Device History Record (DHR)	253
11.4	The Technical Documentation File (TDF)	253
11.5	A Comparison of the Medical Device Records	254
	References	257
Section 3	The Design Phase	259
Chapter 12	Hazard and Risk Analysis	261
	Markus Weber	
12.1	Hazards, Risks, and Mitigation	262
12.2	Hazard Analysis	266
12.3	Risk Analysis	279
12.4	Risk Analysis Matrix	291
12.5	Software Hazard Analysis	294
12.6	Safety Requirements Specification	301
12.7	Hazard Analysis and Quality Control	302
12.8	Conclusion	303
	References	303
Chapter 13	Hardware Design	305
	Richard C. Fries	
13.1	Block Diagram	306
13.2	Redundancy	306
13.3	Component Selection	310

Contents

13.4	Component Derating	314
13.5	Safety Margin	316
13.6	Load Protection	317
13.7	Environmental Protection	317
13.8	Product Misuse	318
13.9	Design for Variation	319
13.10	Design of Experiments	319
13.11	Design Changes	320
13.12	Design Reviews	322
	References	324
Chapter 14	Software Design	327
	Sherman Eagles	
14.1	Fundamentals of Software Engineering Management	328
14.2	Planning Software Development	328
14.3	Choosing the Software Development Process Model	330
14.4	Development Process Models for High Level of Concern	331
14.5	Development Process Models for Low Level of Concern	334
14.6	Choosing a Design Method	335
14.7	Choosing a Programming Language	337
14.8	Estimating and Scheduling	338
14.9	Tracking Progress	339
14.10	Necessary Technical Software Development Activities	340
14.11	Software Requirements Analysis	340
14.12	Software Hazard Analysis	341
14.13	Requirements Traceability	342
14.14	Software Architectural Design	343
14.15	Detailed Design	344
14.16	Implementation (Coding)	346
14.17	Integration	347
14.18	Software Configuration Management	348
14.19	Conclusion	349
	References	350
Chapter 15	Human Factors Engineering	353
	Richard C. Fries	
15.1	What Is Human Factors?	353
15.2	Human Factors Process	361
15.3	Specifying the User Interface	371
15.4	Additional Human Factors Design Considerations	372
15.5	Documentation	375
15.6	Anthropometry	376
15.7	Alarms and Signals	380

15.8	Labeling	383
15.9	Software	385
	References	392

Chapter 16 Biocompatibility..395
Richard C. Fries

16.1	The FDA and Biocompatibility	397
16.2	International Regulatory Efforts	402
16.3	Device Category and Choice of Test Programs	403
16.4	Preparation of Extracts	406
16.5	Biological Control Tests	408
16.6	Tests for Biological Evaluation	409
16.7	Alternative Test Methods	416
	References	416

Chapter 17 Reliability Assurance...419
Richard C. Fries

17.1	Reliability versus Unreliability	420
17.2	Quality versus Reliability	420
17.3	The Definition of Reliability	421
17.4	History of Reliability	423
17.5	Types of Reliability	424
17.6	Device Reliability	429
17.7	Optimizing Reliability	430
17.8	Reliability's Effect on Medical Devices	432
17.9	Initial Reliability Prediction	433
17.10	Design for Variation	448
	References	449

Chapter 18 Product User Guides...451
Margaret Rickard

18.1	Why User Documentation Is Important	452
18.2	It's a Team Effort	453
18.3	How a Manual Evolves	456
18.4	Style Guides	472
18.5	Manual Tips	488
	References	492

Chapter 19 Translation: "It's A Small World After All"..................495
Margaret Rickard

19.1	Defining Translation and Localization	496
19.2	The Importance of Good English	498
19.3	The Translation Process	501

Contents

19.4	Symbols and Graphics	504
19.5	The Importance of Glossaries	507
19.6	Choosing a Translator	508
19.7	It's a Small World	512
	References	513
Chapter 20	Liability	515
	Richard C. Fries	
20.1	Negligence	516
20.2	Strict Liability	517
20.3	Breach of Warranty	518
20.4	Defects	520
20.5	Failure to Warn of Dangers	522
20.6	Plaintiff's Conduct	522
20.7	Defendant's Conduct	523
20.8	Defendant-Related Issues	523
20.9	Manufacturer's and Physician's Responsibilities	524
20.10	Conclusion	525
	References	525
Chapter 21	Intellectual Property	527
	Richard C. Fries	
21.1	Patents	528
21.2	Copyrights	536
21.3	Trademarks	542
21.4	Trade Secrets	547
	References	551
Section 4	**Verification and Validation**	**553**
Chapter 22	Testing	555
	Lisa Henn	
22.1	Purposes	555
22.2	Proper Setup	557
22.3	Running the Test	572
22.4	Analyzing the Outcome	572
22.5	Limits to Analysis	574
22.6	Conclusion	576
	References	576
Chapter 23	Overview of Verification and Validation for Embedded Software in Medical Systems	579
	Andre Bloesch	
23.1	Verification and Validation Planning	579

23.2   Test Development..588
23.3   Test Execution and Reporting........................597
            References..600

Chapter 24 Software Verification and Validation........................601
            Sherman Eagles
24.1   Planning Software Verification and Validation...............602
24.2   Static Verification Techniques...................................604
24.3   Modeling Techniques...609
24.4   Dynamic Testing Techniques...................................610
24.5   Verification Activities..617
24.6   Verifying Safety..620
24.7   Verification Measurement.......................................621
24.8   Software Validation..624
24.9   Conclusion..625
            References..625

Chapter 25 Reliability Evaluation......................................629
            Richard C. Fries
25.1   Standard Tests...629
25.2   Environmental Testing..631
25.3   Accelerated Testing...638
25.4   Sudden Death Testing...642
25.5   The Sudden Death Test..646
            References..655

Chapter 26 Analysis of Test Results....................................657
            Richard C. Fries
26.1   Failure Rate..658
26.2   Mean Time Between Failures (MTBF).......................659
26.3   Reliability..664
26.4   Confidence Level..665
26.5   Confidence Limits...666
26.6   Minimum Life..668
26.7   Graphical Analysis..668
            References..672

Section 5   **The Manufacturing/Field Phase**........................**675**

Chapter 27 Quality System Regulations and Manufacturing.............677
            Richard C. Fries
27.1   History of the Quality System Regulations...................678
27.2   Scope...679

Contents

27.3   General Provisions....680
27.4   Design for Manufacturability....682
27.5   Design for Assembly....683
27.6   The Manufacturing Process....686
     References....690

Chapter 28   Configuration Management....693
     Richard C. Fries
28.1   Configuration Identification....694
28.2   Configuration Audits....698
28.3   Configuration Management Metrics....699
28.4   FDA's View of Configuration Management....700
28.5   Status Accounting....701
     References....702

Chapter 29   The Quality System Audit....705
     Tina Juneau
29.1   Preparation....705
29.2   What to Expect on Audit Day....709
29.3   Surveillance....712
     References....713

Chapter 30   Analysis of Field Data....715
     Richard C. Fries
30.1   Analysis of Field Service Reports....716
30.2   Failure Analysis of Field Units....720
30.3   Warranty Analysis....722
     References....722

Section 6   **Appendices....725**

Appendix 1   *Chi Square Table....727*
Appendix 2   *Percent Rank Tables....729*
Appendix 3   *Glossary....749*

Index   *....771*

Contributors

Andre Bloesch
Manager of Software Validation
Datex-Ohmeda, Inc., Madison, Wisconsin

Sherman Eagles
Senior Principle Software Engineer
Medtronic, Inc., Minneapolis, Minnesota

Paul Fabry
Senior Engineer
Canadian Standards Association, Toronto, Ontario, Canada

Richard C. Fries
Manager of Reliability Engineering
Datex-Ohmeda, Inc., Madison, Wisconsin

Nancy George
President and Senior Consultant
Software Quality Management, Inc., Towson, Maryland

Lisa Henn
Manager of Software Validation
Datex-Ohmeda, Inc., Madison, Wisconsin

Tina Juneau
Quality System Facilitator
Lunar Inc., Madison, Wisconsin

Margaret Rickard
Manager of Technical Communications, Graphics, and Human Factors
Datex-Ohmeda, Inc., Madison, Wisconsin

Markus Weber
President
System Safety, Inc., San Diego, California

Section 1

Standards and Regulations

Chapter 1

FDA Regulations

Richard C. Fries, PE, CRE – Datex-Ohmeda, Inc.
Madison, Wisconsin

Regulation of medical devices is intended to protect consumer's health and safety by attempting to ensure that marketed products are effective and safe. Prior to 1976, the FDA had limited authority over medical devices under the Food, Drug, and Cosmetic Act of 1938. Beginning in 1968, Congress established a radiation control program to authorize the establishment of standards for electronic products, including medical and dental radiology equipment. From the early 1960s to 1975, concern over devices increased and six United States Presidential messages were given to encourage medical device legislation.

In 1969, the Department of Health, Education, and Welfare appointed a special committee (the Cooper Committee) to review the scientific literature associated with medical devices. The Committee estimated that over a 10-year period, 10,000 injuries were associated with medical devices, of which 731 resulted in death. The majority of problems were associated with three device types: artificial heart valves, cardiac pacemakers, and intrauterine contraceptive devices. There activities culminated in passage of the Medical Devices Amendments of 1976.

Devices marketed after 1976 are subject to full regulation unless they are found substantially equivalent to a device already on the market in 1976. By the end of 1981, only about 300 of the 17,000 products submitted for clearance to the FDA after 1976 had been found not substantially equivalent.

1.1   History of Device Regulation

In 1906, the Food and Drug Administration enacted its first regulations addressing public health. While these regulations did not address medical devices per se, they did establish a foundation for future regulations. It was not until 1938, with the passage of the Federal Food, Drug and Cosmetic Act (FFD&C) that the FDA was authorized, for the first time, to regulate medical devices. This act provided for regulation of adulterated or misbranded drugs, cosmetics and devices that were entered into interstate commerce. A medical device could be marketed without being federally reviewed and approved.

In the years following World War II, the FDA focused much of the attention on drugs and cosmetics. Over-the-counter drugs became regulated in 1961. In 1962, the FDA began requesting safety and efficacy data on new drugs and cosmetics.

By the mid-1960s, it became clear that the provisions of the FFD&C Act were not adequate to regulate the complex medical devices of the times to ensure both patient and user safety. Thus, in 1969, the Cooper Committee was formed to examine the problems associated with medical devices and to develop concepts for new regulations.

In 1976, with input from the Cooper Committee, the FDA created the Medical Device Amendments to the FFD&C Act, which were subsequently signed into law. The purpose of the amendments was to ensure that medical devices were safe, effective and properly labeled for their intended use. To accomplish this mandate, the amendments provided the FDA with the authority to regulate devices during most phases of their development, testing, production, distribution and use. This marked the first time the FDA clearly distinguished between devices and drugs. Regulatory requirements were derived from this 1976 law.

In 1978, with the authority granted the FDA by the amendments, the Good Manufacturing Practices (GMP) were promulgated. The GMP represents a quality assurance program intended to control the manufacturing, packaging, storage, distribution and installation of medical devices. This regulation was intended to allow only safe and effective devices to reach the market place. It is this regulation that has the greatest effect on the medical device industry. It allows the FDA to inspect a company's operations and take action on any noted deficiencies, including prohibition of device shipment.

Recent regulations specific to medical devices are the Medical Device Reporting (MDR) regulation of 1984, the Device Reconditioner/ Rebuilder (DRR) regulation of 1988, and the Safe Medical Devices Act of 1992.

1.2 Device Classification

A medical device is any article or health care product intended for use in the diagnosis of disease or other condition or for use in the care, treatment, or prevention of disease that does not achieve any of its primary intended purposes by chemical action or by being metabolized.

From 1962, when Congress passed the last major drug law revision, and first attempted to include devices, until 1976 when device laws were finally written, there were almost constant congressional hearings. Testimony was presented by medical and surgical specialty groups, industry, basic biomedical sciences, and various government agencies, including all the FDA. All of the viewpoints and arguments that we hear today were proposed, and considered in public discussion. Nearly two dozen bills were rejected as either inadequate or inappropriate.

The Cooper Committee concluded that the many inherent and important differences between drugs and devices necessitated a regulatory plan specifically adapted to devices. They recognized that some degree of risk is inherent in the development of many devices, so that all hazards cannot be eliminated, that there is often little or no prior experience on which to base judgements about safety and effectiveness, that devices undergo performance improvement modifications during the course of clinical trials, and that results also depend upon the skill of the user.

They therefore rejected the drug-based approach and created a new and different system for evaluating devices. All devices were placed into classes based upon the degree of risk posed by each individual device and its use. The Pre-Market Notification Process (510(k)) and the Pre-Market Approval Application (PMAA) became the regulatory pathways for device approval. The Investigational Device Exemption (IDE) became the mechanism to establish safety and efficacy in clinical studies for PMAAs.

1.2.1   Class I Devices

Class I devices were defined as not life sustaining, their failure poses no risk to life, and there is no need for performance standards. Basic standards, however, such as premarket notification (510(k)), registration, device listing, good manufacturing practices (GMP), and proper record keeping are all required. Nonetheless, the FDA has exempted many of the simpler Class I devices from some or all of these requirements. For example, tongue depressors and stethoscopes are both Class I devices, both are exempt from GMP, tongue depressors are exempt from 510(k) filing, whereas stethoscopes are not.

1.2.2   Class II Devices

Class II devices were also defined in 1976 as not life sustaining. However, they must not only comply with the basic standards for Class I devices, but must meet specific controls or performance standards. For example, sphygmomanometers, although not essential for life, must meet standards of accuracy and reproducibility.

Premarket notification is documentation submitted by a manufacturer that notifies the FDA that a device is about to be marketed. It assists the agency in making a determination about whether a device is "substantially equivalent" to a previously marketed predecessor device. As provided for in section 510(k) of the Food, Drug, and Cosmetic Act, the FDA can clear a device for marketing on the basis of premarket notification that the device is substantially equivalent to a pre-1976 predecessor device. The decision is based on premarket notification information that is provided by the manufacturer and includes the intended use, physical composition, and specifications of the device. Additional data usually submitted include in vitro and in vivo toxicity studies.

The premarket notification or 510(k) process was designed to give manufacturers the opportunity to obtain rapid market approval of these noncritical devices by providing evidence that their device is "substantially equivalent" to a device that is already marketed. The device must have the same intended use and the same or equally safe and effective technological characteristics as a predicate device.

Class II devices are usually exempt from the need to prove safety and efficacy. The FDA, however, may require additional clinical or laboratory studies. On occasion these may be as rigorous as for an IDE in support of a PMA, although this is rare. The FDA responds with an "order of concurrence" or nonconcurrence with the manufacturer's equivalency claims.

The Safe Medical Device Act of 1990 and the Amendments of 1992 attempted to take advantage of what had been learned since 1976 to give both the FDA and manufacturers greater leeway by permitting down-classification of many devices, including some life supporting and life sustaining devices previously in Class III, provided that reasonable assurance of safety and effectiveness can be obtained by application of "Special Controls" such as performance standards, postmarket surveillance, guidelines and patient and device registries.

1.2.3   Class III Devices

Class III devices were defined in 1976 as either sustaining or supporting life so that their failure is life threatening. For example, heart valves, pacemakers and PCTA balloon catheters are all Class III devices. Class III devices almost always require a PMAA, a long and complicated task fraught with many pitfalls that has caused the greatest confusion and dissatisfaction for both industry and the FDA.

The new regulations permit the FDA to use data contained in four prior PMAs for a specific device, that demonstrate safety and effectiveness, to approve future PMA applications by establishing performance standards or actual reclassification. Composition and manufacturing methods which companies wish to keep as proprietary secrets are excluded. Advisory Medical panel review is now elective.

However, for PMAAs that continue to be required, all of the basic requirements for Class I and II devices must be provided, plus failure mode analysis, animal tests, toxicology studies and then finally human clinical studies, directed to establish safety and efficacy under an IDE.

It is necessary that preparation of the PMA must actually begin years before it will be submitted. It is only after the company has the results of all of the laboratory testing, pre-clinical animal testing, failure mode analysis and manufacturing standards on their final design, that their proof of safety and efficacy can begin, in the form of a clinical study under an IDE.

At this point the manufacturer must not only have settled on a specific, fixed design for the device, but with marketing and clinical consultants must also have decided on what the indications, contraindications, and warnings for use will be. The clinical study must be carefully designed to support these claims.

Section 520(g) of the Federal Food, Drug, and Cosmetic Act, as amended, authorizes the FDA to grant an IDE to a researcher using a device in studies undertaken to develop safety and effectiveness data for that device when such studies involve human subjects. An approved IDE application permits a device that would otherwise be subject to marketing clearance to be shipped lawfully for the purpose of conducting a clinical study. An approved IDE also exempts a device from certain sections of the Act. All new significant risk devices not granted substantial equivalence under the 510(k) section of the Act must pursue clinical testing under an IDE.

An Institutional Review Board (IRB) is a group of physicians and lay people at a hospital who must approve clinical research projects prior to their initiation. The IRB is discussed in detail in Section 6.6.1.

1.3   Registration and Listing

Under section 510 of the Act, every person engaged in the manufacture, preparation, propagation, compounding or processing of a device shall register their name, place of business and such establishment. This includes manufacturers of devices and components, repackers, relabelers, as well as initial distributors of imported devices. Those not required to register include manufacturers of raw materials, licensed practitioners, manufacturers of devices for use solely in research or teaching, warehousers, manufacturers of veterinary devices, and those who only dispense devices, such as pharmacies.

Upon registration, the FDA issues a device registration number. A change in the ownership or corporate structure of the firm, the location, or person designated as the official correspondent must be communicated to the FDA device registration and listing branch within 30 days. Registration must be done when first beginning to manufacture medical devices and must be updated yearly.

Section 510 of the Act also requires all manufacturers to list the medical devices they market. Listing must be done when first beginning to manufacture a product and must be updated every 6 months. Listing includes not only informing the FDA of products manufactured, but also providing the agency with copies of labeling and advertising.

Foreign firms that market products in the United States are permitted but not required to register, and are required to list. Foreign devices that are not listed are not permitted to enter the country.

Registration and listing provides the FDA with information about the identity of manufacturers and the products they make. This information enables the agency to schedule inspections of facilities and also to follow up on problems. When the FDA learns about a safety defect in a particular type of device, it can use the listing information to notify all manufacturers of those devices about that defect.

1.4   Good Laboratory Practices (GLP)

In 1978, FDA adopted Good Laboratory Practices rules and
implemented a laboratory audit and inspection procedure covering every
regulated entity which conducts nonclinical laboratory studies for product
safety and effectiveness. The GLPs were amended in 1984.

The GLP standard addresses all areas of laboratory operations
including requirements for a Quality Assurance Unit to conduct periodic
internal inspections and keep records for audit and reporting purposes,
Standard Operating Procedures (SOPs) for all aspects of each study and for all
phases of laboratory maintenance, a formal mechanism for evaluation and
approval of study protocols and their amendments, and reports of data in
sufficient detail to support conclusions drawn from them. The FDA inspection
program includes GLP compliance, and a data audit to verify that information
submitted to the agency accurately reflects the raw data.

1.5   Good Manufacturing Practices (GMP)

FDA is authorized, under section 520(f) of the Act, to promulgate
regulations detailing compliance with current good manufacturing practices.
GMPs include the methods used in, and the facilities and controls used for, the
manufacture, packing, storage and installation of a device. The GMP
regulations were established as manufacturing safeguards to ensure the
production of a safe and effective device and include all of the essential
elements of a quality assurance program. Because manufacturers cannot test
every device, the GMPs were established as a minimum standard of
manufacturing to ensure that each device produced would be safe. If a product
is not manufactured according to GMPs, even if it is later shown not to be a
health risk, it is in violation of the Act and subject to FDA enforcement action.

The general objectives of the GMPs, not specific manufacturing
methods, are found in Part 820 of the Code of Federal Regulations. The GMPs
apply to the manufacture of every medical device. The proposed new GMP
regulations, scheduled to be released in 1996, gives FDA the authority to
examine the design area of the product development cycle for the first time.
The regulation also parallels very closely the ISO 9000 set of standards.

1.6   Human Factors

In April, 1996, the FDA issued a draft primer on the use of Human Factors in medical device design. The purpose of the document was to improve the safety of medical devices by minimizing the likelihood of user error by systematic, careful design of the user interface, i.e., the hardware and software features that define the interaction between the users and the equipment. The document contains background information about human factors as a discipline, descriptions and illustrations of device problems, and a discussion of human factors methods. It also contains recommendations for manufacturers and health facilities.

As the source for this document, the FDA extensively used the guideline *Human Factors Engineering Guidelines and Preferred Practices for the Design of Medical Devices* published by the Association for the Advancement of Medical Instrumentation as well as interfacing with Human Factors consultants. It is expected that Human Factors requirements will become part of the product submission as well as the GMP inspection.

1.7   Design Control

With the anticipated publication of the new GMP regulations, the FDA will have the authority to cover design controls in their inspections. In preparation for this, the FDA issued a draft guidance document in March, 1996 entitled *Design Control Guidance for Medical Device Manufacturers*. The purpose of the document was to provide readers with an understanding of what is meant by "control" in the context of the requirements. By providing an understanding of what constitutes control of a design process, readers could determine how to apply the concepts in a way that was both consistent with the requirements and best suited for their particular situation.

Three underlying concepts served as a foundation for the development of this guidance:

> - the nature of the application of design controls for any device should be proportional to both the complexity of and the risks associated with that device

- the design process is a multifunctional one that involves other departments beside design and development if it is to work properly, thus involving senior management as an active participant in the process
- the product life cycle concept serves throughout the document as the framework for introducing and describing the design control activities and techniques.

Design control concepts are applicable to process development as well as product development. The extent is dependent upon the nature of the product and processes used to manufacture the product. The safety and performance of a new product is also dependent on an intimate relationship between product design robustness and process capability.

The document covers the areas of:

- risk management
- design and development planning
- organizational and technical interfaces
- design input
- design output
- design review
- design verification
- design validation
- design changes
- design transfer.

These topics are covered in detail in later sections of this book.

1.8   Software

The subject of software in and as a medical device has become an important topic for the FDA. This interest began in 1985 when software in a radiation treatment therapy device was alleged to have resulted in a lethal overdose. The FDA then analyzed recalls by fiscal year to determine how many were caused by software problems. In FY 1985, for example, 20% of all neurology device recalls were attributable to software problems, while 8% of cardiovascular problems had the same cause. This type of analysis, along with

authority to inspect the design area and the qualifications of personnel in all aspects of the product development process.

1.10   Dealing with the FDA

Several recommendations can be made regarding how to deal with the FDA and its regulatory process. None of these bits of advice are dramatic or new, but in the course of observing a firm's interaction with the agency, it is amazing how many times the failure to think of these steps can result in significant difficulties.

Know your district office. This may not be an easy thing to accomplish, since, understandably, there is a great reluctance to walk into a regulatory agency and indicate you are there to get acquainted. As opportunities arise, however, they should not be overlooked. Situations such as responding to a notice of an investigator's observations at the conclusion of an inspection or a notice of adverse findings letter are excellent opportunities to hand deliver a reply instead of simply mailing it. The verbal discussion with the reply may make the content much more meaningful and will allow both sides to learn more about the intent and seriousness with which the subject is being approached.

Prepare for inspections. When the FDA investigator walks into your manufacturing facility or corporate offices, there should be a procedure established that everyone is familiar with as to who is called, who escorts the investigator through the facility, who is available to make copies of records requested, etc. A corollary to this suggestion is to be prepared to deal with adverse inspectional findings or other communications from the agency that indicate the FDA has found violations, a serious health hazard, or other information that requires high-level company knowledge and decision making.

Take seriously FDA audit reports (483's) and letters. Many regulatory actions are processed with no apparent indication that a firm seriously considered the violations noted by the agency.

Keep up with current events and procedures of the FDA. This will minimize the changes or surprise interpretations that could have an effect on a firm's operations and will allow for advance planning for new FDA requirements. The Agency publishes much of its new program information in bulletins and other broad distribution documents, but much more can be learned from obtaining copies of FDA Compliance Policy Guides and Compliance Programs.

Let the FDA know of your firm's opinions on issues, whether they are in the development state at the Agency or are policies or programs established and in operation. The Agency does recognize that the firms it regulates are the true experts in device manufacturing and distribution, and their views are important. The Agency also recognizes that the regulation of manufacturers is not the only bottom line - solving public health problems is equally or more important, and there are generally many ways to solve those problems.

References

Banta, H. David, "The Regulation of Medical Devices," in *Preventive Medicine*. Volume 19, Number 6, November, 1990.

Basile, Edward, "Overview of Current FDA Requirements for Medical Devices," in *The Medical Device Industry: Science, Technology, and Regulation in a Competitive Environment*. New York: Marcel Dekker, Inc., 1990.

Basile, Edward M. and Alexis J. Prease, "Compiling a Successful PMA Application," in *The Medical Device Industry: Science, Technology, and Regulation in a Competitive Environment*. New York: Marcel Dekker, Inc., 1990.

Bureau of Medical Devices, Office of Small Manufacturers Assistance, *Regulatory Requirements for Marketing a Device*. Washington, DC: U.S. Department of Health and Human Services, 1982.

Center for Devices and Radiological Health, *Devic Good Manufacturing Practices Manual.* Washington, DC: U.S. Department of Health and Human Services, 1987.

Food and Drug Administration, *Federal Food, Drug and Cosmetic Act, as Amended January, 1979.* Washington, DC: U.S. Government Printing Office, 1979.

Food and Drug Administration, *Guide to the Inspection of Computerized Systems in Drug Processing.* Washington, DC: Food and Drug Administration, 1983.

Food and Drug Administration, *FDA Policy for the Regulation of Computer Products (Draft).* Washington, DC: Federal Register, 1987.

Food and Drug Administration, *Software Development Activities.* Washington, DC: Food and Drug Administration, 1987.

Food and Drug Administration, *Medical Devices GMP Guidance for FDA Inspectors.* Washington, DC: Food and Drug Administration, 1987.

Food and Drug Administration, *Reviewer Guidance for Computer-Controlled Medical Devices (Draft).* Washington, DC: Food and Drug Administration, 1988.

Food and Drug Administration, *Investigational Device Exemptions Manual.* Rockville MD: Center for Devices and Radiological Health, 1992.

Food and Drug Administration, *Premarket Notification 510(k): Regulatory Requirements for Medical Devices.* Rockville MD: Center for Devices and Radiological Health, 1992.

Food and Drug Administration, *Premarket Approval (PMA) Manual.* Rockville MD: Center for Devices and Radiological Health, 1993.

Food and Drug Administration, *Design Control Guidance for Medical Device Manufacturers.* Draft. Rockville, MD: Center for Devices and Radiological Health, 1996.

Food and Drug Administration, *Do It By Design: An Introduction to Human Factors in Medical Devices*. Draft. Rockville, MD: Center for Devices and Radiological Health, 1996.

Fries, Richard C. et al, "Software Regulation" in *The Medical Device Industry: Science, Technology, and Regulation in a Competitive Environment*. New York: Marcel Dekker, Inc., 1990.

Ginzburg, Harold M., "Protection of Research Subjects in Clinical Research," in *Legal Aspects of Medicine*. New York: Springer-Verlag, 1989.

Gundaker, Walter E., "FDA's Regulatory Program for Medical Devices and Diagnostics," in *The Medical Device Industry: Science, Technology, and Regulation in a Competitive Environment*. New York: Marcel Dekker, Inc., 1990.

Holstein, Howard M., "How to Submit a Successful 510(k)," in *The Medical Device Industry: Science, Technology, and Regulation in a Competitive Environment*. New York: Marcel Dekker, Inc., 1990.

Jorgens III, J. and C. W. Burch, "FDA Regulation of Computerized Medical Devices," *Byte*. Volume 7, 1982.

Jorgens III, J., "Computer Hardware and Software as Medical Devices," *Medical Device and Diagnostic Industry*. May, 1983.

Jorgens III, J. and R. Schneider, "Regulation of Medical Software by the FDA," *Software in Health Care*. April-May, 1985.

Kahan, J. S., "Regulation of Computer Hardware and Software as Medical Devices," *Canadian Computer Law Reporter*. Volume 6, Number 3, January, 1987.

Magee, Stan and Leondard Tripp, *Guide to Software Engineering Standards and Specifications*. Boston, Massachusetts, Artech House, 1997.

Magee, Stan, "ISO/IEC Software Life Cycle Standard 12207," *Datapro Management of Applications Software*. February, 1995.

Munsey, Rodney R. and Howard M. Holstein, "FDA/GMP/MDR Inspections: Obligations and Rights," in *The Medical Device Industry: Science, Technology, and Regulation in a Competitive Environment*. New York: Marcel Dekker, Inc., 1990.

Office of Technology Assessment, Federal Policies and the Medical Devices Industry. Washington, DC: U.S. Government Printing Office, 1984.

Sheretz, Robert J. and Stephen A. Streed, "Medical Devices - Significant Risk vs Nonsignificant Risk," in Journal of the American Medical Association, Volume 272, Number 12, September 28, 1994.

Trull, Frankie L. and Barbara A. Rich, "The Animal Testing Issue," in *The Medical Device Industry: Science, Technology, and Regulation in a Competitive Environment*. New York: Marcel Dekker, Inc., 1990.

U. S. Congress, House Committee on Interstate and Foreign Commerce. Medical Devices. Hearings before the Subcommittee on Public Health and the Environment. October 23-24, 1973. Serial Numbers 93-61 Washington DC: U.S. Government Printing Office, 1973.

Wholey, Mark H. and Jordan D. Hailer, "An Introduction to the Food and Drug Administration and How It Evaluates New Devices: Establishing Safety and Efficacy," in *Cardiovascular and Interventional Radiology*. Volume 18, Number 2, March/April 1995

Chapter 2

Preparing an FDA Submission

Richard C. Fries, PE, CRE – Datex-Ohmeda, Inc.
Madison, Wisconsin

Regulation of medical devices is intended to protect consumer's health. Section 510(k) of the Food, Drug and Cosmetic Act requires those device manufacturers who must register to notify FDA, at least 90 days in advance, of their intent to market a medical device. This is known as Premarket Notification, also called PMN or 510(k). It allows FDA to determine whether the device is equivalent to a device already placed into one of the three classification categories. Thus, "new" devices (not in commercial distribution prior to May 28, 1976) that have not been classified can be properly identified.

Specifically, medical device manufacturers are required to submit a premarket notification if they intend to introduce a device into commercial distribution for the first time or reintroduce a device that will be significantly changed or modified to the extent that its safety or effectiveness could be affected. Such change or modification could relate to the design, material, chemical composition, energy source, manufacturing process, or intended use.

A PMA can be viewed as a compilation of sections and "modules" that together become a complete application. The "PMA Shell" is an outline of those sections that will be necessary to complete the PMA. It will include all modules needed to support filing and approval of a specific medical device. The term "module" will be used to identify a set of elements, tests, information, etc., addressing a selected aspect of the device subject to a PMA. A module may begin as the simple identification of the issue to be addressed and later developed into a detailed listing of the specific test results to be submitted as one report.

What is needed for each module will be decided by agreement between FDA and the module submitter. Discussion and agreement on the shell are needed because modules will be accepted and reviewed individually as sections of a PMA and should therefore include information and analyses with same level of detail as would be included in the PMA. When the PMA is submitted it will consist of the collection of the modules already submitted along with any other information needed to complete the PMA. Ideally, the shell should be constructed during the early stages of the investigational process but it may be established at any time before submission of the PMA.

2.1   Device Classification

A medical device is any article or health care product intended for use in the diagnosis of disease or other condition or for use in the care, treatment, or prevention of disease that does not achieve any of its primary intended purposes by chemical action or by being metabolized.

From 1962, when Congress passed the last major drug law revision, and first attempted to include devices, until 1976 when device laws were finally written, there were almost constant congressional hearings. Testimony was presented by medical and surgical specialty groups, industry, basic biomedical sciences, and various government agencies, including all the FDA. All of the viewpoints and arguments that we hear today were proposed, and considered in public discussion. Nearly two dozen bills were rejected as either inadequate or inappropriate.

The Cooper Committee concluded that the many inherent and important differences between drugs and devices necessitated a regulatory plan specifically adapted to devices. They recognized that some degree of risk is inherent in the development of many devices, so that all hazards cannot be eliminated, that there is often little or no prior experience on which to base judgements about safety and effectiveness, that devices undergo performance improvement modifications during the course of clinical trials, and that results also depend upon the skill of the user.

They therefore rejected the drug-based approach and created a new and different system for evaluating devices. All devices were placed into classes based upon the degree of risk posed by each individual device and its use. The Pre-Market Notification Process (510(k)) and the Pre-Market Approval Application (PMAA) became the regulatory pathways for device approval. The Investigational Device Exemption (IDE) became the mechanism to establish safety and efficacy in clinical studies for PMAAs.

2.1.1   Class I Devices

Class I devices were defined as not life sustaining, their failure poses no risk to life, and there is no need for performance standards. Basic standards, however, such as premarket notification (510(k)), registration, device listing, good manufacturing practices (GMP), and proper record keeping are all required. Nonetheless, the FDA has exempted many of the simpler Class I devices from some or all of these requirements. For example, tongue depressors and stethoscopes are both Class I devices, both are exempt from GMP, tongue depressors are exempt from 510(k) filing, whereas stethoscopes are not.

2.1.2   Class II Devices

Class II devices were also defined in 1976 as not life sustaining. However, they must not only comply with the basic standards for Class I devices, but must meet specific controls or performance standards. For example, sphygmomanometers, although not essential for life, must meet standards of accuracy and reproducibility.

Premarket notification is documentation submitted by a manufacturer that notifies the FDA that a device is about to be marketed. It assists the agency in making a determination about whether a device is "substantially equivalent" to a previously marketed predecessor device. As provided for in section 510(k) of the Food, Drug, and Cosmetic Act, the FDA can clear a device for marketing on the basis of premarket notification that the device is substantially equivalent to a pre-1976 predecessor device. The decision is based on premarket notification information that is provided by the manufacturer and includes the intended use, physical composition, and specifications of the device. Additional data usually submitted include in vitro and in vivo toxicity studies.

The premarket notification or 510(k) process was designed to give manufacturers the opportunity to obtain rapid market approval of these noncritical devices by providing evidence that their device is "substantially equivalent" to a device that is already marketed. The device must have the same intended use and the same or equally safe and effective technological characteristics as a predicate device.

Class II devices are usually exempt from the need to prove safety and efficacy. The FDA, however, may require additional clinical or laboratory studies. On occasion these may be as rigorous as for an IDE in support of a PMA, although this is rare. The FDA responds with an "order of concurrence" or nonconcurrence with the manufacturer's equivalency claims.

The Safe Medical Device Act of 1990 and the Amendments of 1992 attempted to take advantage of what had been learned since 1976 to give both the FDA and manufacturers greater leeway by permitting down-classification of many devices, including some life supporting and life sustaining devices previously in Class III, provided that reasonable assurance of safety and effectiveness can be obtained by application of "Special Controls" such as performance standards, post market surveillance, guidelines and patient and device registries.

2.1.3   Class III Devices

Class III Devices were defined in 1976 as either sustaining or supporting life so that their failure is life threatening. For example, heart valves, pacemakers and PCTA balloon catheters are all Class III devices. Class III devices almost always require a PMAA, a long and complicated task fraught with many pitfalls that has caused the greatest confusion and dissatisfaction for both industry and the FDA.

The new regulations permit the FDA to use data contained in four prior PMAs for a specific device, that demonstrate safety and effectiveness, to approve future PMA applications by establishing performance standards or actual reclassification. Composition and manufacturing methods which companies wish to keep as proprietary secrets are excluded. Advisory Medical panel review is now elective.

However, for PMAs that continue to be required, all of the basic requirements for Class I and II devices must be provided, plus failure mode analysis, animal tests, toxicology studies and then finally human clinical studies, directed to establish safety and efficacy under an IDE.

It is necessary that preparation of the PMA must actually begin years before it will be submitted. It is only after the company has the results of all of the laboratory testing, pre-clinical animal testing, failure mode analysis and manufacturing standards on their final design, that their proof of safety and efficacy can begin, in the form of a clinical study under an IDE.

At this point the manufacturer must not only have settled on a specific, fixed design for his device, but with his marketing and clinical consultants must also have decided on what the indications, contraindications, and warnings for use will be. The Clinical Study must be carefully designed to support these claims.

Section 520(g) of the Federal Food, Drug, and Cosmetic Act, as amended, authorizes the FDA to grant an IDE to a researcher using a device in studies undertaken to develop safety and effectiveness data for that device when such studies involve human subjects. An approved IDE application permits a device that would otherwise be subject to marketing clearance to be shipped lawfully for the purpose of conducting a clinical study. An approved IDE also exempts a device from certain sections of the Act. All new significant risk devices not granted substantial equivalence under the 510(k) section of the Act must pursue clinical testing under an IDE.

An Institutional Review Board (IRB) is a group of physicians and lay people at a hospital who must approve clinical research projects prior to their initiation. The IRB is discussed in detail in Section 2.7.1.

2.2   The Traditional 510(k)

2.2.1   Determining Substantial Equivalency

A new device is substantially equivalent if, in comparison to a legally marketed predicate device, it has the same intended use and 1)has the same technological characteristics as the predicate device or 2)has different technological characteristics and submitted information that does not raise different questions of safety and efficacy and demonstrates that the device is as safe and effective as the legally marketed predicate device. Figure 2-1 is an overview of the substantial equivalence decision making process. Figure 2-2 is a detailed view of the substantial equivalence decision making process.

2.2.2   Preparing a 510(k)

2.2.2.1 Types of 510(k)s

There are several types of 510(k) submissions that require different formats for addressing the requirements. These include:

- Submissions for Identical Devices
- Submissions for Equivalent but not Identical Devices
- Submissions for Complex Devices or for Major differences in Technological Characteristics
- Submissions for Software-Controlled Devices.

The 510(k) for simple changes, or for identical devices should be kept simple and straightforward. The submission should refer to one or more predicate devices, it should contain samples of labeling, it should have a brief

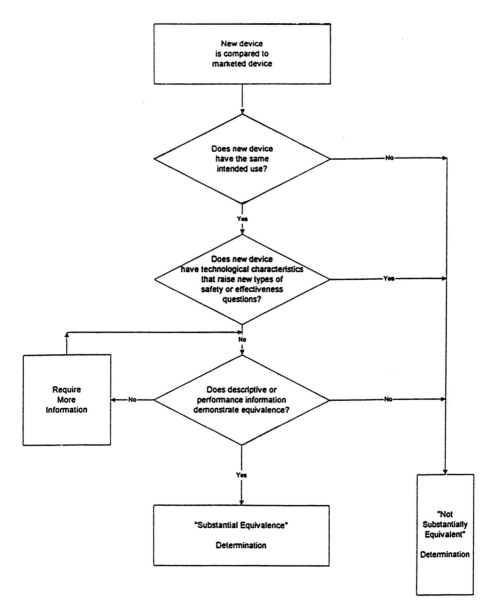

Figure 2-1   The substantial equivalence process.   (From FDA, 1992.)

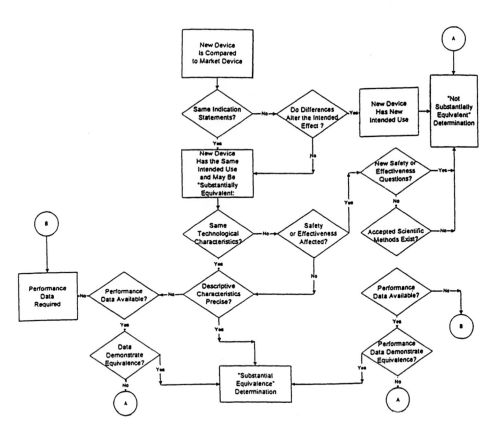

Figure 2-2   Detailed substantial equivalence process. (From FDA, 1992.)

statement of equivalence, and it may be useful to include a chart listing similarities and differences. The group of equivalent but not identical devices includes combination devices where the characteristics or functions of more than one predicate device are relied on to support a substantially equivalent determination. This type of 510(k) should contain all of the information listed above as well as sufficient data to demonstrate why the differing characteristics or functions do not affect safety or effectiveness. Submission of some functional data may be necessary. It should not be necessary, however, to include clinical data-bench or pre-clinical testing results should be sufficient. Preparing a comparative chart showing differences and similarities with predicate devices can be particularly helpful to the success of this type of application.

Submissions for complex devices or for major differences in technological characteristics is the most difficult type of submission, since it begins to approach the point at which the FDA will need to consider whether a 510(k) is sufficient of whether a PMAA must be submitted. The key is to demonstrate that the new features or the new uses do not diminish safety or effectiveness and that there are no significant new risks posed by the device. In addition to the types of information described above, this type of submission will almost always require submission of some data, possibly including clinical data.

As a general rule, it often is a good idea to meet with FDA to explain why the product is substantially equivalent, to discuss the data that will be submitted in support of a claim of substantial equivalence, and to learn the FDA's concerns and questions so that these may be addressed in the submission. The FDA's guidance documents can be of greatest use in preparing this type of submission.

The term software includes programs and or data that pertain to the operation of a computer-controlled system, whether they are contained on floppy disks, hard disks, magnetic tapes, laser disks, or embedded in the hardware of a device. The depth of review by the FDA is determined by the "level of concern" for the device and the role that the software plays in the functioning of the device. Levels of concern are listed as minor, moderate, and major and are tied very closely with risk analysis.

In reviewing such submissions, the FDA maintains that end-product testing may not be sufficient to establish that the device is substantially equivalent to the predicate devices. Therefore, a firm's software development process and/or documentation should be examined for reasonable assurance of safety and effectiveness of the software-controlled functions, including incorporated safeguards. 510(k)s that are heavily software dependent will receive greater FDA scrutiny, and the questions posed must be satisfactorily addressed.

2.2.2.2 The 510(k) Format

The actual 510(k) submission will vary in complexity and length according to the type of device or product change for which substantial equivalency is sought. A submission shall be in sufficient detail to provide an understanding of the basis for a determination of substantial equivalence. All submissions shall contain the following information:

- the submitter's name, address, telephone number, a contact person, and the date the submission was prepared
- the name of the device, including the trade or proprietary name, if applicable, the common or usual name, and the classification name
- an identification of the predicate or legally marketed device or devices to which substantial equivalence is being claimed
- a description of the device that is the subject of the submission, including an explanation of how the device functions, the basic scientific concepts that form the basis for the device, and the significant physical and performance characteristics of the device such as device design, materials used, and physical properties
- a statement of the intended use of the device, including a general description of the diseases or conditions the device will diagnose, treat, prevent, cure, or mitigate, including a description, where appropriate, of the patient population for which the device is intended. If the indication statements are different from those of the predicate or legally marketed device identified above, the

submission shall contain an explanation as to why the differences are not critical to the intended therapeutic, diagnostic, prosthetic, or surgical use of the device and why the differences do not affect the safety or effectiveness of the device when used as labeled
- a statement of how the technological characteristics (design, material, chemical composition, or energy source) of the device compare to those of the predicate or legally marketed device identified above.

510(k) summaries for those premarket notification submissions in which a determination of substantial equivalence is based on an assessment of performance data shall contain the following information in addition to that listed above:

- a brief discussion of the nonclinical tests and their results submitted in the premarket notification
- a brief discussion of the clinical tests submitted, referenced, or relied on in the premarket notification submission for a determination of substantial equivalence. This discussion shall include, where applicable, a description of the subjects upon whom the device was tested, a discussion of the safety and/or effectiveness data obtained with specific reference to adverse effects and complications, and any other information from the clinical testing relevant to a determination of substantial equivalence
- the conclusions drawn from the nonclinical and clinical tests that demonstrate that the device is safe, effective, and performs as well as or better than the legally marketed device identified above.

The summary should be in a separate section of the submission beginning on a new page and ending on a page not shared with any other section of the premarket notification submission, and should be clearly identified as a "501(k) summary."

A 510 (k) statement submitted as part of a premarket notification must state as follows:

> I certify that (name of person required to submit the premarket notification) will make available all information included in this premarket notification on safety and effectiveness that supports a finding of substantial equivalence within 30 days of request by any person. The information I agree to make available does not include confidential patient identifiers.

This statement should be made in a separate section of the premarket notification submission and should be clearly identified as a 510(k) statement.

A class III certification submitted as part of a premarket notification shall state as follows:

> I certify that a reasonable search of all information known or otherwise available to (name of premarket notification submitter) about the types and causes of reported safety and/or effectiveness problems for the (type of device) has been conducted. I further certify that the types of problems to which the (type of device) is susceptible and their potential causes are listed in the attached class III summary, and that this class III summary is complete and accurate.

This statement should be clearly identified as a class III certification and should be made in the section of the premarket notification submission that includes the class III summary.

A 510(k) should be accompanied by a brief cover letter that clearly identifies the submission as a 510(k) premarket notification. To facilitate prompt routing of the submission to the correct reviewing division within FDA, the letter can mention the generic category of the product and its intended use.

When the FDA receives a 510(k) premarket notification, it is reviewed according to a checklist to ensure its completeness. A sample 510(k) checklist is shown in Figure 2-3.

	Critical Elements		
1	Is the product a device?	Yes☐	No☐
2	Is the device exempt from 510(k) by regulation or policy?	Yes☐	No☐
3	Is device subject to review by CDRH (Center for Devices and Radiological Health)?	Yes☐	No☐
4	Are you aware that this device has been the subject of a previous NSE (Not Substantially Equivalent) decision?	Yes☐	No☐
	If yes, does this new 510(k) address the NSE issue(s) (e.g., performance data)?		
5	Are you aware of the submitter being the subject of and integrity investigation? If yes, consult the ODE (Office of Device Evaluation) Integrity Officer.	Yes☐	No☐
6	(ii). Has the ODE Integrity Officer given permission to proceed with the review? (Blue Book Memo #I91-2 and Federal Register 90N-0332, September 10, 1990	Yes☐	No☐
7	Does the submission contain the information required under Sections 510(k) , 513(f) and 513(i) of the Federal, Food, Drug and Cosmetic Act (Act) and Subpart E of Part 807 in Title 21 of the Code of Federal Regulations?:	Yes☐	No☐
8	Device trade or proprietary name?	Yes☐	No☐
9	Device common or usual name or classification name?	Yes☐	No☐
10	Establishment registration number (only applies if establishment is registered)?	Yes☐	No☐
11	Class into which the device is classified under (21 CFR Parts 862 to 892) ?	Yes☐	No☐
12	Classification Panel?	Yes☐	No☐
13	Action taken to comply with Section 514 of the Act?	Yes☐	No☐
14	Proposed labels, labeling and advertisements (if available) that describe the device, its intended use, and directions for use (Blue Book Memo #G91-1)?	Yes☐	No☐
15	A 510(k) summary of safety and effectiveness or a 510(k) statement that safety and effectiveness information will be made available to any person upon request?	Yes☐	No☐
16	For class III devices only, a class III certification and a class III summary?	Yes☐	No☐
17	Photographs of the device?	Yes☐	No☐
18	Engineering drawings for the device with dimensions and tolerances?	Yes☐	No☐
19	The marketed device(s) to which equivalence is being claimed including labeling and description of the device?	Yes☐	No☐
20	Statement of similarities and/or differences with marketed device(s)?	Yes☐	No☐
21	Data to show consequences and effects of a modified device(s)?	Yes☐	No☐
22	Additional Information that is necessary under 21 CFR 807.87(h):	Yes☐	No☐
23	Submitter's name and address?	Yes☐	No☐
24	Contact person, telephone number and fax number?	Yes☐	No☐
25	Representative/Consultant if applicable?	Yes☐	No☐
26	Table of Contents with pagination?	Yes☐	No☐
27	Address of manufacturing facility/facilities and, if appropriate, sterilization site(s)?	Yes☐	No☐
28	Additional Information that may be necessary under 21 CFR 807.87(h):	Yes☐	No☐
29	Comparison table of the new device to the marketed device(s)?	Yes☐	No☐
30	Action taken to comply with voluntary standards?	Yes☐	No☐
31	Performance data	Yes☐	No☐
	marketed device?	Yes☐	No☐
	bench testing?	Yes☐	No☐
	animal testing?	Yes☐	No☐
	clinical data?	Yes☐	No☐
	new device ?	Yes☐	No☐
	bench testing?	Yes☐	No☐
	animal testing?	Yes☐	No☐
	clinical data?	Yes☐	No☐
32	Sterilization information?	Yes☐	No☐
33	Software information?	Yes☐	No☐
34	Hardware information?	Yes☐	No☐
35	If this 510(k) is for a kit, has the kit certification statement been provided?	Yes☐	No☐
36	Is this device subject to issues that have been addressed in specific guidance document(s)?	Yes☐	No☐
	If yes, continue review with checklist from any appropriate guidance documents.		
	If no, is 510(k) sufficiently complete to allow substantive review?		
37	Truthfulness certification?	Yes☐	No☐
38	Others as required?	Yes☐	No☐

Figure 2.3   Sample FDA checklist.   (From Fries, 1997.)

2.3   Special 510(k)

Under this option, a manufacturer who is intending to modify their own legally marketed device will conduct the rrisk analysis and the necessary verification and validation activities to demonstrate that the design outputs of the modified device meet the design input requirements. Once the manufacturer has ensured the satisfactory completion of this process, a *Special 510(k); DeviceModification* may be submitted. While the basic content requirements of the 510(k) will remain the same, this type of submission should also reference the cleared 510(k) numbe4r and contain a *Declaration of Conformity* with design control requirements.

Under the Quality System Regulation, manufacturers are responsible for performing internal audits to assess their conformance with design controls. A manufacturer could, however, use a third party to provide a supporting assessment of the conformance. In this case, the third party will perform a conformance assessment for the device manufacturer and provide the manufacturer with a statement to this effect. The marketing application should then include a declaration of conformity signed by the manufacturer, while the statement from the third party should be maintained in the Device Master Record. As always, responsibility for conformance with design control requirements rests with the manufacture.

In order to provide an incentive for manufacturers to choose this option, the Office of Device Evaluation (ODE) intends to process Special 510(k)s within 30 days of receipt by the Document Mail Center. The Special 510(k) option will allow the Agency to review modifications that do not affect the device's intended use or alter the device's fundamental scientific technology within this abbreviated time frame. The agency does not believe that modifications that affect the intended use or alter the fundamental scientific technology of the device are appropriate for review under this type of application, but rather should continue to be subject to the traditional 510(k) procedures.

To ensure the success of the of the Special 510(k) option, there must be a common understanding of the types of device modifications that may gain marketing clearance by this path. Therefore, it is critical that industry and agency staff can easily determine whether a modification is appropriate for submission by this option. To optimize the chance that this option will be accepted and promptly cleared, manufacturers should evaluate each modification against the considerations described below to ensure that the particular change does not:

- affect the intended use
- alter the fundamental scientific technology of the device.

2.3.1 Special 510(k) Content

A Special 510(k) should include the following:

- a coversheet clearly identifying the application as a "Special 510(k); Device Modification"
- the name of the legally marketed (unmodified) device and the 510(k) number under which it was cleared
- items required under paragraph 807.87, including a description of the modified device and a comparison to the cleared device, the intended use of the device, and the proposed labeling for the device
- a concise summary of the design control activities. This summary should include 1) an identification of the risk analysis method(s) used to assess the impact of the modification on the device and its components as well as the results of the analysis, 2) based on the risk analysis, an identification of the verification and/or validation activities required, including methods or tests used and the acceptance criteria applied, 3) a declaration of conformity with design controls. The declaration of conformity should include:

    - A statement that, as required by the risk analysis, all verification and validation activities were performed by the designated individual(s) and the results demonstrated that the predetermined acceptance criteria were met
    - A statement that the manufacturing facility is in conformance with the design control procedure

requirements as specified in 21 CFR 820.30 and
the records are available for review.

The above two statements should be signed by the designated individual(s)
responsible for those particular activities.

2.4   Abbreviated 510(k)

Device manufacturers may choose to submit an Abbreviated 510(k)
when:

- a guidance document exists
- a special control has been established, or
- FDA has recognized a relevant consensus standard.

An Abbreviated 510(k) submission must include the required elements
identified in 21 CFR 807.87. In addition, manufacturers submitting an
Abbreviated 510(k) that relies on a guidance document and/or special control(s)
should include a summary report that describes how the guidance document
and /or special control(s) were used during device development and testing.
The summary report should include information regarding the manufacturer's
efforts to conform with the guidance document and/or special control(s) and
should outline any deviations. Persons submitting an Abbreviated 510(k) that
relies on a recognized standard should provide the information described below
(except for the summary report) and a declaration of conformity to the
recognized standard.

In an Abbreviated 510(k), a manufacturer will also have the option of
using a third party to assess conformance with the recognized standard. Under
this scenario, the third party will perform a conformance assessment to the
standard for the device manufacturer and should provide the manufacturer with
a statement to this effect. Like a Special 510(k), the marketing application
should include a declaration of conformity signed by the manufacturer, while
the statement from the third party should be maintained in the Device Master
Record pursuant to the Quality System Regulation. Responsibility for
conformance with the recognized standard, however, rests with the
manufacturer, not the third party.

The incentive for manufacturers to elect to provide summary reports on the use of guidance documents and/or special controls or declarations of conformity to recognized standards will be an expedited review of their submissions. While abbreviated submissions will compete with traditional 510(k) submissions, it is anticipated that their review will be more efficient than that of traditional 510(k) submissions, which tend to be data intensive. In addition, by allowing ODE reviewers to rely on a manufacturer's summary report on the use of a guidance document and/or special controls and declarations of conformity with recognized standards, review resources can be directed at more complicated issues and thus should expedite the process.

2.4.1   Abbreviated 510(k) Content

An Abbreviated 510(k) should include:

- a coversheet clearly identifying the application as an Abbreviated 510(k)
- items required under paragraph 807.87, including a description of the device, the intended use of the device, and the proposed labeling for the device
- for a submission that relies on a guidance document and/or special control(s), a summary report that describes how the guidance and/or special control(s) were used to address the risks associated with the particular device type.
- for a submission that relies on a recognized standard, a declaration of conformity to the standard
- data/information to address issues not covered by guidance documents, special controls, and/or recognized standards
- indications for use enclosure.

2.5   Declaration of Conformity to a Recognized Standard

Declarations of conformity to recognized standards should include the following information:

- an identification of the applicable recognized consensus standards that were met
- a specification, for each consensus standard, that all requirements were met, except for inapplicable requirements or deviations noted below
- an identification for each consensus standard, of any manner(s) in which the standard may have been adopted for application to the device under review, (e.g., an identification of an alternative series of tests that were performed)
- an identification for each consensus standard of any requirements that were not applicable to the device
- a specification of any deviations from each applicable standard that were applied
- a specification of the differences that may exist, if any, between the tested device and the device to be marketed and a justification of the test results in these areas of difference
- the name and address of any test laboratory or certification body involved in determining the conformance of the device with the applicable consensus standards and a reference to any accreditations of those organizations.

2.6   PMA Application

Premarket Approval (PMA) is an approval application for a Class III medical device, including all information submitted with or incorporated by reference. The purpose of the regulation is to establish an efficient and thorough device review process to facilitate the approval of PMAs for devices that have been shown to be safe and effective for their intended use and that otherwise meet the statutory criteria for approval, while ensuring the disapproval of PMAs for devices that have not been shown to be safe and effective or that do not otherwise meet the statutory criteria for approval.

2.6.1   The PMA Application Process

The first step in the PMAA process is the filing of the investigational device exemption (IDE) application for significant risk devices. The IDE is reviewed by the FDA and once accepted, the sponsor can proceed with clinical trials.

2.6.2   Contents of a PMAA

Section 814.20 of 21 CFR defines what must be included in an application, including:

- name and address
- application procedures and table of contents summary
- complete device description
- reference to performance standards
- nonclinical and clinical investigations
- justification for single investigator
- bibliography
- sample of device
- proposed labeling
- environmental assessment
- other information.

The summary should include indications for use, a device description, a description of alternative practices and procedures, a brief description of the marketing history, and a summary of studies. This summary should be of sufficient detail to enable the reader to gain a general understanding of the application. The PMAA must also include the applicant's foreign and domestic marketing history as well as any marketing history of a third party marketing the same product.

The description of the device should include a complete description of the device, including pictorial presentations. Each of the functional components or ingredients should be described, as well as the properties of the device relevant to the diagnosis, treatment, prevention, cure, or mitigation of a disease or condition. The principles of the device's operation should also be explained. Information regarding the methods used in, and the facilities and controls used for the manufacture, processing, packing, storage, and installation of the device should be explained in sufficient detail so that a person generally familiar with current good manufacturing practices can make a knowledgeable judgment about the quality control used in the manufacture of the device.

To clarify which performance standards must be addressed, applicants may ask members of the appropriate reviewing division of the Office of Device Evaluation (ODE) or consult FDA's list of relevant voluntary standards or the Medical Device Standards Activities Report.

2.7   Investigational Device Exemptions

The purpose of the Investigational Device Exemption (IDE) regulation is to encourage the discovery and development of useful devices intended for human use while protecting the public health. It provides the procedures for the conduct of clinical investigations of devices. An approved IDE permits a device to be shipped lawfully for the purpose of conducting investigations of the device without complying with a performance standard or having marketing clearance.

2.7.1   Institutional Review Boards (IRBs)

Any human research is covered by Federal regulation will not be funded unless it has been reviewed by an IRB. The fundamental purpose of an IRB is to ensure that research activities are conducted in an ethical and legal manner. Specifically, IRBs are expected to ensure that each of the basic elements of informed consent, as defined by regulation, are included in the document presented to the research participant for signature or verbal approval.

The deliberations of the IRB must determine that:

- the risks to subjects is equitable
- the selection of subjects is equitable

- informed consent will be sought from each prospective subject or their legally authorized representative
- informed consent will be appropriately documented

- where appropriate, the research plan makes adequate provision for monitoring the data collected to ensure the safety of the subjects
- where appropriate, there are adequate provisions to protect the privacy of subjects and to maintain the confidentiality of data.

It is axiomatic that the IRB should ensure that the risks of participation in a research study should be minimized. The IRB must determine that this objective is to be achieved by ensuring that investigators use procedures that are consistent with sound research design and that do not necessarily expose subjects to excessive risk. In addition, the IRB needs to ensure that the investigators, whenever appropriate, minimize risk and discomfort to the research participants by using, where possible, procedures already performed on the subjects as part of routine diagnosis or treatment.

The Institutional Review Board is any board, committee, or other group formally designated by an institution to review, to approve the initiation of, and to conduct periodic review of biomedical research involving human subjects. The primary purpose of such review is to ensure the protection of the rights and welfare of human subjects.

An IRB must comply with all applicable requirements of the IRB regulation and the IDE regulation in reviewing and approving device investigations involving human testing. An IRB has the authority to review and approve, require modification, or disapprove an investigation. If no IRB exists or if FDA finds an IRB's review to be inadequate, a sponsor may submit an application directly to FDA.

An investigator is responsible for:

- ensuring that the investigation is conducted according to the signed agreement, the investigational plan, and applicable FDA regulations

- protecting the rights, safety, and welfare of subjects
- control of the devices under investigation.

An investigator is also responsible for obtaining informed consent and maintaining and making reports.

2.7.2   IDE Format

There is no preprinted form for an IDE application, but the following information must be included in an IDE application for a significant risk device investigation. Generally, an IDE application should contain the following:

- name and address of sponsor
- complete report of prior investigations
- description of the methods, facilities, and controls used for the manufacture, processing, packing, storage, and installation of the device
- an example of the agreements to be signed by the investigators and a list of the names and addresses of all investigators
- certification that all investigators have signed the agreement, that the list of investigators includes all investigators participating in the study, and that new investigators will sign the agreement before being added to the study
- list of the names, addresses, and chairpersons of all IRBs that have or will be asked to review the investigation and a certification of IRB action concerning the investigation
- the name and address of any institution (other than those above) where a part of the investigation may be conducted
- the amount, if any, charged for the device and an explanation of why sale does not constitute commercialization
- a claim for categorical exclusion or an environmental assessment
- copies of all labeling for device

- copies of all informed consent forms and all related information materials provided to subjects

- any other relevant information that FDA requests for review of the IDE application.

2.8   Software Classification

When a computer product is a component, part, or accessory of a product recognized as a medical device in its own right, the computer component is regulated according to the requirements for the parent device unless the component of the device is separately classified. Computer products that are medical devices and not components, parts or accessories of other products that are themselves medical devices are subject to one of three degrees of regulatory control depending on their characteristics. These products are regulated with the least degree of control necessary to provide reasonable assurance of safety and effectiveness. Computer products that are substantially equivalent to a device previously classified will be regulated to the same degree as the equivalent device. Those devices that are not substantially equivalent to a preamendment device or that are substantially equivalent to a Class III device are regulated as Class III devices.

Software classification, as listed in the FDA draft policy of 1987, follows a similar pattern to devices. Medical software is divided into three classes with regulatory requirements specific to each:

Class I software is subject to the Act's general controls relating to such matters as misbranding, registration of manufacturers, record keeping, and good manufacturing practices. An example of Class I software would be a program that calculates the composition of infant formula.

Class II software is that for which general controls are insufficient to provide reasonable assurance of safety and effectiveness and for which performance standards can provide assurance. This is exemplified by a computer program designed to produce radiation therapy treatment plans.

Class III software is that for which insufficient information exists to ensure that general controls and performance standards will provide reasonable assurance of safety and effectiveness. Generally, these devices are represented to be life-sustaining or life-supporting and may be intended for a use that is of substantial importance in preventing impairment to health. They may be implanted in the body or present a potential unreasonable risk of illness or injury. A program that measures glucose levels and calculates and dispenses insulin based upon those calculations without physician intervention would be a Class III device.

References

Banta, H. David, "The Regulation of Medical Devices," in *Preventive Medicine.* Volume 19, Number 6, November, 1990.

Basile, Edward, "Overview of Current FDA Requirements for Medical Devices," in *The Medical Device Industry: Science, Technology, and Regulation in a Competitive Environment.* New York: Marcel Dekker, Inc., 1990.

Basile, Edward M. and Alexis J. Prease, "Compiling a Successful PMA Application," in *The Medical Device Industry: Science, Technology, and Regulation in a Competitive Environment.* New York: Marcel Dekker, Inc., 1990.

Bureau of Medical Devices, Office of Small Manufacturers Assistance, *Regulatory Requirements for Marketing a Device.* Washington, DC: U.S. Department of Health and Human Services, 1982.

Center for Devices and Radiological Health, *Devic Good Manufacturing Practices Manual.* Washington, DC: U.S. Department of Health and Human Services, 1987.

Food and Drug Administration, *Federal Food, Drug and Cosmetic Act, as Amended January, 1979.* Washington, DC: U.S. Government Printing Office, 1979.

Food and Drug Administration, *Guide to the Inspection of Computerized Systems in Drug Processing*. Washington, DC: Food and Drug Administration, 1983.

Food and Drug Administration, *FDA Policy for the Regulation of Computer Products (Draft)*. Washington, DC: Federal Register, 1987.

Food and Drug Administration, *Software Development Activities*. Washington, DC: Food and Drug Administration, 1987.

Food and Drug Administration, *Medical Devices GMP Guidance for FDA Inspectors*. Washington, DC: Food and Drug Administration, 1987.

Food and Drug Administration, *Reviewer Guidance for Computer-Controlled Medical Devices (Draft)*. Washington, DC: Food and Drug Administration, 1988.

Food and Drug Administration, *Investigational Device Exemptions Manual*. Rockville MD: Center for Devices and Radiological Health, 1992.

Food and Drug Administration, *Premarket Notification 510(k): Regulatory Requirements for Medical Devices*. Rockville MD: Center for Devices and Radiological Health, 1992.

Food and Drug Administration, *Premarket Approval (PMA) Manual*. Rockville MD: Center for Devices and Radiological Health, 1993.

Food and Drug Administration, *Design Control Guidance for Medical Device Manufacturers*. Draft. Rockville, MD: Center for Devices and Radiological Health, 1996.

Food and Drug Administration, *Do It By Design: An Introduction to Human Factors in Medical Devices*. Draft. Rockville, MD: Center for Devices and Radiological Health, 1996.

Food and Drug Administration, *The New 510(k) Paradigm: Alternate Approaches to Demonstrating Substantial Equivalence in Premarket*

Notifications. Rockville, MD: U.S. Department of Health and Human Services, March 20, 1998.

Food and Drug Administration, *Guidances for the Medical Device Industry on PMA Shell Development and Modular Review.* Rockville, MD: U.S. Department of Health and Human Services, November 6, 1998.

Fries, Richard C. et al, "Software Regulation" in *The Medical Device Industry: Science, Technology, and Regulation in a Competitive Environment (Norman Estrin, ed.).* New York: Marcel Dekker, Inc., 1990.

Fries, Richard C., *Reliable Design of Medical Devices.* New York: Marcel Dekker, Inc., 1997.

Ginzburg, Harold M., "Protection of Research Subjects in Clinical Research," in *Legal Aspects of Medicine.* New York: Springer-Verlag, 1989.

Gundaker, Walter E., "FDA's Regulatory Program for Medical Devices and Diagnostics," in *The Medical Device Industry: Science, Technology, and Regulation in a Competitive Environment.* New York: Marcel Dekker, Inc., 1990.

Holstein, Howard M., "How to Submit a Successful 510(k)," in *The Medical Device Industry: Science, Technology, and Regulation in a Competitive Environment.* New York: Marcel Dekker, Inc., 1990.

Jorgens III, J. and C. W. Burch, "FDA Regulation of Computerized Medical Devices," *Byte.* Volume 7, 1982.

Jorgens III, J., "Computer Hardware and Software as Medical Devices," *Medical Device and Diagnostic Industry.* May, 1983.

Jorgens III, J. and R. Schneider, "Regulation of Medical Software by the FDA," *Software in Health Care.* April-May, 1985.

Kahan, J. S., "Regulation of Computer Hardware and Software as Medical Devices," *Canadian Computer Law Reporter.* Volume 6, Number 3, January, 1987.

Munsey, Rodney R. and Howard M. Holstein, "FDA/GMP/MDR Inspections: Obligations and Rights," in *The Medical Device Industry: Science, Technology, and Regulation in a Competitive Environment*. New York: Marcel Dekker, Inc., 1990.

Office of Technology Assessment, Federal Policies and the Medical Devices Industry. Washington, DC: U.S. Government Printing Office, 1984.

Sheretz, Robert J. and Stephen A. Streed, "Medical Devices - Significant Risk vs Nonsignificant Risk," in *Journal of the American Medical Association*. Volume 272, Number 12, September 28, 1994.

Trull, Frankie L. and Barbara A. Rich, "The Animal Testing Issue," in *The Medical Device Industry: Science, Technology, and Regulation in a Competitive Environment*. New York: Marcel Dekker, Inc., 1990.

U. S. Congress, House Committee on Interstate and Foreign Commerce. Medical Devices. Hearings before the Subcommittee on Public Health and the Environment. Octover 23-24, 1973. Serial Numbers 93-61 Washington DC: U.S. Government Printing Office, 1973.

Wholey, Mark H. and Jordan D. Hailer, "An Introduction to the Food and Drug Administration and How It Evaluates New Devices: Establishing Safety and Efficacy," in *CardioVascular and Interventional Radiology*. Volume 18, Number 2, March/April 1995.

Chapter 3

European Standards and Regulations

Richard C. Fries, PE, CRE – Datex-Ohmeda, Inc.
Madison, Wisconsin

The drive toward the creation of a single European economic entity began in 1957 with the signing of the Treaty of Rome. In 1986, the Single European Act established the goal of achieving a single market by 1992 to include 12 member states and approximately 350 million people. Common legislation, the so-called European Directives, were scheduled to cover the entire market. The intention of the European Community (EC) 1992 process was to streamline the approval process for products marketed in the 12 member states. Conceivably, the five member nations of the European Free Trade Association would also recognize the European Directives, even though these nations do not belong to the new common market.

Nearly 300 European Commission Directives have been approved to support implementation of a unified internal market. These directives are not detailed, but rather contain information regarding general *essential requirements*. European regional standards setting bodies are responsible for

establishing the voluntary standards, which elaborate on the essential
requirements.

The European Union was known as the European Community until
the Maastricht Treaty took effect in 1993. Present members include:

> Austria
> Belgium
> Denmark
> France
> Finland
> Germany
> Greece
> Ireland
> Italy
> Luxembourg
> The Netherlands
> Portugal
> Spain
> Sweden
> The United Kingdom.

In 1994, the Agreement on a European Economic Area took effect, adding
Iceland, Liechtenstein, and Norway to the single market, although they did not
join the European Union. These 18 countries comprise a market approximately
the size of the North American Free Trade Agreement.

Standards serve as an essential component in assuring the complete
freedom of trade in merchandise across national borders. Standard bodies in
the member states are obliged to adopt European standards and withdraw
conflicting national standards. Harmonized, European-wide standards in key
product sectors are now replacing the thousands of differing national standards
that existed within member states. Today, the European standardization system
has almost 5,000 standards and produces approximately five new standards per
working day.

3.1   The European Regulatory Scene

The production and adoption of software standards is very much the responsibility of international and national standards organizations and, in the case of the European context, bodies set up to represent a number of national organizations. Progressively, it is becoming the case that standards are developed by the international bodies and then adopted by the national bodies. Appendix 3 lists the addresses and telephone numbers of the various international standards bodies. Some of the international bodies include:

BSI. The British Standards Institute is the United Kingdom's national standards making organization. In performing its duties, it collaborates with industry, government agencies, other standard bodies, professional organizations, etc.

CEN. The Comité Européen de Normalisation (European Committee for Standardization) is composed of members drawn from the European Union (EU) and the European Free Trade Association (EFTA). The role of CEN is to produce standards for use within Europe and effectively covers the area addressed by ISO.

CENELAC. The Comité Européen de Normalisation Electronique (European Committee for Electrotechnical Standardization) is made up of representatives from the national Electrotechnical committees, the majority of whom are represented on the IEC. Its responsibilities are for electrical and electronic standards within Europe and it has close links with the activities of the IEC.

CISPR. The International Special Committee on Radio Interference is a committee under the auspices of the IEC and run through a Plenary Assembly consisting of delegates from all the member bodies, including the United States. The committee is headquartered in Geneva, Switzerland and is composed of seven subcommittees, including:

- Radio Interference Measurement and Statistical Methods
- Interference from Industrial, Scientific and Medical Radio Frequency Apparatus

- Interference from Overhead Power Lines, High Voltage Equipment and Electric Traction Systems
- Interference Related to Motor Vehicles and Internal Combustion Engines
- Interference Characteristics of Radio Receivers
- Interference from Motor, Household Appliances, Lighting Apparatus and the like
- Interference from Information Technology Equipment

DIN. The Deutsches Institut für Normung (German Standardization Institute) is the committee that sets German standards.

DOH. The Department of Health has the same responsibility in England that the FDA has in the United States. DOH sets forth standards for medical devices and has established a Good Manufacturing Practice for Medical Equipment, similar to that of the FDA. DOH is headquartered in London. DOH currently has reciprocity with the FDA, meaning the FDA will accept DOH inspection data as their own and DOH will accept FDA inspection data. This is particularly applicable for companies with facilities in both England and the United States.

IEC. The International Electrotechnical Commission was established in 1906 with the responsibility for developing international standards within the electrical and electronics field. By agreement with the International Standards Organization, the IEC has sole responsibility for these standards.

ISO. The International Standards Organization was established in 1947 and its members are drawn from the national standards bodies of its members. ISO is responsible for standardization in general, but with the exception of electrical and electronic standards which are the responsibility of the IEC.

3.2   European Directives

In the period up to 1992, and subsequently, the European Parliament has enacted a series of measures intended to put the single market into practice. Some of these directives have been aimed at removing barriers of a purely customs/excise nature, while others have concentrated on transport arrangements to ensure the free movement of goods. A series of directives, produced under the heading of "New Approach Directives," are intended to provide controls on product design, with the principal objective being to provide a level playing field for product safety requirements across the European Union.

The primary function of these directives is to ensure that products are sufficiently well designed and built to be fit for the purpose for which they are sold, and that reasonable precautions are taken to protect the user against injury while the product is being used. Recent directives have included provisions for medical devices and electromagnetic compatibility.

In the past, the European Union relied on harmonized legislation to enforce common production standards, without reference to voluntary standards or a marking system. Under this old approach, directives contained such a high degree of detail on the technical specifications of products, it sometimes required a decade or more to complete the technical work.

Now, the new approach directives specify only the *essential requirements* to be met by products and that the technical specifications governing the production and marketing of products meeting the essential requirements be laid down by the relevant European standardization bodies.

3.3   European Standardization Bodies

Under this approach, the European Commission mandated that the private sector be responsible for development of European technical standards. Three regional standards organizations were assigned the task:

- The European Committee for Standardization (CEN),
- The European Committee for Electrotechnical Standardization (CENELEC),
- The European Telecommunications Standards Institute (ETSI).

CEN, CENELEC, and ETSI constitute a European forum for standardization that organizes participation of all parties concerned in the development and standardization programs. These parties include national government authorities, the Commission of European Communities (commonly known as the European Commission) the European Free Trade Association, public bodies, manufacturers, trade unions, users, and consumers. These parties come together in hundreds of technical groups to prepare European standards through procedures that guarantee respect for the principles of openness and transparency, consensus, national commitment, technical coherence at the national and European level, and correct integration with other international work. Consequently, the development of standards within the national bodies of the European Union essentially ceased and work was transferred into the European standards organizations.

Many multinational manufacturers have globalized their product development efforts. Until recently, they have regarded the FDA as the agency with the most experience in regulating medical devices. The EC 1992 process splits the burden of stringent regulation between the United States and the European Commission. Many of these multinational manufacturers have grown accustomed to dealing with U.S. bureaucracy, but now will have to work also with the incipient EC bureaucracy in Brussels. Unraveling the complex European process is extremely difficult. Change is rapid and what is established as fact this week, may be overturned or obsolete next week.

These complex changes and the bureaucracy being created in Brussels are being driven by seven major groups of organizations. The groups consist of the following:

- the European Commission,
- standing committees,
- standards organizations,
- Notified Bodies,
- Board of Health,
- Ethical Committee.

The European Commission, one of the three major branches of the European government, is the primary force of change. Another branch, the European Parliament, debates the directives proposed by the Commission. The third branch, the Court of Justice, will adjudicate any differences that arise between parties within the European Community.

The three medical device directives create standing committees, which after the European Commission, constitute the second major force behind the European regulatory changes. Each directive creates two committees, which could be combined into one major standing committee that would address differences between essential requirements outlined in all the directives and international or European normalized standards. The second standing committee, which might vary depending upon the directive, would address specific issues relevant to that directive. What have been termed *competent authorities*, namely the boards of health of the 12 member states, constitute another major force behind these changes.

Notified Bodies compose yet another force for change. In reality, these are the test houses that are designated by individual member states' board of health. Some states may have more than one test house, and smaller countries may have none. Those member states that do not designate a Notified Body will delegate their medical device issues to member states that have larger and more resourceful boards of health and Notified Bodies.

Ethical committees at EC medical institutions also play an important role in evaluating investigational devices. Many European teaching institutions already have ethics committees properly constituted and duly functioning. Many non-teaching institutions, however, do not have such committees and will be required to form them.

These organizational forces are, and will remain, highly interactive. Many institutions are working diligently at what they perceive to be their mandate. From the United States perspective, the European process is producing a great deal of activity and, in some cases, significant action. It is clear that many organizations are working to change the legislative and regulatory environment for medical devices in Europe.

3.4   European Standards Development Process

Through their standardization work, CEN, CENELEC, and ETSI aim to remove any differences of a technical nature, either between the national standards of the member states or between measures applied at the national level to certify conformity, that could give rise to technical barriers to trade. In the areas of technology, European Standards are prepared following specific requests from the European Commission and the European Free Trade Association.

3.4.1   New Work

The Dresden Agreement, between CENELEC and IEC, gives IEC the "Right of First Refusal" for work proposed in CENELEC. According to the Vienna Agreement, CEN must determine whether it is possible to give preference to ISO to develop a new project, noting that a completed standards project must be available within specific timeframes. ISO has three months to respond to any such request received from CEN. CEN must also consider its various procedural options and, if the CEN technical committee decides to propose the work item to ISO, work will commence following the normal procedures in one of the following scenarios:

- new work falling within the scope of an existing ISO technical committee and subcommittee
- new work requiring an extension of the scope of an existing ISO technical committee
- new work proposed that falls into a field(s) not yet covered in ISO.

3.4.2   Development

Most European Standards not taken from one of the international standardization organizations are developed in working groups reporting to technical committees or subcommittees of the regional European standards organizations. Access to this process by U.S. interests has been acquired in four ways:

- Under the Vienna and Dresden Agreements, the relevant ISO or IEC/RCs or SCs can appoint a representative, preferably no more than two, to the parallel European activity, including working groups

- ANSI can officially request that an American be allowed to attend a working group meeting(s) as an observer
- Interests with representatives in Europe can become members of a European country's delegation and participate directly
- Informal agreements between U.S. interests and their counterparts in CEN or CENELEC working groups allow participation.

3.4.3 Public Enquiry

Public enquiry is a six month time period during which the European members can offer national body comments. This is not a voting stage. Under the Vienna and Dresden Agreements, CEN and CENELEC have agreed to accept comments on preliminary European Standards (prEN) and preliminary Harmonized Documents (prHD) from ISO and IEC member bodies. ANSI, as the U.S. member body, announces availability of all prENs and prHDs in ANSI's Standards Action and via their site on the world wide web. Enquiry drafts can be purchased from ANSI's Customer Services Department and comments submitted via staff in ANSI's Standards Facilitation Department. U.S. comments are sent to the offices of the respective Central Secretariat in Brussels and are referred to the applicable technical committee for response. Replies to U.S. comments are received in due course by ANSI and referred back to the originator in the United States.

3.4.4 Formal Vote

CEN, CENELEC, and ETSI are populated at the formal vote stage by member countries, not by individuals. National delegations have weighted votes, applied for by the national body and confirmed by the General Assemblies of the respective organizations.

The United States, as a non-member nation, does not have a vote. If ANSI were to be a member and have a vote in these organizations, the United States would be obligated by the respective Operating Procedures to adopt and implement approved ENs at the national level and to withdraw any conflicting national standard. U.S. interests have indicated that they are unwilling to accept as a matter of course the outright adoption as national standards of all documents developed and approved by the European standardization bodies.

Further, within the European regional bodies, the U.S. would have only one vote, even if weighted to some extent. Through ANSI, the U.S. has considerably more options in lining up support for issues arising under the purview of the ISO and IEC. In the international arena, even though it is still one country - one vote, ANSI can call upon allies in the Pan American Standards Commission (COPANT) and the Pacific Area Standards Congress (PASC) for supporting votes from outside Europe.

ANSI does, however, publish notice of the two month formal vote stage in Standards Action. The formal vote documents, which in most cases become the approved European Standard, are available for sale through ANSI's Customer Services Department.

3.4.5   Publication

ETSI publishes its final documents following approval by its constituents. Member countries are responsible for publishing European Standards approved by CEN and CENELEC. ANSI obtains and sells ENs upon request.

3.5   Other European Standards Considerations

3.5.1   Primary Questionnaire Procedure

In order to test the market need for a standard, a Primary Questionnaire (PQ) has been developed. The PQ procedure permits CEN or CENELEC to determine whether enough interest exists in harmonization on the subject proposed, the existing degree of national harmonization on the reference document in question, and whether the document would be acceptable as an EN, HD, or ENV. The PQ procedure serves the same purpose as the six-month enquiry procedure and concerns entirely new documents being offered to CEN or CENELEC.

3.5.2   Dual Regional and International Work

If European regional activities are already underway and the international community attempts to begin a similar activity, the Europeans may resist the suggestion for a new international committee. As an alternative, the European regional body may suggest that they will "fast-track" their work into ISO or IEC, as appropriate, at the enquiry stage (DIS or CDV, respectively), thereby providing non-Europeans with an opportunity to cast a national body position during the fast-track DIS or CDV ballot. The problem, however, is that comments will be forwarded back to the regional body for response. This scenario provides relatively little input for non-Europeans to participate in the development of the project.

When faced with this situation, the affected U.S. industry sector, normally working through a trade association or professional society and via ANSI, must actively persuade other non-European countries of the necessity of doing the work in an international organization like ISO or IEC. The United States should be extremely confident that it has the required number of allies guaranteed to support the formation of a new ISO or IEC TC or SC prior to ANSI or USNC submission of the proposal for a new area of technical work.

3.5.3   Parallel Voting

According to the Lugano Agreement, only DIS (Draft International Standards) were processed for parallel voting both within IEC and CENELEC. Now with the approval of the Dresden Agreement, IEC working drafts will also be sent to CENELEC for parallel review and comment. This procedure makes it more likely that the draft standard will be accepted not only internationally, but also as an identical European standard.

The Vienna Agreement also provides for parallel voting at the DIS and FDIS (Final Draft International Standard) level. If mutual agreement is reached, the International Standard (IS) and EN would be published concurrently. The submitting organization is responsible for responding to comments during voting.

3.5.4   Unique Acceptance Procedure

The Unique Acceptance Procedure (UAP) may be applied in any type
of document, whatever its origin, in order to achieve rapid approval of an EN
or HD, if it is reasonable to suppose that the document is acceptable at the
European level. For a reference document, the UAP combines the
questionnaire procedure and the formal vote.

If CEN or CENELEC modify an international standard, ISO or IEC
must either agree to incorporate the changes into a new international standard,
or the regional bodies shall adopt the revised text as a regional, but not
international, standard.

3.6   Conformity Assessment and Testing

The European Commission has supported its program of directives for
the elimination of technical barriers to trade with a selection of harmonized
conformity modules and with the use of a harmonized European mark, the CE
mark.

The purpose of the directives is not to ban any products from the
European Union single market, unless the product is very poorly made or is
unsafe. For most reputable manufacturers, complying with the essential
protection requirements of the directives is not particularly onerous and
companies that have always taken a responsible attitude to the performance and
design of their products will have few problems complying with the directives.

3.6.1   The CE Mark

CE marking does not indicate conformity to a standard, but rather
indicates conformity to the legal requirements of EU directives. Many of the
EU directives require manufacturers to have a Certified Quality System
conforming to ISO 9000 in operation and to use the assistance of a Notified
Body in order that the manufacturer can legitimately apply the CE marking to
their product.

As there may be difficulties in the administrative requirements, a new way of working for some manufacturers and suppliers, particularly small businesses, may be required. Manufacturers may well find it cost effective to seek outside help in the early stages of complying with the directives, in order to save time and prevent expensive mistakes. However, it is important to be aware that it is rarely necessary to commit to an expensive program of testing and certification. Unless the directives applying to the product specifically require the involvement of a third party for product approval or quality system assessment, the manufacturer can affix the mark without having to involve test house, consultant or anyone else.

The CE mark (Figure 3-1) must be affixed to the product, its instructional manual, or its packaging. It must be at least 5 mm high. It is not intended to be a mark of quality. Rather, it is intended to indicate to the authorities responsible for enforcing the directives that the product's manufacturer claims compliance with the directives that apply to the product.

The act of fixing the mark to the product, and signing the Declaration of Conformity, constitutes a declaration by the manufacturer that the product meets the requirements of all the directives that apply to it. The onus is very much on the manufacturer to take responsibility for this actually being true. Marking a product which is not fully in accordance with the requirements of the applicable directives is an offense in its own right, and would also contravene related consumer safety and trade description legislation.

3.6.2   The Keymark

The purpose of the "Keymark" (Figure 3-2) is to make available to European industry a voluntary harmonized service that provides for the independent third-party testing of products and to ensure compliance with the requirements of the relevant European Standards developed by CEN or CENELEC. The Keymark also requires confirmation of the manufacturer's quality management system. To ensure that quality is maintained, both the manufacturer and the product will be subject to regular assessment.

Contrary to the mandatory "CE" mark, use of the Keymark is voluntary. The Keymark may replace many, if not all, of the numerous

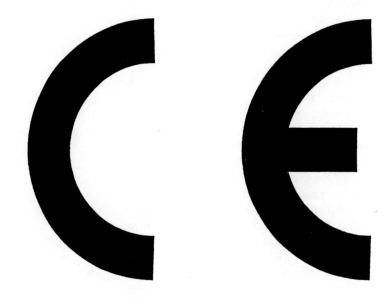

Figure 3-1   The CE mark. (From Fries, 1998.)

national certification marks for products which are sold throughout Europe. It is expected that there will be a reduction in costs related to certification, which will impact the consumer at another level.

The U.S. will monitor use of the mark to ensure that it does not become de facto mandatory as, for example, in procurements.

3.7   European Organization for Testing and Certification

The European Organization for Testing and Certification (EOTC) was established in April, 1990 by the European Commission, the European Free Trade Association, and the European Standards Bodies. Articles of Association were signed by the 22 founding members on December 3, 1992, and the EOTC attained a legal status under Belgian law in April, 1993. EOTC members are testing and calibration laboratories with help and input from certification

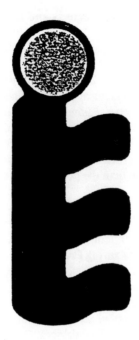

Figure 3-2   The Keymark. (From Fries, 1998.)

bodies, manufacturers, and trade associations. The customer base of EOTC is composed of suppliers, manufacturers, purchasers, and users of goods and services and all those who benefit from the development of mutual recognition in any sector.

The EOTC acts as a focal point for conformity assessment issues in Europe, but does not itself test or certify products or services. Testing is performed by recognized Agreement Groups consisting of test laboratories or certification bodies.

3.8   Examples of European Directives and Regulations

3.8.1   The ISO Guidance Documents for ISO 9001 and 9002

ISO Technical Committee 210 has recently developed two guidelines relating ISO 9001 and 9002 to medical devices. The 1994 version of ISO 9001 and 9002 are intended to be general standards defining quality system requirements. ISO 13485 provides particular requirements for suppliers of medical devices that are more specific than the general requirements of ISO 9001. ISO 13488 provides particular requirements for suppliers of medical devices that are more specific than the general requirements of ISO 9002.

In conjunction with ISO 9001 and 9002, these International Standard define requirements for quality systems relating to the design, development, production, installation and servicing of medical devices. They embrace all the principles of the Good Manufacturing Practices (GMPs) used in the production of medical devices. They can only be used in conjunction with ISO 9001 and 9002 and are not a stand alone standards.

They specify the quality system requirements for the production and, where relevant, installation of medical devices. They are applicable when there is a need to assess a medical device supplier's quality system or when a regulatory requirement specifies that this standard shall be used for such assessment. As part of an assessment by a third party for the purpose of regulatory requirements, the supplier may be required to provide access to confidential data in order to demonstrate compliance with one of these standards. The supplier may be required to exhibit these data, but is not obliged by the standard to provide copies for retention.

Particular requirements in a number of clauses of these standards are covered in detail in other International Standards. Suppliers should review the requirements and consider using the relevant International Standards in these areas.

To assist in the understanding of the requirements of ISO 9001, 9002, ISO 13485, and 13488, an international guidance standard is being prepared. The document provides general guidance on the implementation of quality systems for medical devices based on ISO 13485. Such quality systems include those of the EU Medical Device Directives and the GMP requirements currently in preparation in Canada, Japan, and the U. S. It may be used for systems based on ISO 13488 by the omission of sub-clause 4.4.

The guidance given in this document is applicable to the design, development, production, installation and servicing of medical devices of all kinds. The document describes concepts and methods to be considered by medical device manufacturers who are establishing and maintaining quality systems. this document describes examples of ways in which the quality system requirements can be met, and it is recognized that there may be alternative ways that are better suited to a particular device/manufacturer. It is not intended to be directly used for assessment of quality systems.

3.8.2   ISO 14000 Series

ISO formed Technical Committee 207 in 1993 to develop standards in the field of environmental management tools and systems. The work of ISO TC 207 encompasses seven areas:

- management systems
- audits
- labeling
- environmental performance evaluation
- life cycle assessment
- terms and definitions
- environmental aspects in product standards.

The ISO 14000 standards are not product standards, nor do they specify performance or pollutant/effluent levels. They specifically exclude test methods for pollutants and do not set limit values regarding pollutants or effluents.

The 14000 standards are intended to promote the broad interests of the public and users, be cost-effective, non-prescriptive and flexible, and be more easily accepted and implemented. The goal is to improve environmental protection and quality of life.

ISO 14000 provides for the basic tenets of an environmental management system (EMS). An environmental management system is the management system which addresses the environmental impact of a company's processes and product on the environment. The EMS provides a formalized structure for ensuring that environmental concerns are addressed and met, and works to both control a company's significant environmental effects and achieve regulatory compliance.

The certification process for ISO 14000 has six steps:

- quality documentation review
- initial visit, preassessment or checklist
- on-site audit
- follow-up audits to document corrective action
- periodic audits to document compliance
- renewal audit every 3-5 years.

Currently, there is limited correlation between ISO 14000 and ISO 9000, but the requirements of the two series may become more harmonized in the future. Under certain conditions, the ISO 14000 audit and the ISO 9000 audit can be combined into one. It has been estimated that the cost of complying to ISO 14000 would be comparable to that for certification to ISO 9000. The registration process itself could take up to 18 months to complete.

It is expected that ISO 14000 will be in print and official by mid-summer, 1996. Many European countries have already accepted the draft version as their EMS standard and have begun issuing accreditation. The Japanese Ministry of International Trade and Industry is asking companies to prepare new environmental management plans that conform with ISO 14000 by the end of 1996.

In the US, ANSI has established a national program to accredit ISO 14000 registrars, auditor certifiers, and training providers. The ISO 14000 registrars are likely to come from the registrars currently performing certifications in ISO 9000.

The creation of a universal single set of EMS standards will help companies and organizations to better manage their environmental affairs, and show a commitment to environmental protection. It should also help them avoid multiple registrations, inspections, permits, and certifications of products exchanged among countries. In addition, it should concentrate worldwide attention on environmental management. The World Bank and other financial institutions may qualify their loans to less developed countries and being to use the 14000 standards as an indicator of commitment to environmental protection.

In the U.S., implementation of ISO 14000 could become a condition of business loans to companies that are not even involved in international trade. Insurance companies may lower premiums for those who have implemented the standard. It may become a condition of some supplier transactions, especially in Europe and with the U.S. government. Evidence of compliance could become a factor in regulatory relief programs, the exercise of prosecutorial and sentencing discretion, consent decrees and other legal instruments, and multilateral trade agreements. U.S. government agencies considering the ISO 14000 standards include:

- the Environmental Protection Agency
- the Department of Defense
- the Department of Energy
- the Food and Drug Administration
- the National Institute of Standards and Technology
- the Office of the U.S. Trade Representative
- the Office of Science, Technology and Policy.

3.9   Medical Informatics

The real world is perceived as a complex system characterized by the existence of various parallel autonomous processes evolving in a number of separate locations, loosely coupled, cooperating by the interchange of mutually understandable messages. Due to the fact that medical specialties, functional areas, and institutions create, use and rely on interchanged information, they should share a common basic understanding in order to cooperate in accordance with a logical process constrained under an administrative organization, a medical heuristics and approach to care.

A health care framework is a logical mapping between the real world, in particular the health care environment, and its health care information systems architecture. This framework, representing the main health care subsystems, their connections, rules, etc. is the basis for an evolutionary development of heterogenous computer-supported health care information and communications systems. A key feature of the framework is its reliance on the use of abstractions. In this way, the framework, at its most abstract level, reflects the fundamental and essential features of health care processes and information, and can be seen as applicable to all health care entities. It defines the general information structure and enables the exchangeability of the information.

The European health care framework will maintain and build upon the diversity of national health care systems in the European countries. A harmonized description/structure of planning documentation will be provided to ensure comparisons between European countries.

The main rationale for a standardized health care information framework is:

- to act as a contract between the users and procures on the one hand and the developers and providers of information systems on the other
- to ensure that all applications and databases are developed to support the health care organization as a whole as opposed to just a single organization or department
- to obtain economies of scale, originating from enhanced portability, as health care information systems are expensive to develop and to maintain, and tend to be installed on an international basis
- to define a common basic understanding that allows all health care information systems to interchange data.

To this end, CEN/CENELAC has tasked a committee with creating the Health Care Framework model.

3.10 The Global Harmonization Task Force

The Global Harmonization Task Force was formed in September, 1992 with the goal of facilitating the mutual recognition of quality system approvals relating to medical devices. The Task Force was sponsored by the European Commission and is made up of delegates from industry and government in Australia, Canada, Europe, Japan, Mexico, and the United States. At its first meeting, the Task Force set as its goal the assurance that the internationally recognized ISO 9000 series of quality system standards was interpreted in each country's law in an equivalent way.

To date, many countries have welcomed the comments and advice of the Task Force without the existence of a formal structure or formal obligations. The comments of the Task Force on national draft regulations have been considered in detail by the countries concerned with regard to current regulations. Nevertheless, there is a need for more discussion on how to give greater political impact to the Task Force's documents.

3.10.1 Objectives of the Task Force

The Global Harmonization Task Force has taken on the following objectives:

- to examine differing supplementary requirements to ISO 9001/9002 and agree or propose textual changes to bring them into alignment.
- to examine the need for new documents or programs that would help in the uniform application and inspection of quality systems and identify the steps needed to create them.

Three new study groups were initially formed to help the task force in meeting its objectives. The responsibilities of each group were:

Study Group I: Comparison of Regulatory Schemes

The Group will consider regulatory systems in the United States, Canada, Japan, and the European Community for selection of medical devices. The purpose will be to evaluate and compare all aspects of product approval processes.

<u>Study Group II</u>: Harmonization of the FDA/GMP and EN 46001

The Group will work toward aligning the United States' GMP system and Europe's prEN 46001.

<u>Study Group III</u>: Guidance Documents

The Group will aim to harmonize all existing or draft guidance quality system documents into one general guidance document for manufacturers and inspectors of medical devices. Appendices may have to be harmonized for specific issues, such as sterilization, software, and clean rooms.

The Global Harmonization Task Force attempts to fulfill its goals by taking on the following tasks:

- examining the supplementary requirements to ISO 9001 and 9002 and agreeing or proposing textual changes to bring them into alignment
- examining available or draft guidance documents to quality system standards for use by manufacturers and or inspectors, and agreeing or proposing steps to bring them into alignment
- examining available or draft documents addressing issues related to quality systems and agreeing or proposing steps to bring them into alignment
- examining the need for new documents or programs that would facilitate the uniform application and inspection of quality systems and identifying the steps needed to bring them into existence
- recognizing the need for and developing the procedure for the establishment of an internationally harmonized nomenclature system for medical devices.

3.10.2   Philosophy of the Task Force

Work on a global vigilance system for medical devices will be based on the philosophy and structure of the European system.   While national quality systems differ, there are areas of common ground where harmonization could be achieved.   Harmonization of requirements is regarded as a feasible first step toward the ultimate goal of mutual recognition.

3.10.3   Current Activities

The Global Harmonization Task Force currently has four active study groups:

Study Group 1	Regulatory Systems
Study Group 2	Post-Market Surveillance
Study Group 3	Quality Systems
Study Group 4	Quality Systems Auditing

Working Group 1 is involved with examining medical device regulatory systems in use in the major trading countries/regions to identify features of those systems which have a common basis, but different applications, identifying features peculiar to individual systems, which may present obstacles to uniform regulation, making proposals to the Task Force for harmonization activities relating to these features, and suggesting priorities.

Working Group 2 is involved with working on the harmonization of requirements for reporting adverse events, device nomenclature, and requirements for exchange of regulatory data.

Working Group 3 is involved with issuing guidance on the implementation of quality systems, and working on guidance for design control and process validation.

Working Group 4 is involved with developing guidance on the auditing of quality systems for the design and manufacture of medical devices.

References

American National Standards Institute (ANSI), *American Access to the European Standardization Process*. New York: American National Standards Institute, 1996.

Association for the Advancement of Medical Instrumentation, *ISO/DIS 13485, Medical Devices - Particular Requirements for the Application of ISO 9001*. Arlington, VA: Association for the Advancement of Medical Instrumentation, 1995.

Association for the Advancement of Medical Instrumentation, *ISO/DIS 13488, Medical Devices - Particular Requirements for the Application of ISO 9002*. Arlington, VA: Association for the Advancement of Medical Instrumentation, 1995.

Association for the Advancement of Medical Instrumentation, *First Draft of Quality Systems - Medical Devices - Guidance on the Application of ISO 13485 and ISO 13488*. Arlington, VA: Association for the Advancement of Medical Instrumentation, 1995.

Banta, H. David, "The Regulation of Medical Devices," in *Preventive Medicine*. Volume 19, Number 6, November, 1990.

Cascio, Joe, editor, *The ISO 114000 Handbook*. Milwaukee, WI: The American Society for Quality Control, 1996.

CEN/CENELAC, *Directory of the European Standardization Requirements for Health Care Informatics and Programme for the Development of Standards*. Brussels, Belgium: European Committee for Standardization, 1992.

CEN/CENELAC, *Directory of the European Standardization Requirements for Health Care Informatics and Programme for the Development of Standards*. Brussels, Belgium: European Committee for Standardization, 1992.

CEN/CENELAC, *EN 46001*. Brussels, Belgium: European Committee for Standardization, 1995.

CEN/CENELAC, *EN 46002*. Brussels, Belgium: European Committee for Standardization, 1995.

"Changes ahead for Global Harmonisation Task Force," in *Clinica World Medical Device And Diagnostic News*. October 21, 1996.

Department of Trade and Industry, *Guide to Software Quality Management System Construction and Certification Using EN 29001*. London: DISC TickIT Office, 1987.

"Differences in quality systems reviewed," in *Clinica World Medical Device And Diagnostic News*. November 24, 1993.

Donaldson, John, "U.S. Companies Gear Up for ISO 14001 Certification," in *In Tech*. Volume 43, Number 5, May, 1996.

"European vigilance to be model for global system," in *Clinica World Medical Device And Diagnostic News*. March 18, 1996.

Fries, Richard C., *Reliable Medical Device Design*. New York: Marcel Dekker, Inc., 1997.

Fries, Richard C., *Medical Device Quality Assurance and Regulatory Compliance*. New York: Marcel Dekker, Inc., 1998.

"Global Harmonisation Task Force sets its agenda," in *Clinica World Medical Device And Diagnostic News*. February 17, 1993.

"Global harmonisation of medical device regulation," in *Clinica World Medical Device And Diagnostic News*. October 6, 1993.

"Harrmonisation of US device-approved regulations," in *Clinica World Medical Device And Diagnostic News*. July 31, 1995.

"Harmonizing quality system auditing stresses interest conflicts," in *Europe Drug & Device Report.* Volume 6, Number 9, April 29, 1996.

"Harmonization efforts will bring more data to FDA," in *Devices & Diagnostics Letter.* Volume 23, Number 43, November 8, 1996.

International Standard Organization, *Quality Management and Quality Assurance Standards - Part 3: Guidelines for the Application of ISO 9001 to the Development, Supply and Maintenance of Software.* Geneva, Switzerland: International Organization for Standardization, 1991.

"International device harmonization a double-edged sword," in *Europe Drug & Device Report.* Volume 6, Number 23, December 9, 1996.

Meeldijk, Victor, *Electronic Components: Selection and Application Guidelines.* New York: John Wiley & Sons, Inc., 1996.

Schaefer, Jack, "Europe 1992: Organizational Structure, Administrative Procedures, and Proposed Regulations," in *Medical Design and Material.* Volume 1, Number 2, February, 1991.

Shaw, Roger, "Safety Critical Software and Current Standards Initiatives," in *Computer Methods and Programs in Biomedicine.* Volume 44, Number 1, July, 1994.

"Stepwise approach to global harmonisation," in *Clinica World Medical Device And Diagnostic News.* July 10, 1995.

Tabor, Tom and Ira Feldman, *ISO 14000: A Guide to the New Environmental Management Standards.* Milwaukee, WI: The American Society for Quality Control, 1996.

"U.S. and EU industry split over new ISO device committee," in *Europe Drug & Device Report.* Volume 4, Number 16, August 8, 1994.

Working Group #4, *Draft of Proposed Regulatory Requirements for Medical Devices Sold in Canada.* Ottawa, Ontario Canada: Environmental Heal Directorate, 1995.

Chapter 4

The Medical Device Directives

Richard C. Fries, PE, CRE – Datex-Ohmeda, Inc.
Madison, Wisconsin

The European Community's program on the Completion of the Internal Market has, as the primary objective for medical devices, to assure Community-wide free circulation of products. The only means to establish such free circulation, in view of quite divergent national systems, regulations governing medical devices, and existing trade barriers, was to adopt legislation for the Community, by which the health and safety of patients, users and third persons would be ensured through a harmonized set of device related protection requirements. Devices meeting the requirements and sold to members of the Community are identified by means of a CE mark.

The Active Implantable Medical Devices Directive adopted by the Community legislator in 1990 and the Medical Devices Directive in 1993 cover more than 80% of medical devices for use with human beings. After a period of transition, i.e., a period during which the laws implementing a Directive co-exist with pre-existing national laws, these directives exhaustively govern the conditions for placing medical devices on the market. Through the agreements on the European Economic Area (EEA), the relevant requirements and procedures are the same for all European Community (EC) member states and European Free Trade Association (EFTA) countries that belong to the EEA, an economic area comprising more than 380 million people.

4.1   Definition of a Medical Device

The various Medical Device Directives define a medical device as:

"any instrument, appliance, apparatus, material or other
article, whether used alone or in combination, including
the software necessary for its proper application, intended by the
manufacturer to be used for human beings for the purpose of:

- diagnosis, prevention, monitoring, treatment or alleviation of disease
- diagnosis, monitoring, alleviation of or compensation for an injury or handicap
- investigation, replacement or modification of the anatomy or of a physiological process
- control of conception;

and which does not achieve its principal intended action in
or on the human body by pharmacological, immunological or
metabolic means, but which may be assisted in its function
by such means."

One important feature of the definition is that it emphasizes the "intended use" of the device and its "principal intended action." This use of the term *intended* gives manufacturers of certain products some opportunity to include or exclude their product from the scope of the particular Directive.

Another important feature of the definition is the inclusion of the term *software*. The software definition will probably be given further interpretation, but is currently interpreted to mean 1) software intended to control the function of a device is a medical device, 2) software for patient records or other administrative purposes is not a device, 3) software which is built into a device, e.g., software in an electrocardiographic monitor used to drive a display, is clearly an integral part of the medical device or 4) a software update sold by the manufacturer, or a variation sold by a software house, is a medical device in its own right.

4.2   The Medical Device Directives Process

The process of meeting the requirements of the Medical Device Directive is a multi-step approach, involving the following activities:

- analyze the device to determine which directive is applicable
- identify the applicable Essentials Requirements List
- identify any corresponding Harmonized Standards
- confirm that the device meets the Essential Requirements/Harmonized Standards and document the evidence
- classify the device
- decide on the appropriate conformity assessment procedure
- identify and choosing a notified body
- obtain conformity certifications for the device
- establish a Declaration of Conformity
- apply for the CE mark.

This process does not necessarily occur in a serial manner, but iterations may occur throughout the cycle. Each activity in the process will be examined in detail.

4.3   Choosing the Appropriate Directive

Because of the diversity of current national medical device regulations, the Commission decided that totally new Community legislation covering all medical devices was needed. Software or a medical device containing software may be subject to the requirements of the Active Implantable Medical Device Directive or the Medical Device Directive.

Three directives are envisaged to cover the entire field of medical devices:

Active Implantable Medical Device Directive (AIMDD)

This directive applies to a medical device which depends on a source of electrical energy or any source of power other than that directly generated by the human body or gravity, which is intended to be totally or partially introduced, surgically or medically, into the human body or by medical intervention into a natural orifice, and which is intended to remain after the procedure. This directive was adopted in June, 1990, implemented in January, 1993 and the transition period ended January, 1995.

Medical Device Directive (MDD)

This directive applies to all medical devices and accessories, unless they are covered by the Active Implantable Medical Device Directive or the In Vitro Diagnostic Medical Device Directive. This directive was adopted in June, 1993, was implemented in January, 1995 and the transition period ends June, 1998.

In Vitro Diagnostic Medical Device Directive (IVDMDD)

This directive applies to any medical device that is a reagent, reagent product, calibrator, control kit, instrument, equipment or system intended to be used in vitro for the examination of samples derived from the human body for the purpose of providing information concerning a physiological state of health or disease or congenital abnormality, or to determine the safety and compatibility with potential recipients. This directive is currently in preparation.

4.4   Identifying the Applicable Essential Requirements

The major legal responsibility the Directives place on the manufacturer of a medical device requires the device meet the Essential Requirements set out in Annex I of the Directive which applies to them, taking into account the intended purpose of the device. The Essential Requirements are written in the form of 1) general requirements which always apply and 2) particular requirements, only some of which apply to any particular device.

The general requirements for the Essential Requirements List take the following form:

- the device must be safe. Any risk must be acceptable in relation to the benefits offered by the device
- the device must be designed in such a manner that risk is minimized
- the device must perform in accordance with the manufacturer's specification
- the safety and performance must be maintained throughout the indicated lifetime of the device.
- the safety and performance of the device must not be affected by normal conditions of transport and storage.
- any side effects must be acceptable in relation to the benefits offered.

The particular requirements for the Essential Requirements List address the following topics:

- chemical, physical, and biological properties
- infection and microbial contamination
- construction and environmental properties
- devices with a measuring function
- protection against radiation
- requirements for devices connected to or equipped with an energy source
- protection against electrical risks
- protection against mechanical and thermal risks
- protection against the risks posed to the patient by energy supplies or substances
- information supplied by the manufacturer.

The easiest method of assuring the Essential Requirements are met is to establish a checklist of the Essential Requirements from Appendix I of the appropriate Directive, which then forms the basis of the technical dossier. Figure 4-1 is an example of an Essential Requirements checklist.

Product: _____

Essential Requirements	A or N/A	Standards	Activity	Test Clause	Pass/Fail	Document Location
I. General Requirements						
1. The device must be designed and manufactured in such a way that, when used under the conditions and for the purposes intended, they will not compromise the clinical condition or the safety of patients, users, and where applicable, other persons. The risks associated with devices must be reduced to an acceptable level compatible with a high level of protection for health and safety.	A	Internal	Hazard Analysis Safety review			Project file Project file
2. The solutions adopted by the manufacturer for the design and construction of the devices must comply with safety principles and also take into account the generally acknowledged state of the art.	A	Internal	Specification reviews Design reviews Safety review			Project file Project file Project file
3. The devices must achieve the performance intended by the manufacturer, i.e., be designed and manufactured in such a way, that they are suitable for some or more of the functions referred to in Article 1(2)(a) as specified by the manufacturer.	A	Internal Internal	Specification reviews Validation testing		 P	Project file Project file

Figure 4-1   Sample of an essential requirements list. (From Fries, 1995.)

The Essential Requirements checklist includes:

- a statement of the Essential Requirements
- an indication of the applicability of the Essential Requirements to a particular device
- a list of the standards used to address the Essential Requirements
- the activity that addresses the Essential Requirements,
- the clause(s) in the standard detailing the applicable test for the particular Essential Requirement
- an indication of whether the device passed/or failed the test
- a statement of the location of the test documentation or certificates.

4.5   Identification of Corresponding Harmonized Standards

A "harmonized" standard is a standard produced under a mandate from the European Commission by one of the European standardization bodies, such as CEN (the European Committee for Standardization) and CENELEC (the European Committee for Electrotechnical Standardization), and which has its reference published in the *Official Journal of the European Communities*.

The Essential Requirements are worded such that they identify a risk and state that the device should be designed and manufactured so that the risk is avoided or minimized. The technical detail for assuring these requirements is to be found in Harmonized Standards. Manufacturers must therefore identify the Harmonized Standards corresponding to the Essential Requirements which apply to their device.

With regard to choosing such standards, the manufacturer must be aware of the hierarchy of standards which have been developed:

- Horizontal Standards: generic standards covering fundamental requirements common to all, or a very wide range of medical devices
- Semi-Horizontal Standards: group standards which deal with requirements applicable to a group of devices

- Vertical Standards: product-specific standards which give requirements to one device or a very small group of devices.

Manufacturers must give particular attention to the horizontal standards since, because of their general nature, they apply to almost all devices. As these standards come into use for almost all products, they will become extremely powerful.

Semi-horizontal standards may be particularly important as they have virtually the same weight as horizontal standards for groups of devices, such as orthopedic implants, IVDs, or X-ray equipment.

Vertical standards might well be too narrow to cope with new technological developments when a question of a specific feature of a device arises.

Table 4-1 lists some common harmonized standards for medical devices and medical device electromagnetic compatibility standards.

4.6   Assurance that the Device Meets the Essential Requirements and Harmonized Standards

Once the Essential Requirements List has been developed and the harmonized standards chosen, the activity necessary to address the Essential Requirements List must be conducted. Taking the activity on the Essential Requirements checklist from Figure 4-1, the following activity may be conducted to assure the requirements are met.

Essential Requirement 1.

This requirement is concerned with the device not compromising the clinical condition or the safety of patient, users, and where applicable, other persons. The methods used to meet this requirement are the conduction of a hazard analysis and a safety review.

Standard	Areas Covered
EN 60 601 Series	Medical Electrical Equipment
EN 29000 Series	Quality Systems
EN 46000 Series	Quality Systems
EN 55011 (CISPR 11)	EMC/Emission
EN 60801 Series	EMC/Immunity
EN 540	Clinical Investigation of Medical Devices
EN 980	Symbols on Medical Equipment
IEC 601-1-2	Medical Device Emission and Immunity
IEC 801-2	Electrostatic Discharge
IEC 801-2	Immunity to Radiated Radio Frequency Electromagnetic Fields
IEC 801-4	Fast Transients/Burst
IEC 801-5	Voltage Surge Immunity

Table 4-1   Important Harmonized and EMC Standards (From Fries, 1995.)

Hazard Analysis

A hazard analysis is the process, continuous throughout the product development cycle, that examines the possible hazards that could occur due to equipment failure and helps the designer to eliminate the hazard through various control methods. The hazard analysis is conducted on hardware, software, and the total system during the initial specification phase and is updated throughout the development cycle. The hazard analysis is documented on a form similar to that shown in Figure 4-2.

Potential Hazard	Generic Cause	Specific Cause	Probability	Severity	Control Mode	Control Method	Comments	Review Comments

Figure 4-2   Sample hazard analysis form. (From Fries, 1995.)

The hazard analysis addresses the following issues:

Potential Hazard	Identifies possible harm to patient, operator, or system.
Generic Cause	Identifies general conditions that can lead to the associated Potential Hazard.
Specific Cause	Identifies specific instances that can give rise to the associated Generic Cause.
Probability	Classifies the likelihood of the associated Potential Hazard according to Table 4-2.
Severity	Categorizes the associated Potential Hazard according to Table 4-3.
Control Mode	Means of reducing the probability and/or severity of the associated Potential Hazard.
Control Method	Actual implementation to achieve the associated Control Mode.
Comments	Additional information, references, etc.
Review Comments	Comments written down during the review meeting.

When the hazard analysis is initially completed, the probability and severity refer to the potential hazard prior to its being controlled. As the device is designed to minimize or eliminate the hazard, and control methods are imposed, the probability and severity will be updated.

Safety Review

An organization separate from R&D, such as Quality Assurance, reviews the device to assure it is safe and effective for its intended use. The device, when operated according to specification, must not cause a hazard to the user or the patient. In the conduction of this review, the following may be addressed:

Classification Indicator	Classification Rating	Classification Meaning
1	Frequent	likely to occur often
2	Occasional	will occur several times in the life of the system
3	Reasonably Remote	likely to occur sometime in the life of the system
4	Remote	unlikely to occur, but possible
5	Extremely Remote	probability of occurrence indistinguishable from zero
6	Physically Impossible	

Table 4-2.   Hazard Analysis Probability Classification   (From Fries, 1995)

- pertinent documentation such as drawings, test reports, and manuals
- a sample of the device
- a checklist specific to the device, which may include:

> voltages
> operating frequencies
> leakage currents
> dielectric withstand
> grounding impedance
> power cord and plug
> electrical insulation
> physical stability
> color coding
> circuit breakers and fuses
> alarms, warnings and indicators
> mechanical design integrity.

Severity Indicator	Severity Rating	Severity Meaning
I	Catastrophic	may cause death or system loss
II	Critical	may cause severe injury, severe occupational illness, or severe system loss
III	Marginal	may cause minor injury, minor occupational illness, or minor system loss
IV	Negligible	will not result in injury, illness, or system damage

Table 4-3.   Hazard Analysis Severity Classification (From Fries, 1995.)

Essential Requirement 2

This requirement is concerned with the device complying with safety principles and the generally acknowledged state of the art. The methods used to meet this requirement are peer reviews and the safety review.

Peer Review

Peer review of the Product Specification, Design Specification, Software Requirements Specification and the actual design are conducted using qualified individuals not directly involved in the development of the device. The review is attended by individuals from Design, Reliability, Quality Assurance, Regulatory Affairs, Marketing, Manufacturing, and Service. Each review is documented with issues discussed and action items. After the review, the project team assigns individuals to address each action item and a schedule for completion.

<u>Safety Review</u>

This was discussed under Essential Requirement 1.

<u>Essential Requirement 3</u>

This requirement is concerned with the device achieving the performance intended by the manufacturer.

The methods used to meet this requirement are the various specification reviews and the validation of the device to meet these specifications.

<u>Specification Reviews</u>

This was discussed under Essential Requirement 2.

<u>Validation Testing</u>

This activity involves assuring that the design and the product meet the appropriate specifications that were developed at the beginning of the development process. Testing is conducted to address each requirement in the specification and the test plan and test results documented. It is helpful to develop a requirements matrix to assist in this activity.

<u>Essential Requirement 4</u>

This requirement is concerned with the device being adversely affected by stresses which can occur during normal conditions of use.

The methods used to meet this requirement are environmental testing, Environmental Stress Screening (ESS), and Use/Misuse evaluation;

Environmental Testing

Testing is conducted according to Environmental Specifications listed for the product. Table 4-4 lists the environmental testing to be conducted and the corresponding standards and methods employed. Test results are documented.

Environmental Stress Screening

The device is subjected to temperature and vibration stresses beyond that which the device may ordinarily see in order to precipitate failures. The failure may then be designed out of the device before it is produced. ESS is conducted according to a specific protocol which is developed for the particular device. Care must be taken in preparing the protocol to avoid causing failures which would not ordinarily be anticipated. Results of the ESS analysis are documented.

Use/Misuse Evaluation

Whether through failure to properly read the operation manual or through improper training, medical devices are going to be misused and even abused. There are many stories of product misuse, such as the hand-held monitor that was dropped into a toilet bowl, the physician that hammered a 9 volt battery in backwards and then reported the device was not working, or the user that spilled a can of soda on and into a device.

Practically, it is impossible to make a device completely immune to misuse, but it is highly desirable to design around the misuse situations than can be anticipated. These include:
- excess application of cleaning solutions
- physical abuse
- spills
- excess weight applied to certain parts of the device
- excess torque applied to controls or screws
- improper voltages, frequencies, or pressures
- interchangeable electrical or pneumatic connections.

Each potential misuse situation should be evaluated for its possible result on the device and a decision made on whether the result can be designed out.

Environmental Test	Specification Range	Applicable Standard
Operating temperature	5 to 35○C	IEC 68-2-14
Storage temperature	-40 to +65○C	IEC 68-2-1-Ab IEC 68-2-2-Bb
Operating humidity	15 to 95% RH non-condensing	IEC 68-2-30
Operating pressure	500 to 797 mm Hg	IEC 68-2-13
Storage pressure	87 to 797 mm Hg	IEC 68-2-13
Radiated electrical emissions	System: 4dB margin Subsystem: 15 dB	CISPR 11
Radiated magnetic emissions	System: 4dB margin Subsystem: 6dB	VDE 871
Linc conducted emissions	System: 2dB margin Subsystem: 2dB	CISPR 11 VDE 871
Electrostatic discharge	Contact: 7 KV Air: 10 KV	EN 60601-2 EN 1000-4-2
Radiated electric field immunity	5 V/m @ 1KHz	EN 60601-2 EN 1000-4-3
Electrical fast transient immunity	Power mains: 2.4 KV Cables > 3m: 1.2 KV	EN 60601-2 EN 1000-4-4
Stability		UL 2601
Transportation		NSTA Preshipment
Transportation		NSTA Overseas

Table 4-4   List of Environmental Testing (From Fries, 1995.)

Activities similar to these are carried out to complete the remainder of the Essential Requirements checklist for the device.

4.7   Classification of the Device

It is necessary for the manufacturer of a Medical Device to have some degree of proof that a device complies with the Essential Requirements before the CE marking can be applied. This is defined as a "conformity assessment procedure." For devices applicable to the AIMDD, there two alternatives for the conformity assessment procedure. For devices applicable to the IVDMDD, there is a single conformity assessment procedure. For devices applicable to the MDD, there is no conformity assessment procedure that is suitable for all products, as the Directive covers all medical devices. Medical devices are therefore divided into four classes, which have specific conformity assessment procedures for each of the four classes.

It is crucial for manufacturers to determine the class into which each of their devices falls. This demands careful study of the Classification Rules given in Annex IX of the Directive. As long as the intended purpose, the implementing rules and the definitions are clearly understood, the classification process is straightforward and the rules, which are laid out in a logical order, can be worked out in succession from Rule 1. If the device is used for more than one intended purpose, then it must be classified according to the one which gives the highest classification.

The rules for determining the appropriate classification of a medical device include:

Rule	Type of Device	Class
1-4	Non-invasive devices are in Class I except:	
	use for storing body fluids	IIa
	connected to an active medical device in Class IIa or higher	IIa
	modification of body fluids	IIa/IIb
	some wound dressings	IIa/IIb

Rule	Type of Device	Class
5	Devices invasive with respect to body orifices:	
	transient use	I
	short-term use	IIa
	long-term use	IIb
6-8	Surgically-invasive devices:	
	re-usable surgical instruments	I
	transient or short-term use	IIa
	long-term use	IIb
	contact with CCS or CNS	III
	devices which are absorbable or have a biological effect	IIb/III
	devices which deliver medicines	IIb/III
	devices applying ionizing radiation	IIb
13	Devices incorporating medicinal products	III
14	Contraceptive devices	IIb/III
15	Chemicals used for cleaning or disinfecting:	
	medical devices	IIa
	contact lenses	IIb
16	Devices specifically intended for recording X-ray images	IIa
17	Devices made from animal tissues	III
18	Blood bags	IIb

In the cases of active devices, the rules are based mainly on the purpose of the device, i.e., diagnosis or therapy, and the corresponding possibility of absorption of energy by the patient:

Rule	Type of Device	Class
9	Therapeutic devices administering or exchanging energy	IIa
	if operating in a potentially hazardous way	IIb
10	Diagnostic devices:	
	supplying energy other than illumination	IIa
	imaging radiopharmaceuticals in vivo	IIa
	diagnosing/monitoring vital functions	IIa
	monitoring vital functions in critical care conditions	IIb
	emitting ionizing radiation	IIb
11	Active devices administering/removing medicines/body substances	IIa
	if operating in a potentially hazardous way	IIb
12	All other active devices	I

In order to use the classification system correctly, manufacturers must have a good understanding of the implementing rules and definitions.

The key implementing rules include:

- application of the Classification Rules is governed by the intended purpose of the device
- if the device is intended to be used in combination with another device, the Classification Rules are applied separately to each device
- accessories are classified in their own right, separately from the device with which they are used
- software, which drives a device or influences the use of a device, falls automatically in the same class as the device itself.

4.8   Decision on the Appropriate Conformity Assessment Procedure

<u>Medical Device Directive</u>

There are six conformity assessment Annexes to the Medical Device Directive. Their use for the different classes of devices is specified in Article 11 of the Directive.

<u>Annex II</u>

This Annex describes the system of full quality assurance covering both the design and manufacture of devices.

<u>Annex III</u>

This Annex describes the type examination procedure according to which the manufacturer submits full technical documentation of the product, together with a representative sample of the device to a Notified Body.

<u>Annex IV</u>

This Annex describes the examination by the Notified Body of every individual product, or one or more samples from every production batch, and the testing which may be necessary to show the conformity of the products with the approved/documented design.

<u>Annex V</u>

This Annex describes a production quality system which is to be verified by a Notified Body as assuring that devices are made in accordance with an approved type, or in accordance with technical documentation describing the device.

<u>Annex VI</u>

This Annex describes a quality system covering final inspection and testing of products to ensure that devices are made in accordance with an approved type, or in accordance with technical documentation.

Annex VII

This Annex describes the technical documentation that the manufacturer must compile in order to support a declaration of conformity for a medical device, where there is no participation of a Notified Body in the process.

The class to which the medical device is assigned has an influence on the type of conformity assessment procedure chosen.

Class I

Compliance with the Essential Requirements must be shown in technical documentation compiled according to Annex VII of the Directive.

Class IIa

The design of the device and it compliance with the Essential Requirements must be established in technical documentation described in Annex VII. However, for this Class, agreement of production units with the technical documentation must be assured by a Notified Body according to one of the following alternatives:

sample testing	Annex IV
an audited production quality system	Annex V
an audited product quality system	Annex VI

Class IIb

The design and manufacturing procedures must be approved by a Notified Body as satisfying Annex II, or the design must be shown to conform to the Essential Requirements by a type examination (Annex III) carried out by a Notified Body.

Class III

The procedures for this class are similar to Class IIb, but significant differences are that when the quality system route is used, a design dossier for each type of device must be examined by the Notified Body. Clinical data relating to safety and performance must be included in the design dossier or the documentation presented for the type examination.

Active Implantable Medical Device Directive

For devices following the AIMDD, Annexes II through V cover the various conformity assessment procedures available. There are two alternative procedures:

Alternative 1

A manufacturer must have in place a full quality assurance system for design and production and must submit a design dossier on each type of device to the Notified Body for review.

Alternative 2

A manufacturer submits an example of each type of his device to a Notified Body, satisfactory production must be assured by either the quality system at the manufacturing site must comply with EN 29002 + EN 46002 and must be audited by a Notified Body, or samples of the product must be tested by a Notified Body.

In Vitro Diagnostic Medical Devices Directive

For devices adhering to the IVDMDD, the conformity assessment procedure is a manufacturer's declaration. In Vitro devices for self testing, must additionally have a design examination by a Notified Body, or be designed and manufactured in accordance with a quality system.

In choosing a conformity assessment procedure it is important to remember that:

- it is essential to determine the classification of a device before deciding on a conformity assessment procedure

- it may be more efficient to operate one conformity assessment procedure throughout a manufacturing plant, even though this procedure may be more rigorous than strictly necessary for some products
- tests and assessments carried out under current national regulations can contribute towards the assessment of conformity with the requirements of the Directives.

4.9   Type Testing

A manufacturer of Class IIb or Class III medical devices can choose to demonstrate that his device meets the Essential Requirements by submitting to a Notified Body for a type examination as described in Annex III of the Directive. The manufacturer is required to submit technical documentation on his device together with an example of the device. The Notified Body will then carry our such tests as it considers necessary to satisfy itself, before issuing the EC Type Examination Certificate.

Type testing of many kinds of medical devices, particularly electromedical equipment, is required under some current national regulations. Manufacturers who are familiar with this process and who have established relations with test houses which are, or will be, appointed as Notified Bodies, are likely to find this a more attractive procedure than the design control procedures of EN29001/EN46001. Existing products which have already been type tested under current national procedures are likely to meet most of the Essential Requirements and may require little or no further testing. Testing by one of the nationally recognized test houses may also gain entitlement to national or proprietary marks which can be important in terms of market acceptance.

A major issue in type examination is the handling of design and manufacturing changes. Annex III states that the manufacturer must inform the Notified Body of any significant change made to an approved product, and that the Notified Body must give further approval if the change could affect conformity with the Essential Requirements. The meaning of *significant change* must be negotiated with the Notified Body but clearly for certain products or for manufacturers with a large number of products, the notification and checking of changes could impose a serious burden.

When a change could have an effect on the compliance with the Essential Requirements, the manufacturer should make his own assessment, including tests, to determine that the device still complies and submit up-dated drawings and documentation, together with the test results. The Notified Body must be informed of all changes made as a result of an adverse incident.

When the assessment is that the changes are not liable to have an effect, they should be submitted to the Notified Body "for information only." The manufacturer must, in such cases, keep records of the change and of the rationale for the conclusion that the change could not have an effect.

4.10   Identification and Choice of a Notified Body

Identifying and choosing a Notified Body is one of the most critical issues facing a manufacturer. A long-term and close relationship should be developed and time and care spent in making a careful choice of a Notified Body should be viewed as an investment in the future of the company.

Notified bodies must satisfy the criteria given in Annex XI of the Medical Device Directive, namely:

- independence from the design, manufacture or supply of the devices in question
- integrity
- competence
- staff who are trained, experienced, and able to report
- impartiality of the staff
- possession of liability insurance
- professional secrecy.

In addition, the bodies must satisfy the criteria fixed by the relevant Harmonized Standards. The relevant Harmonized Standards include those of the EN 45000 series dealing with the accreditation and operation of certification bodies.

The tasks to be carried out by Notified Bodies include:

- audit manufacturers; quality systems for compliance with Annexes II, V and VI
- examine any modifications to an approved quality system
- carry out periodic surveillance of approved quality systems
- examine design dossiers and issue EC Design Examination Certificates
- examine modifications to an approved design
- carry out type examinations and issue EC Type Examination Certificates
- examine modifications to an approved type
- carry out EC verification
- take measures to prevent rejected batches from reaching the market
- agree with the manufacturer time limits for the conformity assessment procedures
- take into account the results of tests or verifications already carried out
- communicate to other Notified Bodies (on request) all relevant information about approvals of quality systems issued, refused, and withdrawn
- communicate to other Notified Bodies (on request) all relevant information about EC Type Approval Certificates issued, refused, and withdrawn.

Notified bodies must be located within the European Community in order that effective control may be applied by the Competent Authorities that appointed them, but certain operations may be carried out on behalf of Notified Bodies by subcontractors who may be based outside the European Community. Competent Authorities will generally notify bodies on their own territory, but they may notify bodies based in another Member State provided that they have already been notified by their parent Competent Authority.

There are several factors to be taken into account by a manufacturer in choosing a Notified Body, including:

- experience with medical devices
- range of medical devices for which the Notified Body has skills
- possession of specific skills, e.g., EMC or software
- links with subcontractors and subcontractor skills
- conformity assessment procedures for which the body is notified
- plans for handling issues, such as clinical evaluation
- attitude to existing certifications
- queue times/processing times
- costs
- location and working languages.

Experience with medical devices is limited to a small number of test houses and their experience is largely confined to electromedical equipment. Manufacturers should probe carefully the competence of the certification body to assess their device. Actual experience with a product of a similar nature would be reassuring. The certification body should be pressed to demonstrate sufficient understanding of the requirements, particularly where special processes are involved (e.g., sterilization) and/or previous experience.

Certain devices demand specific skills which may not be found in every Notified Body. Clearly, the Notified Body must have, or be able to obtain, the skills required for the manufacturer's devices.

Many Notified Bodies will supplement their in-house skills by the use of specialist subcontractors. This is perfectly acceptable as long as all the rules of subcontracting are followed. Manufacturers should verify for themselves the reputation of the subcontractor and the degree of supervision applied by the Notified Body.

The main choice open to manufacturers is full Quality System certification or Type Examination combined with one of the less rigorous Quality System certifications. Some Notified Bodies have a tradition of either product testing or systems evaluation and it therefore makes sense to select a Notified Body with experience in the route chosen.

A clinical evaluation is required for some medical devices, especially Class III devices and implants. Although this will be a key aspect of demonstrating conformity, it will be important for manufacturers to know how the Notified Body intends to perform this function.

In preparing the Medical Device Directives, the need to avoid re-inventing the wheel has been recognized. In order to maximize this need, companies whose products have already been certified by test houses which are likely to become Notified Bodies may wish to make use of the organizations with whom they have previously worked. It will be important to verify with the Notified Body the extent to which the testing previously performed is sufficient to meeting the Essential Requirements.

At the time of this writing, most Notified Bodies seem to be able to offer fairly short lead times. The time for actually carrying out the examination or audit should be questioned.

It must be remembered that manufacturers will have to pay Notified Bodies for carrying out the conformity assessment procedures. There will certainly be competition and this may offer some control over costs. Although it will always be a factor, the choice of a Notified Body should not be governed by cost alone bearing in mind the importance of the exercise.

For obvious reasons of expense, culture, convenience and language there will be a tendency for European manufacturers to use a Notified Body situated in their own country. Nevertheless, this should not be the principal reason for selection and account should be taken of the other criteria discussed here. For manufacturers outside the European Community, the geographical locations is less important. Of greater significance to them, particularly United States companies, is the existence of overseas subsidiaries or subcontractors of some of the Notified Bodies. Manufacturers should understand that the Notified Body must be a legal entity established within the Member State that has notified it. This does not prevent the Notified Body subcontracting quite significant tasks to a subsidiary.

Article 11.12 states that the correspondence relating to the conformity assessment procedures must be in the language of the Member State in which the procedures are carried out and/or in another Community language acceptable to the Notified Body. Language may thus be another factor affecting the choice of Notified Body, although most of the major certification bodies will accept English and other languages.

The most significant factor of all is likely to be existing good relations with a particular body. Notified Bodies will be drawn from existing test and certification bodies and many manufacturers already use such bodies, either as part of a national approval procedure, or as part of their own policy for ensuring the satisfactory quality of their products and processes.

Another consideration which could become significant is that of variations in the national laws implementing the Directives. Notified Bodies will have to apply the law of the country in which they are situated and some differences in operation could be introduced by this means.

4.11   Establishing a Declaration of Conformity

Of all documents prepared for the Medical Device Directives, the most important may be the declaration of conformity. Every device, other that a custom-made or clinical investigation device, must be covered by a declaration of conformity.

The general requirement is that the manufacturer must draw up a written declaration that the products concerned meet the provisions of the Directive that apply to them. The declaration must cover a given number of the products manufactured. A strictly literal interpretation of this wording would suggest that the preparation of a declaration of conformity is not a once-and-for-all event with an indefinite coverage, but rather a formal statement that products which have been manufactured and verified in accordance with the particular conformity assessment procedure chosen by the manufacturer do meet the requirements of the Directive. Such an interpretation would impose severe burdens on manufacturers, and the Commission is understood to be moving to a position where a declaration of conformity can be prepared in respect of future production of a model of device for which the conformity assessment procedures have been carried out. The CE marking of individual devices after manufacture can then be regarded as a short-form expression of the declaration of conformity in respect of that individual device. This position is likely to form part of future Commission guidance.

Even so, the declaration remains a very formal statement from the manufacturer and accordingly, must be drawn up with care. The declaration must include the serial numbers or batch numbers of the products it covers and manufacturers should give careful thought to the appropriate coverage of a declaration. In the extreme, it may be that a separate declaration should be prepared individually for each product or batch.

A practical approach is probably to draw up one basic declaration which is stated to apply to the products whose serial (batch) numbers are listed in an Appendix. The Appendix can then be added to at sensible intervals. A suggested format is shown if Figure 4-3.

4.12 Application of the CE Mark

The CE marking (Figure 4-4) is the symbol used to indicate that a particular product complies with the relevant Essential Requirements of the appropriate Directive, and as such, that the product has achieved a satisfactory level of safety and thus may circulate freely throughout the Community.

It is important to note that it is the manufacturer or his authorized representative who applies the CE marking to the product, and not the Notified Body. The responsibility for ensuring that each and every product conforms to the requirements of the Directive is that of the manufacturer and the affixing of the CE marking constitutes the manufacturer's statement that an individual device conforms.

The CE marking should appear on the device itself, if practicable, on the instructions for use, and on the shipping packaging. It should be accompanied by the identification number of the Notified Body which has been involved in the verification of the production of the device. It is prohibited to add other marks which could confuse or obscure the meaning of the CE marking.

The XXXX noted in Figure 4-4 is the identification number of the notified body.

4.13 Conclusion

Compliance with the EC Directives will imply major changes for medical device manufacturers. Such changes relate to the requirements to be

DECLARATION OF CONFORMITY

We: Company Name
                       Company Address

Declare that the product(s) listed below:

Product to be declared

Hereby conform(s) to the European Council Directive 93/42/EEC, Medical Device
Directive, Annex II, Article 3. This declaration is based on the Certification of the
Full Quality Assurance System by NAME OF NOTIFIED BODY, Notified Body #
XXXX.

Name (*Print or type*) : _____
Title   : _____
Signature   : _____
Date   : _____

Figure 4-3   Sample declaration of conformity. (From Fries, 1997.)

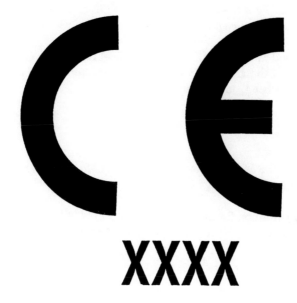

Figure 4-4   Example of CE mark. (From Fries, 1997.)

met in view of the design and manufacture of medical devices as well as to the procedures to be followed by manufacturers prior to and after placing medical devices on the European market. Manufacturers who wish to market are faced with a quite far-reaching and rather complex decision-making process.

References

The Active Implantable Medical Devices Directive. 90/385/EEC, 20 June, 1990.

The Medical Devices Directive. 93/42/EEC, 14 June, 1993.

Draft Proposal for a Council Directive on In Vitro Diagnostic Medical Devices, Working Document. III/D/4181/93, April, 1993.

Fries, R.C. and M. Graber, "Designing Medical Devices for Conformance with Harmonized Standards," *Biomedical Instrumentation & Technology.* Volume 29, Number 4, July/August, 1995.

Fries, Richard C., *Reliable Design of Medical Devices.* New York: Marcel Dekker, Inc., 1997.

Higson, G.R., *The Medical Devices Directive-A Manufacturer's Handbook.* Brussels: Medical Technology Consultants Europe Ltd., 1993.

SWBC, Organization for the European Conformity of Products, *CE-Mark: The New European Legislation for Products.* Milwaukee, WI: ASQC Quality Press, 1996.

Chapter 5

The Basics of ISO 9001

Tina Juneau – Lunar Inc.
Madison, Wisconsin

The ISO 9000 set of standards is used to develop the elements necessary to maintain an efficient quality system at any company. They can be used by manufacturing and service industries alike because they are not specific to any given product. The standards focus on controlling the process an organization uses to develop and produce their products rather than dictating specific requirements for the finished product.

The series really encompass a set of five standards:

ISO 9000-1	Provides guidelines for selection and use of the remaining standards.
ISO 9001	The most comprehensive of the standards. Covers Design, Development, Production, Installation and Servicing.

ISO 9002	Covers Production Installation and Servicing.
ISO 9003	Least comprehensive. Only covers Final Inspection.
ISO 9004-1	A Guide to Quality Management Elements

There are 20 elements or clauses that make up the core of the ISO 9001 standard. The differences in 9001 – 9003 are illustrated in Table 5-1.

5.1   Historical Perspective

Increasing development in world trade made a common set of universally accepted quality standards inevitable. Using guidelines already established by military and defense industries several companies began to implement quality management systems in the early 1970's. As use of these systems grew, many of the companies got together in the late 1970's to review the various approaches used. The result was the first publication of BS 5750:1979 which allowed for the first time a common base for auditing.

In the years that followed considerable input from the US, Canada and the UK led to the ISO 9000 series published in 1987. Within 5 years more than 55 countries had adopted their own equivalent national standard. The US adopted ANSI/ASQC Q90, the UK had BS 5750, and the European Community Standard was EN 29000. In order to address some of the inadequacies in the original publication the ISO 9000 series was revised in 1994.

5.2   ISO 9001 Revision Year 2000

At time of this printing, draft copies of the ISO 9001 year 2000 revision were under review. These proposed changes result in a standard that is more focused on the customer's needs and that make the standard easier to use. The proposed revision consolidates the ISO 9001, 9002 and 9003 standards to one that allows the organization to omit requirements that are not applicable. In addition, the 20 original elements have been restructured to a more generic process based improvement cycle. The 20 current elements of the ISO 9001 standard are still recognizable in the proposed draft and organizations need not

ISO 9001	ISO 9002 *All of ISO 9001 except:*	ISO 9003 *All of ISO 9002 except:*
4.1 Management Responsibilities		
4.2 Quality System	Design Control	Purchasing
4.3 Contract Review		Process Control
4.4 Design Control		Servicing
4.5 Document Control		
4.6 Purchasing		
4.7 Control of Customer Supplied Product		
4.8 Product Identification and Traceability		
4.9 Process Control		
4.10 Inspection and Testing		
4.11 Inspection Measuring and Test Equipment (Calibration)		
4.13 Nonconforming Product		
4.14 Corrective and Preventive Action		
4.15 Handling, Storage, Packaging, Preservation and Delivery		
4.16 Control of Quality Records		
4.17 Internal Audits		
4.18 Training		
4.19 Servicing		
4.20 Statistical Techniques		
Total # of Clauses = 20	19	16

Table 5-1   ISO 9001 Elements

worry about changing the current structure of their system. Neither version imposes any type of structure or organizational requirements on the quality system.

5.3   Requirement Synopses

5.3.1   Management Responsibilities

5.3.1.1 What the Standard Requires

Executive Management needs to document a quality policy that identifies objectives for quality and states their commitment to quality. This policy needs to be understood by all levels of the organization.

The organization needs to define and document the responsibility, authority and interrelation of personnel who manage, perform and verify work affecting quality. The organization must ensure that resources, including trained personnel, are available.

Executive Management needs to appoint a member of management as the Management Representative. The Management Representative is responsible to ensure the quality system is implemented and maintained, that reports on the status of the quality system are presented to executive management for review and to make improvements to the system.

Executive Management needs to review the quality system at defined intervals to ensure it is suitable and is meeting the requirements of the standard and the organizations own requirements. Records of this review must be maintained.

5.3.1.2 How to Meet the Intent

Many companies opt to post the quality policy throughout the facility or distribute quality cards printed with the quality policy. You must ensure that each employee is made familiar with the policy and understands how their position contributes to meeting the policy. This can be done though general employee training, job descriptions or verbally by managers.

Establishing job descriptions and documenting the organization chart can be an easy way to show job interrelations, and most companies will already have this information available, however, there are other ways to meet this intent. Flow charts or responsibility matrices can just as easily meet this requirement.

It is essential that management review needs and ensure adequate resources and personnel are available to maintain compliance to the quality system. Often the Internal Audit process can help identify areas of concern and possible needs for additional resources. To ensure that needs are communicated to Management copies of the reports should be distributed to the Management's Representative.

When external parties are involved, the management representative is most often the organization's liaison who acts as guide and contact for all quality system audits. Internally the Management Representative may act as the contact for quality system related questions and problems.

Often, quarterly, bi-annual or annual management review meetings are held to specifically focus on the status of the quality system. These meetings can cover a wide range of topics from review of internal audit findings and corrective actions, to supplier management, suitability of the quality policy, customer complaints, etc. Goals directly involving the quality system are usually set at this time and then distributed to the organization.

5.3.1.3 Likely Auditor Actions

Auditors will want to speak to members of senior management and the management representative. Minutes of management reviews will likely be looked at, as will organization charts, job descriptions or other descriptions of job interrelations. Resource management and evidence of management's commitment to the quality system will be assessed.

As the audit continues to other elements and areas of the organization the auditors will ensure that employees are aware of the management representative and the quality policy. Auditors will be looking at the level of compliance to other elements of the standard to ensure adequate resources have been applied to implement and maintain the quality system.

5.3.2   Quality System

5.3.2.1   What the Standard Requires

The organization must prepare a quality manual that covers the requirements of the standard. The quality manual should reference or include the procedures that detail how the requirements will be met. The quality manual must also identify the structure of the documentation that makes up the quality system.

The organization must prepare documented procedures for all required elements of the standard and ensure that the quality system, including the documented procedures, is effectively implemented. The organization needs to define and document how the requirements for quality will be met.

5.3.2.2   How to Meet the Intent

To meet the elements of this clause a simple quality manual is established for many organizations. A short statement confirming compliance and referencing lower level documentation which further describe the procedures for maintaining compliance are documented for each element of the standard.

The most common structure for the documented quality system can be seen as a pyramid. At the top is the quality manual that describes the company's policies for each element of the standard. The next tier is the procedures that describe who is responsible, what the requirements are and when they are performed. Below the procedures are work instructions that outline specific instructions for completing a task. The final level contains forms and records that provide evidence that the quality system was carried out effectively.

Documented procedures that are required by the standard need to be maintained according to the organizations document control process. These procedures need to be available to employees. Documented procedures are usually made available through procedure binders located throughout the facility, by issuing documents directly to employees, or having documentation available on a company Intranet.

5.3.2.3 Likely Auditor Actions

Auditors will often verify that you have established a quality manual and structured documentation system prior to their visit. Once on-site their goal is to verify compliance to the documented system. This is done throughout the audit as they verify that the elements described in the quality manual and procedures have been implemented and are effective.

5.3.3 Contract Review

5.3.3.1 What the Standard Requires

The organization needs to document the procedures for contract review including how contract review activities are coordinated. Before acceptance of a contract or order or submission of a tender the organization must ensure that: all requirements are defined and documented, or verbally agreed upon; all differences are resolved; and the organization is sure that it can meet the requirements of the order.

If changes are made to the contract once it has been accepted the changes must be communicated to all parties involved. Records of contract review must be maintained.

5.3.3.2 How to Meet the Intent

Procedures should explain how an order is taken, what information is required, and how the ability to fill the order is confirmed prior to acceptance. The procedure should indicate how and who needs to be informed of changes to all contracts so that appropriate actions may be taken.

Many companies keep a file for each customer, order or other applicable control measure. Files may contain customer information, contract agreements, quotes, change documentation, etc. It is important that the documentation clearly shows what the customer requirements were, and any change history to the order. It is also important that the organization be able to verify that those requirements were met.

5.3.3.3 Likely Auditor Actions

Auditors may follow the entire process of contract review from start to finish or take several orders at various stages of review and verify that all requirements for the current stage are met. Auditors may also select the contract review information from a particular order and verify that the requirements were met by looking at the associated final inspection or shipping documentation.

5.3.4   Design Control

5.3.4.1 What the Standard Requires

The organization must document procedures of how they will control and verify that specified requirements are met when designing product. The organization needs to plan all design and development activities. Plans need to describe the activities involved, define responsibilities for the implementation and ensure that those individuals responsible for the activities are qualified and have adequate resources. All plans should be updated as the design evolves.

Lines of communication between all parties involved in the design and development process must be established and information relevant to the project needs to be readily distributed.

Input requirements for all design and development projects must be identified, documented and reviewed for adequacy. Inputs include requirements of any standards or regulations that may be applicable and take into consideration results of any contract review activities. Any conflicting requirements need to be resolved.

Design output needs to be expressed in terms that can be verified against design input. At appropriate times during the design process formal reviews of the design results need to be planned, conducted and documented.

Design output must be verified to meet the design input requirements at appropriate stages of the design. This verification must be documented. After successful verification of the design, the product must be validated to show that it meets the user needs and/or requirements. Changes to the design must be identified, documented, reviewed and approved before they are implemented.

5.3.4.2 How to Meet the Intent

All members of the design and development project should be identified in the project plan. The plan should indicate how information will be communicated and distributed (through weekly progress reports, meetings, conference calls, etc.) This is especially important when outside design houses or consultants are involved. Ensure that the lines of communication are defined and that all parties know their role in distributing information to the group.

When holding a design review ensure that all persons involved in the design stage being reviewed are involved. Any specialists, if needed, should participate. In many cases formal design reviews are scheduled at the end of each design stage during the initial project planning. This ensures that all tasks are complete prior to advancing the project. Documentation should clearly show who was involved, which elements of the design were reviewed, and any decisions made and actions taken.

Verification documentation must show that your design output does in fact meet your input. In other words, you got what you wanted. While validation of the product ensures that the overall product meets the customer needs – that what you wanted actually works and is what the customer wants. Verification and Validation (V&V) tests should be documented so those tests could be easily reproduced.

5.3.4.3 Likely Auditor Actions

Auditors will usually choose to follow an entire project through the design process by examining the design history and verifying that all elements have been met. Auditors will look at preliminary design specifications and plans and want to be able to see, through your design history documentation, how you ended up with the final product.

5.3.5 Document and Data Control

5.3.5.1 What the Standard Requires

The organization needs to define and document how they will control documents and data. Prior to their use, documents and data need to be reviewed and approved. The organization must develop a master list or equivalent form of control to indicate the current revision status of each document. The control over documentation must also ensure that all documents are available where they are needed, that invalid or obsolete documents are removed, and that when retention of obsolete documents is required that they are suitable identified.

Once implemented, changes to documents and data must be reviewed and approved by the same functions that originally granted approval for use. This change review should be based on pertinent background information and where practical the nature of the changes should be identified.

5.3.5.2 How to Meet the Intent

Documentation and data that need to be controlled by procedures includes any required by the standard and where applicable, external documents such as standards or customer drawings. Electronic or hard copy versions of documents and data are acceptable.

A central or departmental control center can easily develop a matrix, database or other control measure to indicate all active documentation and its revision level. This control center can also gather required approvals prior to release and remove or ensure others remove invalid or obsolete material.

A strong change control system is the backbone of successful document control. Again a control center whether central or departmental can easily gather required approvals by routing change proposals or facilitating change control meetings. In most cases a simple before/after or redline copy of documentation can easily show the nature of the change. Simple change request forms may document reasons for change, documentation involved, required approvals, and implementation information. Because document control affects so many different areas of the organization it is usually the area where the highest number of problems are found.

5.3.5.3 Likely Auditor Actions

During the course of the audit, auditors will ensure that documentation is available where it is needed. They will also verify that the documentation being used is the valid or active version and that it is under proper control. Auditors will look for unapproved changes on documentation. They will ensure that obsolete documentation has been removed from all points of issue.

5.3.6   Purchasing

5.3.6.1 What the Standard Requires

The organization needs to establish a procedure to ensure that purchased product conforms to specified requirements. Suppliers to the organization should be evaluated and selected on the basis of their ability to meet the requirements. The organization must determine the type and extent of control to exercise over subcontractors and maintain records of acceptable subcontractors.

Documentation of purchasing activities should contain all information necessary to ensure that the correct product is ultimately received. Most purchase orders adequately describe product and all requirements that the order and product must meet for quality and standards compliance.

If the organization wishes to verify product ordered at the supplier's premise, the arrangements and method of product release must be adequately described in the purchasing documentation.

The organization must allow for their customers to verify purchased product at their site or their supplier's site when specified in the customer's contract. This verification of product does not preclude the organizations need for effective supplier control, nor does it mean that the organization will not reject unacceptable product.

5.3.6.2 How to Meet the Intent

Documented procedures should detail the process for adding a supplier to the organizations approved supplier list, how those suppliers are monitored, and the requirements necessary to retain the approved supplier status. Considerations for the control exercised over various suppliers may be detailed. Varying degrees of control may be based upon supplier history, quality, timeliness or other factors important to the organization. Procedures should document the methods in place to monitor suppliers and detail action taken when suppliers do not meet the organization's requirements.

5.3.6.3 Likely auditor actions

Auditors will review the supplier approval process and review documentation for new suppliers to ensure that they were approved based on the organization's criteria. Records will be reviewed to ensure that existing suppliers have maintained compliance. Where suppliers have failed to meet the criteria the corrective action taken against the supplier will be reviewed. Auditors will likely sample purchase order records to ensure that the product is received from an approved suppler.

5.3.7   Control of Customer Supplied Product

5.3.7.1 What the Standard Requires

If your customer supplies you with product for use, you must protect it from damage. When a customer supplies the organization with product to be incorporated into the customer's product, the organization must have documented procedures in place to ensure that the customers product will be adequately verified, stored, and maintained. The organization must document and report to the customer if at any time the customer's product is lost damaged or is unusable. Although the organization must verify the product supplied, it does not clear the customer from providing acceptable product.

5.3.7.2 How to Meet the Intent

If the organization has adequate procedures in place for the handling and control over their own product, any customer-supplied product may be handled under those same controls.

5.3.7.3 Likely Auditor Actions

Auditors will review contracts where the customer supplied product to the organization. They will ensure that any damage to the product was documented and reported to the customer.

5.3.8 Product Identification and Traceability

5.3.8.1 What the Standard Requires

The organization must document procedures, where appropriate, to identify product from receipt through production, delivery and installation. Where the organization must maintain records of traceability documented procedures should identify the control over identification of individual product or batches.

5.3.8.2 How to Meet the Intent

First it is important that the organization determine which products need traceability maintenance. This may be individual components, final production product or both. Once determined, items may be traced by serial numbers or some other unique identifier in a logbook, database, inventory system or other means and eventually tied to a customer, batch or lot number. Product can be identified in any way that works for the organization. This may mean Part numbers identifying contents of a bin, serial numbers assigned to components, or system or control numbers assigned to final product.

5.3.8.3   Likely Auditor Actions

Auditors will ensure that the organization can produce traceability information where it is applicable. They may trace a part through the system from time of receipt to delivery to ensure that adequate controls were used to ensure the part is identified and can be easily relocated if needed.

5.3.9   Process Control

5.3.9.1   What the standard requires

The organization must determine which production, installation and servicing processes directly affect quality. Once identified the organization must ensure that those processes are carried out under controlled conditions. Controlled conditions include the following: documented procedures are available where needed, appropriate equipment and work environment are provided, compliance to standards, plans or procedures can be ensured, process parameters and product characteristics are monitored and controlled, appropriate approvals are received for new processes and equipment, criteria for work is defined, and equipment is properly maintained. Qualified operators and specially controlled processes must be in place if requirements for product acceptability can not be fully verified or tested prior to use. The organization needs to specify requirement for the qualification of process operations, equipment and personnel.

5.3.9.2   How to Meet the Intent

Although there are many requirements under this section the implementation can come down to two important questions and the ability to prove them. First, how do personnel in the production, installation and service areas know what to do and how to do it? And second, how do those personnel know that results of the work they have performed and the equipment they used are acceptable? Usually documented work instructions, drawings or other flow diagrams can illustrate what to do and how to do it. It is then just a matter of proving acceptability through various records as the organization determines necessary.

5.3.9.3 Likely Auditor Actions

Auditors will make sure that key processes have been defined and documented in the production, installation and servicing areas. They will want to make sure the employees are able to identify the work instructions, procedures or manuals where the process is documented. Where applicable auditors will ensure that equipment is properly maintained and that the equipment was proved capable of the process prior to production use.

5.3.10   Inspection and Testing

5.3.10.1 What the Standard Requires

Documented procedures need to detail the inspection and test activities and records that will verify that specified requirements have been met. Inspection and testing covers Receiving, Inprocess and Final inspection and test.

Incoming product may not be used or processed until it has been verified according to plans or procedures to meet all prearranged requirements. The organization should consider the control required at receiving inspection based upon the control placed over the supplier and their history of conformance.

Product can only be released to production under urgent circumstances providing that it is clearly identified and recorded in order to permit immediate recall and replacement if it is found to be in nonconformance to the specified requirements.

While product is in process the organization should perform inspections and tests according to plans and/or procedures. Until the required inspections and tests are complete the organization must ensure the product is not released.

Final inspection and testing are performed according to plans or procedures to verify the continued conformance of the finished product to specified requirements. Final inspection and testing of the finished product should include verification of conformance for all receiving and in-process tests. Finished product must not be released until all testing has proven to be completed satisfactorily and authorization for release is received.

Records providing evidence that the product has completed all required inspections and tests are required. The results of the inspections and tests must be clearly shown, and records must identify the authority responsible for release of the product. Where product has failed to meet the defined acceptance criteria the procedures for nonconforming product will apply.

5.3.10.2 How to Meet the Intent

The organization must identify from Receiving through In-Process and on to Final Inspection what inspections and tests are necessary to prove that the product meets the requirements and define the acceptance criteria. When product does not meet the criteria, apply the nonconforming materials procedures. At final inspection verify that all previous tests are complete and that proper authorization for release is received. Finally the organization must maintain the records to prove that all required inspections and tests were performed and the product met the acceptance criteria.

5.3.10.3 Likely Auditor Actions

Throughout the manufacturing and tests areas auditors will look at the tests that are required to be done, and verify that there are records to prove that the product has met the established criteria. Auditors will examine final inspection documentation to ensure that proper approvals are documented and that all required records are maintained to prove that testing is complete.

5.3.11   Control of Inspection Measuring and Test Equipment

5.3.11.1 What the Standard Requires

Documented procedures must be maintained for how inspection, measuring and test equipment (including test software) will be controlled and calibrated. The organization must ensure that any measurements taken are within the equipment's capabilities. Test software or test hardware must be proven to be capable of verifying the acceptability of the product prior to use in any application and their suitability must be rechecked at prescribed intervals. When required the organization must make the data pertaining to inspection measuring and test equipment available to the customer or customer's representative.

Control over equipment needs to ensure the following:

- accuracy of measurements is determined and equipment selected is capable of performing necessary accuracy and precision
- equipment that can affect product quality is calibrated at defined intervals to national or international standards. If no such standards exist the basis for the calibration must be defined and documented
- equipment which will be calibrated is defined, including type, unique identification, location, frequency, check method, acceptance criteria, and actions to take if results are unsatisfactory
- equipment must show calibration status
- records of the calibration are maintained
- equipment that is found to be out-of-calibration has documentation proving the validity of previous inspections and tests
- equipment is used under proper environmental conditions
- equipment is handled and stored to ensure accuracy when used
- test software and hardware are protected against adjustments which may invalidate the calibration setting.

5.3.11.2 How to Meet the Intent

A simple database or equipment log can be established to show all equipment that requires calibration. The log may include such information as serial numbers, location, previous and next calibration date, and calibration schedule. This type of log will ensure that all equipment is monitored to ensure that it maintains its calibration.

Records for equipment should prove that calibration tests were performed. These tests may be done by an outside vendor or by in house personnel. It is important the records show the test values for the equipment prior to tests and after tests are performed. This ensures that equipment has maintained its calibration during use.

If equipment was found to be out of calibration at the time of the scheduled tests, there must be documentation on file showing that the production tests performed with the equipment are still valid.

5.3.11.3 Likely Auditor Actions

Auditors will likely record information about various pieces of equipment as they are in the test areas and then look to verify that proper records are on file. Auditors will also look to see that any equipment that was out of calibration when brought in for testing has previous tests verified.

5.3.12   Inspection and Test Status

5.3.12.1 What the Standard Requires

Quality plans or documented procedures must define how the status of product will be identified throughout production, installation and servicing to ensure that only product which has passed inspections and tests is dispatched, used or installed.

5.3.12.2 How to Meet the Intent

Status of inspections and tests may be defined by tags, location, associated paperwork or other means as the organization sees fit. In most cases the inspections and tests performed will produce the status indicators necessary and material can be segregated, or documentation updated to indicate status of materials.

5.3.12.3 Likely Auditor Actions

Auditors will be sure that they can easily tell the status of parts and product during the audit. This will most likely be done as part of auditing the inspection and test process. Auditors will expect parts and product labeled or otherwise identified with current status. Checksheets, routing documentation or segregated materials will be verified to match stated status.

5.3.13   Control of Nonconforming Product

5.3.13.1 What the Standard Requires

Documented procedures must describe the process to ensure that product which does not conform to specified requirements is not used or installed. The procedures should explain how nonconforming material will be identified, documented, evaluated, segregated (when practical), dispositioned and how this information is communicated.

Documented procedures should define the review process for nonconforming material. The responsibility for the review and the authority for determining disposition of nonconforming product must be defined. Determination may be made to

- rework the product to meet the specification
- accept the product with or without repair
- regrade the product for alternative applications
- reject or scrap the product.

When required in the customer's contract the organization must report any decision to use or repair product that does not meet specified requirements.

5.3.13.2 How to Meet the Intent

Employees at each stage of the process need to know what to do with product that does not meet the requirements. In most cases, this material is tagged or placed in a quarantine area to ensure it is not used. Many companies have a group of people designated with authority to disposition the material. Other companies allow the person that identified the non-conformance to disposition the material.

It is important that the re-inspection of any rework follow documented procedures or plans. This may be documented on the same forms or using the same system which recorded the original nonconformance.

5.3.13.3 Likely Auditor Actions

Auditors will ensure that materials, which are nonconforming, are identified according to the organization's procedures. They will ensure that documentation explains the material disposition and that an authorized person performed it.

5.3.14   Corrective and Preventive Action

5.3.14.1 What the Standard Requires

Documented procedures must describe the corrective and preventive action process. Action taken must be appropriate for the magnitude of problems found. Changes to procedures, which result from corrective or preventive actions, should be implemented and recorded.

Procedures for corrective action must include information relating to: handling of customer complaints and product nonconformities, how product, process and quality system nonconformities will be investigated and recorded, how actions to be taken will be determined, and how to ensure that actions taken have been effective.

Procedures for preventive action must include: all appropriate sources of information be used to detect, analyze and eliminate potential nonconformity, how problems requiring preventive action will be handled, how to ensure preventive actions are effective, and how relevant information will be submitted to management.

5.3.14.2 How to Meet the Intent

Documented procedures need to describe the various inputs into the corrective and preventive action programs, how reports are investigated, and how the actions taken are reviewed for effectiveness. Procedures for corrective actions should ensure that the root cause of the problem is identified and that any action taken will further prevent the problem for recurring. Appropriate sources, which may reveal a need for preventive actions, should be monitored and any actions taken reviewed for effectiveness at preventing the problem from occurring.

5.3.14.3 Likely Auditor Actions

Auditors will look at various functions that feed information into the corrective action system. They will ensure that each report is recorded and investigated. Auditors will examine the action plans and follow-up activities to ensure that the corrective or preventive action was effective. This may be done through a documentation audit of the corrective/preventive action files, or by further examination within the organization.

5.3.15   Handling, Storage, Packaging, Preservation and Delivery

5.3.15.1 What the Standard Requires

Procedures for handling, storage, packaging, preservation and delivery must be in place. Product must be handled to prevent damage or deterioration. Storage areas must be adequate to prevent damage and deterioration. Methods of input and retrieval to storage areas must be defined. Stock should be assessed at appropriate intervals to detect deterioration.

Packing, packaging and marking must be controlled to ensure conformance to specified requirements. Preservation and segregation controls should be put in place where necessary. Product must be protected after final inspection and test. If delivery is part of the customer's contract, protection must extend through delivery.

5.3.15.2 How to Meet the Intent

Documented procedures for this clause are often in the form of work instructions or specifications. The organization needs to address shelf life, and storage conditions as well as identify how product suitability will be monitored. Procedures need to be in place to ensure that packaging is controlled to meet product and customer requirements. Requirements for delivery need to be established and communicated to ensure safety and protection of product. Finally, authorization for input or removal of product from warehouse locations should be defined.

5.3.15.3 Likely Auditor Actions

Auditors will look at product storage locations and ensure materials are properly handled. First impression can make a big difference here. Cleanliness, and organization of an area says a great deal about the general controls in place. Auditors will look at product that is ready to be shipped and verify that all requirements are in place. Auditors may also verify that shipping materials have been verified to be adequate to ship product without damage.

5.3.16   Control of Quality Records

5.3.16.1 What the Standard Requires

Procedures must be established that identify required quality records and explain their collection, indexing, access, filing, storage, maintenance and disposition. Required quality records include those from the organization as well as any records provided by suppliers. Records must be stored to protect them from loss or damage. They must be readily retrievable for the organization and when required by the contract for the customer or customer's representative.

5.3.16.2 How to Meet the Intent

Records generated as a result of quality system related activities must be identified. This may be achieved by listing the required information regarding the records within related procedures, or by a separate document which identifies all records with relevant information. Because these records provide proof of product acceptability they are often already maintained under the organization's standard business practices.

5.3.16.3 Likely Auditor Actions

In each area were records are maintained the auditors will be looking at this element. If it is difficult to produce a file or record it will raise questions about the system. Auditors will look at the filing or storage systems to ensure needs are being met and talk to the persons responsible to see that they understand the requirements for protection and retention.

5.3.17   Internal Quality Audits

5.3.17.1 What the Standard Requires

Procedures that explain the planning and implementation of internal quality audits must be established. Audits need to be carried out by persons independent o the area audited, and should be scheduled on the basis of status and importance of the activity. Results of audits need to be recorded and presented to those responsible for the area. Once presented timely action to correct deficiencies is required. Follow up activities need to verify and record that corrective action was implemented and effective.

5.3.17.2 How to Meet the Intent

An audit schedule must be established. The frequency of audits needs to be based on the status and importance of the activity. During the development of the system it is likely that audits are performed more frequently. As the system matures audits may be performed less frequently, although it is standard practice to audit each element of the standard at least once during a 12-month period. Any nonconformances to the system must be reported to management. It is usual for internal audits to conduct follow-up for corrective action implementation during subsequent visits to the area.

5.3.17.3 Likely Auditor Actions

Auditors will review the audit schedule and ensure that audits are conducted as planned by the organization. They will look for results of audits to be reported to management and used as part of the management review process. Where non-conformances were identified the auditors will look for corrective action to be taken and ensure it is effectively implemented.

5.3.18   Training

5.3.18.1 What the Standard Requires

Procedures to describe the process for identifying training needs and providing training for all personnel affecting quality are required. Personnel should be qualified on the basis of education, training and/or experience. Records of training need to be maintained.

5.3.18.2 How to Meet the Intent

Management must determine what training is necessary and ensure that personnel receive it. A simple matrix identifying required training could easily meet this element.

5.3.18.3 Likely Auditor Actions

During the course of the audit names of people who are interviewed or that appear on records will be recorded. Training files for these individuals will then be reviewed to ensure that training for the required tasks is complete. Auditors may also discuss training with employees to examine their knowledge of the quality system.

5.3.19   Servicing

5.3.19.1 What the Standard Requires

Documented procedures of how service is performed, verified and reported are required where servicing is a specified requirement.

5.3.19.2 How to meet the intent

If your company services it's product, then you will need to document how service is performed. Most likely your company will have service manuals already in place. This documentation normally describes how service is performed and verified. Service records or reports will document the problem identified, actions taken to correct it and any tests that were done to ensure the product functions correctly. Organizations must realize that although the requirements listed under the Servicing section are very brief, they must follow all the elements of the standard as they apply to the area.

5.3.19.3 Likely Auditor Actions

Auditors will look at recently completed service and verify that records show that all requirements were met. Interaction with field representatives and international organizations may be looked at as applicable.

5.3.20   Statistical Techniques

5.3.20.1 What the Standard Requires

If statistical techniques are needed to establish, control and verify process capability and product characteristics then the organization must establish documented procedures to control their application.

5.3.20.2 How to Meet the Intent

Identify areas where statistical methods are needed and implement procedures that govern their use. Areas such as Receiving Inspection and Process Controls are likely candidates if sampling methods are used to determine the quantity needed to be tested or to identify process improvements.

5.3.20.3 Likely Auditor Actions

Auditors will ensure that procedures are followed for areas where these methods are used. Auditors may look at procedures used to monitor and control production processes and how they identify product performance issues.

References

Fries, Richard C., *Reliable Design of Medical Devices*. New York: Marcel Dekker, Inc., 1997.

ISO 9001, *Quality systems - Model for quality assurance in design, development, production, installation and servicing*. Switzerland: International Organization for Standardization, 1994.

ISO 9001:2000, *Quality Management Systems, First Committee Drafts*. Milwaukee, WI: American Society for Quality. 1998.

Steudel, H.J & Associates, Inc,. *What every employee needs to know about ISO 9000*. Madison, WI: 1995.

Chapter 6

Design of Medical Devices for the Canadian Market

Paul Fabry – Canadian Standards Association
Toronto, Canada

All Medical Devices sold in Canada must be in compliance with the *Food and Drugs Act, Medical Device Regulations*, published in July, 1998, Registration SOR/98-282 7 May, 1998. The *Medical Devices Regulations* prepared by the Medical Device Bureau, Health Protection Branch, set out the requirements governing the sale, importation, and advertisement of medical devices. The goal of the Regulations is to ensure that medical devices distributed in Canada are both safe and effective. In developing these Regulations, emphasis was placed on developing requirements, which are harmonious with those of Canadian international trading partners and eliminating, to the greatest extent possible, requirements unique to Canada. Harmonization allows meaningful negotiations toward Mutual Recognition Agreements (MRA) to occur, thereby eliminating barriers to trade. MRAs, once operational, will allow devices to be assessed in one jurisdiction and placed on the market in all other jurisdictions party to the agreement without further assessment.

The *Medical Devices Regulations* are administrated by theTherapeutic Products Programme (TPP), which recognizes and strongly endorses the importance of harmonization as a key factor of these Medical Devices Regulations. Harmonization of requirements to the greatest extent possible with the European Union and United States, would facilitate mutual recognition agreements (MRAs) with both these jurisdictions, which in turn would lead to elimination of duplication of third party audits and significant cost savings to industry and regulators. Canada has signed an MRA with the EU, and the *Medical Device Regulations* are similar with the EU *Medical Device Directive* (MDD). The groundwork is also being laid to facilitate similar agreement with the FDA. In the broader international scheme Canada is participating in the Global Harmonization Task Force (GHTF).

All of these activities, schemes, and agreements would eventually lead the designer to design the product which would comply with the single standard and the single regulation, which would be acceptable worldwide. The *Medical Device Regulations* are harmonized as closely as possible with those of the EU and the US. However, it must be noted that the systems of administration and enforcement are different. The intent of this chapter is to highlight, explain, and provide the rationale for these unique requirements in Canada.

6.1   Fundamental Safety and Effectiveness Principles

The design of medical devices imported or sold in Canada must meet the following principles, appropriate to the device, on which regulatory requirements would be based:

- Devices must not, when used under the conditions and for the purposes intended, compromise the clinical condition or the safety of patients, or the safety and health of users or, where applicable, other persons, provided that any risk which may be associated with their use constitute acceptable risks when weighed against the benefits to the patient and are compatible with a high level of protection of health and safety.

- A manufacturer must take measures reasonable and prudent to ensure that the design and manufacture of a device conforms to safety principles, taking into account the generally acknowledged state of the art. The measures should, with respect to the use of the device: identify and eliminate or reduce risks as far as possible (inherently safe design and construction), where appropriate take adequate protection measures, including alarms, if necessary, in relation to risks that cannot be eliminated, inform users of the residual risks due to any shortcomings of the protection measures adopted, and minimize the danger from any potential failure during the lifetime of the device.
- The device must perform as intended by the manufacturer, and must be effective for the medical conditions, purposes or uses for which it is recommended or intended.
- The characteristics and performance of the device must not be adversely affected to such a degree that the clinical conditions and safety of patients and, where applicable, of other persons, are compromised during the lifetime of the device as indicated by the manufacturer, when the device is subjected to the stresses which can occur during normal conditions of use.
- The performance of a device shall not be compromised by transport or conditions of storage, taking into account the instructions and information provided by the manufacturer.
- Device materials should be compatible with each other and with materials (biological and non-biological). They may contact during normal use and should not pose unnecessary risks to patients, users and other persons.
- The design, manufacture and packaging of a device should minimize risk to patients, users, and other persons from, for example:

    - flammability or explosion,
    - chemical or microbial contamination and residues,
    - radiation emissions,
    - electrical, mechanical, and thermal hazards,

- fluids leaking from the device, or the ingress of fluids into the device.

- Sterile devices must have been manufactured and sterilized by an appropriate validated method and under appropriately controlled environment conditions.
- Devices intended to be used as part of a system must be compatible with other components of the total system.
- Devices with a measuring function must be designed to perform with a degree of accuracy and stability suitable for the intended purpose.
- Devices, which are or contain software, must be designed to perform as intended, and the performance must be tested and validated.
- Every device must be accompanied by the information needed to use it safely and effectively, taking into account the training and knowledge of the potential users.

The above fundamental safety and effectiveness principles are considered to be equivalent to the Essential Requirements in the *Medical Device Directive*, (Council Directive 93/42/EEC of June 1993), taking into account the differences between the use of the term *effectiveness* in the Canadian Regulations and the use of the term *performance* in the European Directive. The Therapeutic Product Program (TPP) interprets effectiveness to mean that the device will produce the effect represented or intended by the manufacturer relative to the medical conditions, purposes or uses for which the device is recommended or intended.

The TPP has also adopted the spirit and intent of the United States FDA 510(k) safety and effectiveness principles. The TPP consider the European principles too lengthy and has condensed them. Furthermore, whereas the European document uses performance, the TPP must key on the term effectiveness to be consistent with its mandate. The FDA 510(k) does not iterate their principles in the same detail nor identify their principles in one common location.

6.2   Device Classification

The Medical Devices Regulations distinguish medical devices under a risk-based classification system. Devices are grouped into four classes, with Class I representing the lowest risk devices and Class IV representing the highest risk devices. Where a medical device can fit into multiple classes, it is placed in the highest applicable class. Detailed rules to classify medical devices are set out in Schedule I of the Medical Devices Regulations. Factors that are used to classify medical devices include:

- the invasiveness or non-invasiveness of the device and its contact with the user;
- if invasive, the part of the user's body that is penetrated;
- the purpose of the device;
- whether the device is active, i.e., whether its operation depends on a source of energy other than energy generated by the human body or gravity; and
- whether the device is an *in vitro* diagnostic device.

Dental or surgical instruments and devices placed in the oral or nasal cavities, as far as the pharynx or in the ear canal up to the eardrum are examples of Class I devices. Devices used to disinfect or sterilize other devices and non-invasive calibrators are examples of Class II devices. Surgically invasive devices that are intended to be absorbed by the body or that are intended to remain in the body for thirty (30) days or more are examples of Class III devices. Surgically invasive devices used to diagnose, monitor, correct or control a defect of the central cardiovascular system, of the central nervous system or of fetus *in utero* are examples of Class IV devices.

6.3   Labeling

For the designer familiar with the European Union *Medical Device Directive*, it is evident from the described Canadian classification system, that both systems are almost identical. Furthermore the EU MDD classification system is based on FDA 510(k) classification system of Classes I, II, and III, where Class II is split into two Classes, Class IIa and Class IIb.

The unique requirements in the Medical Device Regulations are labeling, since Canada is a bilingual country. The intent of this labeling requirement is to ensure that medical devices are accompanied by certain information to allow:

a)   the proper selection and use by health care professionals and the general public, and

b)   the facilitation of post-market traceability of the device through the distribution network.

Every medical device is required to bear a label, which would include the following particulars:

- information sufficient to identify the device, which must include the name of the device and which may also include the model number, catalogue number and the control number;
- the name and address of the manufacturer, importer or distributor of the device;
- the net weight, length, volume, numerical count, or other expressions of the contents of the package where this is not readily apparent;
- the word *sterile*, if the manufacturer intends the device to be sold sterile;
- the expiration date where applicable, this date to be dependent on the least stable component or shortest-lived component;
- the medical conditions, purposes or uses for which the device is recommended or intended, unless these are obvious to the user;
- the direction for use, except for devices which can be used safely without such directions;
- information identifying special storage conditions.

Devices, which are sold to the general public, are required to bear an outer label, which must display all of the above particulars. Where this is not practical, the direction for use is permitted to appear on another part of the label (e.g., package insert). The required information must be in either of the two official languages in addition to any other language, with the following exceptions:

- warnings and contraindications (one component of the direction for use), for all devices must be in both official languages, and
- the complete directions for use for a device available at a self-service display must be in both official languages.

Where the directions for use for a device are supplied in only one of the two official languages, the direction for use are required to be made available, in a timely manner, in the other official language, upon request of the person who purchased the device.

All information, which is required to be on the label, must be legible, prominently, and permanently displayed. The intended user must express all information, which is required to be on the label, in terms understandable. There are specific labeling requirements for devices sold for clinical investigation, custom devices, and devices sold on compassionate grounds. These requirements are specified in the respective section of the Medical Devices Regulations in Part 2 and Part 3. Assessment of conformity with the labeling requirements is undertaken through pre-market submission for Class III and IV devices. Labeling for Class I and II devices is assessed on a post-market surveillance basis.

6.4   Standards and the Design Process

In the process in designing of medical equipment the knowledge, use and application of applicable standards are essential. The safety, efficacy and performance of the medical device must be introduced during the design process, using all know and applicable standards. The Medical Devices Regulations do not include any standards except *National Standard of Canada CAN/CSA – ISO 13485-98, Quality systems – Medical Devices- Particular requirements for the application of ISO 9001*, and *National Standard of Canada CAN/CSA – ISO 13488- 98, Quality systems –Medical Devices- Particular requirements for the application of ISO 9002*, as amended from time to time.

Policy Documents are used to reference internationally recognized standards, which the TPP consider as being minimum acceptable standards for meeting the Safety and Effectiveness requirements set out in the *Medical Devices Regulations*. Policy Documents are developed for any risk class of device. The TPP uses standards in Policy Documents as a basis for enforcement action based on the following:

- All devices must meet the Safety and Effectiveness requirements set out in the Medical Devices Regulations.
- Standards are a means of stating minimum acceptable requirements respecting the safety and effectiveness requirements applicable to a device or group of devices.
- Where a standard is referenced in a Policy Document by the TPP, the TPP would deem that the manufacturer has demonstrated that their device complies with the applicable safety and effectiveness requirements covered by the standard, where compliance with the standard is demonstrated. A statement to this effect is placed in the *Medical Devices Regulations*.

Where a standard is referenced in a Policy Document and the manufacturer uses an alternate standard, the manufacturer must provide justification that the standard that is used provides equivalent assurance of safety and effectiveness. Standards set out in the Policy Document prescribe an acceptable means of meeting the Safety and Effectiveness requirements set out in the *Medical Devices Regulations*. The option remains open to a manufacturer to propose any alternate means, but the burden of proof required to establish acceptability of the alternate means rest with the manufacturer.

The TPP is not in a position to equip itself with the test equipment and personnel necessary to conduct all the different manufacturer's test methods. Therefore, whenever the TPP would conduct compliance testing, the TPP would use the test method or methods as set out in the Policy Document. Where a manufacturer has chosen to use a standard referenced in a Policy Document, and compliance testing to the device by the TPP to that standard demonstrates that the device does not meet the standard, the TPP would take any necessary enforcement action to resolve the issue. The TPP's action would be based on the fact that compliance with the standard demonstrates that the applicable provisions of the Safety and Effectiveness requirements have been met.

A second case would be where a manufacturer has chosen not to use a standard referenced in a Policy Document, and has demonstrated to the TPP that the standard which they do use provides an equivalent assurance of safety and effectiveness as the standard referenced in a Policy Document. With this case, where compliance testing of the device by the TPP to the standard referenced in the Policy Document demonstrated that the device does not meet the standard, the TPP would discuss with the manufacturer the results of the testing and try to resolve any concerns which are raised as a result of the compliance testing. The TPP is referencing internationally recognized standards such as IEC and ISO where possible and use of uniquely Canadian standards is minimized. The Policy Documents are similar to the FDA Policy on Recognition of Standards.

6.5   Implant Registration

To enhance the ability of a manufacturer to locate devices for recall and post-market surveillance purposes the Medical Devices Regulations cover the implant registration, which requires the manufacturer to provide two patient registration cards as a part of the device labeling for all devices subject to implant registration. The registration system records the following information:

- Information sufficient to identify the device which may include the name of the device, the model number, catalogue number, and control number.
- The name and address of the manufacturer of the device.
- The name and address of any additional contact for the collection of implant registration information.
- The name and address of the implanting practitioner.
- The date the device was implanted.
- The name and address of the health care facility where the device was implanted.
- The patient's name and address or the identification number used by the health care facility to identify the patient.

The implant registration applies to most Class IV implants and to some Class III implants.

6.6   *In Vitro* Diagnostic Devices (IVDDs)

The *Medical Devices Regulations* also covers all IVDDs devices such as reagents, articles, instruments, apparatus, equipment, or system intended for *in vitro* diagnostic use. "Diagnostic" in the interpretation of the Medical Devices Regulations means the examination of specimens for the purpose of providing information concerning a physiological state, state of health or disease or congenital abnormality. The inclusion of IVDDs in the Medical Devices Regulations is a different concept from European Union MDD, where the IVDDs are covered by the separate directive.

For a copy of the *Medical Devices Regulations* as published in the *Canada Gazette Part II*, please contact: Canada Communications Group, Publishing, Ottawa, Ontario, K1A 0S9, telephone (819) 956-4802 or Facsimile (819) 994-1498. Please, quote issue no., *Canada Gazette Part II,* Volume 132 # 11, dated 27 May, 1998.

All application forms, guideline documents and copies of Medical Devices Regulations are available also by downloading them from the Therapeutic Products Web site:

http://www.hc-sc.gc.ca/hpb-dgps/therapeut/
The above Medical Devices Regulations, as administrated by the Therapeutic Products Programme (TPP) on behalf of Federal Health Protection Branch of Health and Welfare Canada, are also supplemented by some other regulations administrated by the Provinces of Canada, which the designer of the medical devices must be familiar.

6.7   Electrically Operated Medical Devices

In Canada, provincial legislation provides for regulation of the sale and use of electrically operated equipment, including the medical devices, with the object of assuring public safety. Typically, the regulations require that the provincial authority approve equipment which is sold or used. Each province administers its regulations through an appropriate inspection agency. The agency may be specialized for electrical safety matters alone or may deal with these and other safety matters as well.

For the bulk of electrical equipment sold in Canada a CSA Monogram or other mark issued by an organization which is accredited by the Standards Council of Canada on the equipment, is considered to be evidence that is approved. This approval by third party (Certification Organization) is mandatory. In some cases, the provincial authority under a procedure usually referred to as special inspection, may approve equipment, which is not approved by the Certification Organization. In such instances, the approval applies only to the specific pieces of equipment examined and labeled by the provincial authority, or its agent, for instance, CSA International.

The standards used for certification of the medical electrical devices are listed in the *Catalogue of Information Products* of CSA International under Health Care Technology section, which comes under the requirements of *Canadian Electrical Code*, Part II-General Requirements. *The Canadian Electrical Code*, Part I establishes safety standards for the installation and maintenance of electrical equipment, and the Section 24 Patient Care Areas covers the requirements for providing a safe environment for patients, who need frequently additional protection from electric shock. Section 24 addresses only those requirements that arise from considerations of safety that should be unique to patient areas in hospitals. This Section applies to the installation of:

- electrical wiring and equipment within patient care areas of hospitals; and
- those portions of electrical systems of hospitals designated as essential electrical systems.

This Section also intends to establish the minimum requirements for the proper and safe design of a building electrical system for hospitals, thus providing the additional protection needed by the patients.

The other unique Section of the *Canadian Electrical Code*, Part I is Section 52, Diagnostic Imaging Installations. This Section applies to the installation of x-ray and other diagnostic imaging equipment operating at any frequency, and is supplementary to, or amendatory of, the general requirements of the *Canadian Electrical Code*, Part I. Rationale for Section 52 is that x-ray or computerized tomography equipment in operation generates very high voltages and dangerous radiation. Special Rules are required to ensure that the electrical installation of such electrical equipment is safe, and these may differ from or be supplementary to other general *Canadian Electrical Code*, Part I, requirements.

The most important standard from the *Canadian Electrical Code*, Part II standards in the Health Care Technology field is:

> *CSA Standard CAN/CSA – C22.2 No. 601.1, Medical Electrical Equipment, Part 1: General Requirements for Safety.*

It is based upon the identically titled second edition *of IEC* (International Electrotechnical Commission*) Standard 601-1*. Some compromises have been made in order to integrate special national needs and this has been achieved by concept of Canadian Deviations to the original IEC requirements. The Canadian Deviations are presented in the pages preceding the original text from *IEC 601 Standard*. Most of the deviations reflect the requirements of the *Canadian Electrical Code, Part I,* while others are based on issues relating to improved patient safety. Items of medical electrical equipment used and offered for sale in Canada must meet the requirements of these deviations, insofar as they apply.

The following are the main Canadian Deviations to IEC 601-1 Standard:

Sub-clause 2.4.1 *High Voltage.*
- Sub-clause 6.6 (b) *Identification of Medical Gas Cylinders and Connections.*
- Clause 45 *Pressure Vessel and Parts Subject to Pressure.*
- Sub-clause 56.3 (a) *Construction of Connectors.*
- Sub-clause 57.2 *Mains Connectors, Appliance Inlets and the like.*
- Sub-clause 57.3 (b) *Power Supply Cords – Types.*
- Sub-clause 59.1 *Internal Wiring.*

CSA Standard CAN/CSA – C22.2 No. 601.1 has two Amendments:

- *CAN/CSA –C22.2 No 601.1S1-94* (Adopted IEC 601-1, Amendment 1)

- *CAN/CSA – C22.2 No 601.1B-98* (Adopted IEC 601-1, Amendment 2)

There are no Canadian Deviations for these two Amendments.

The following Collateral Standards were also published with no Canadian Deviations:

- *CAN/CSA –C22.2 No 601.1.1*

- *CAN/CSA – C22.2 No. 601.1.2*

- *CAN/CSA – C22.2 No. 601.1.3.*

There are 34 particular standards published in C22.2 No. 601.2 Series with no Canadian Deviations, except in *CAN/CSA – C22.2 No. 601.2.2 High Frequency Surgical Equipment* and *CAN/CSA – C22.2 No. 601.2.4 Cardiac Defibrillators and Cardiac Defibrillators Monitors.*

All the above standards in *CAN/CSA – C22.2 No. 601* Series are used by the Certification Organizations as mandatory documents to certify and approve products as required by the Provincial Regulations. There are however under Health Care Technology program a numerous standards published covering subjects such as:

- Cardiovascular Implants
- Cardiac Pacemakers
- Oxygen Monitors
- Biological Evaluation of Medical Devices
- Sterilization of Health Care Products
- Electrical Safety in Patient Care Areas
- Anaesthetic Machines for Medical Use

- Critical Care Ventilators
- Medical Gases
- Pressure Regulators, Gauges, and Flow- Metering Devices for Medical Gases
- Steam Sterilization for Hospitals
- Wheelchairs
- Haemodialyzers, Haemofilters, and Haemoconcentrators

Compliance with many of these standards can be used as evidence of compliance with the safety and effectiveness principles as required in the Medical Device Regulations, and they are listed in Policy Documents. Except in the area of Anaesthetic Machines and Ventilators there is no formal certification program established and manufacturer may self declare the compliance. The Anaesthetic Machine and relating devices must conform to *CSA Standard Z168.3* as required by *Guidelines to the Practice of Anaesthesia of the Canadian Anaesthetists' Society.*

6.8   Medical Devices Incorporating Plumbing Features

Medical devices such as hydromassage, hydrotherapy and haemodialysis units, which incorporate plumbing features, must be in compliance with the *National Plumbing Code of Canada*. The Code contains the requirements for the design and installation of plumbing systems, and is adopted and enacted for legal use by any jurisdiction authority in Canada.

6.9   Summary

All medical devices sold and used in Canada must be designed to comply with the *Medical Devices Regulations* and must be licensed from February 1, 1999. In an addition the electrically powered medical devices must be approved either by the way of Special Inspection or be Certified by an acceptable Certification Organization such as CSA International, to satisfy the Provincial Safety Regulations. Battery powered medical devices must be formally approved only in the Province of British Columbia.

References

Extract Canada Gazette. Part II, May 27, 1998
Department of Health,

Medical Devices Regulations.

1999 Catalogue, Information Products, CSA International.

Canadian Electrical Code, Part I.

Canadian Electrical Code, Part II, Life Sciences Standards.

Chapter 7

Pacific Rim Standards and Regulations

Richard C. Fries, PE, CRE – Datex-Ohmeda, Inc.
Madison, Wisconsin

The far-reaching economic and political turmoil that has rocked Asia for the past few years continues to have profound repercussions both in the countries of the region and throughout the rest of the world. Touched off by a devaluation of the Thai currency and expanding in a ripple effect that grew to tidal-wave proportions, the crisis roiled world financial markets, plunged national economies into recession, and threatened the existence of a new middle class created as a result of rapid economic growth. For foreign companies, including medical device firms, that had looked to Asia both as a site for expanding manufacturing operations and as a market of enormous potential, the crisis was a rude awakening.

In addition, there is the question of what is being done in Asia with regard to standards and regulation. Is the area moving toward harmonization?

All developed nations are rapidly moving toward the same level of sophistication when it comes to the evaluation of medical devices, be they Class I, II, or III. The European Union (EU) has created a regulatory mechanism that ensures the highest level of safety for patients, while quickly moving beneficial products to the market. The EU has already established a very credible review system for medical devices through efforts such as basing the process on quality system standards, using the world-class, globally recognized ISO 9000 series of standards. In fact, as countries update their regulatory procedures, most are following the lead of Europe.

The EU is aggressively pursuing mutual recognition agreements (MRAs) with many non-EU partners, including Switzerland, Canada, Australia, and some Asian countries. Even without an MRA with the EU, some Asian countries, notably China, are unilaterally adopting an EU-style regulatory approach.

7.1   Australia

Australia is currently running an MRA with the European Union, as is New Zealand. The entry requirements are similar to those of the European Union, but a license is required along with a formal application.

7.1.1   General Information

The Therapeutic Goods Act of 1989 regulates the supply of therapeutic goods in Australia with the intention of protecting health care workers and the Australian public by ensuring the safety, quality, and efficacy of therapeutic goods. Unless specifically exempt or excluded, therapeutic goods may not be supplied to the Australian market or exported unless they are listed or registered in the Australian Register of Therapeutic Goods (ARTG). Therapeutic goods are defined as:

> an instrument, apparatus, appliance, material, or other article, whether for use alone or in combination, together with any accessories or software required for its proper functioning, which does not achieve its principal intended action by pharmacological, chemical, immunological, or metabolic

means, although it may be assisted in its function by such means.

Importers, manufacturers, exporters, or modifiers of these devices are considered the *sponsor* for the product and are responsible for entry of the product in the ARTG before it may be supplied in Australia or exported from Australia. The TGA monitors products being supplied in a number of ways and those who knowingly contravene the Act are liable to prosecution.

Products that are not excluded from the operation of the Act are regulated in three categories with respect to the operation of Part 3 of the Act:

- Registrable
- Listable
- Exempt.

The products must be registered in the Australian Register of Therapeutic Goods and must undergo extensive pre-market evaluation before they can be supplied in Australia.

The products must be listed in the ARTG, but do not have to undergo extensive pre-market evaluation before supply. The sponsor must provide the following to the Therapeutic Goods Administration (TGA):

- a complete *Therapeutic Devices Application* form
- a label (either a sample or a draft) that complies with the Therapeutic Goods order for labeling (*TGO 37*)
- package inserts/promotional material that comply with sections 4 and 7 of the Therapeutic Goods Advertising Code
- documented evidence of Good Manufacturing Practice for goods specified in Schedule 6 and a license for manufacture, unless exempt
- test certificates for a batch to be supplied in Australia for condoms, diaphragms, and non-sterile bandages and dressings.

The products are exempt from Part 3, but are still covered by labelling and advertising provisions of the Act.

7.1.2   Application

Applications must be filed by the sponsor, which must be an Australian entity, on a *Therapuetic Devices Application* form that is self-explanatory in relation to the information sought. If the application is the initial one to the TGA, it must be accompanied by an *Enterprise Details* form containing relevant sponsor details and nominating and authorized person. The fees for registrable devices are higher and vary depending on the type of product and the extent of evaluation that is required.

At present, listing applications take approximately 4 weeks to process. Upon receipt, applications are acknowledged by the TGA Business Management Unit and identified by a Therapeutic Goods Application Identification Number (TGAIN). This reference number should be listed in subsequent inquiries about the application.

7.1.3   Proposed New Regulatory Requirements for Medical Devices

The current medical devices regulatory system under the Therapeutic Goods Act of 1989, introduced in 1991, was the first comprehensive national system and replaced a mixture of federal and state responsibilities. Since 1991, a number of significant events have occurred:

- Australia has actively pursued international harmonization as a principal member of the medical device Global Harmonization Task Force
- the European Community approach to medical device regulation has become recognized as a de facto world standard
- a number of shortcomings have been identified with the present Australian system.

The Australian government thought it was time to consider amending the medical device regulatory system.

The purpose of the new proposal is to overcome the identified shortcomings and improve the quality of medical device regulation for the Australian community. This is to be achieved by developing an internationally harmonized medical device regulatory system based on:

- international best practice
- the alignment of Australia's requirements for quality, safety and performance with those of the EC
- the recommendations of the medical device GHTF.

Australia has in general, fewer and/or less stringent regulations for many types of devices than is proposed. The proposal provides for the introduction of

- some minimum requirements for exempt Class I devices
- a more comprehensive pre-market assessment of new technologies high risk active devices and implantable devices
- the extension of quality system requirements to more devices
- the adoption of more international standards
- more powerful mechanisms for requiring sponsors to monitor and report device problems.

This will create a more comprehensive, internationally harmonized and performance based system for the regulation of medical devices in Australia.

Medical device regulation should ensure that the product is safe, is of high quality and performs to the specifications intended by the manufacturer under stated conditions. The common elements of the regulatory systems of the major industrial countries include:

- a device classification scheme with different investigational and premarket requirements, based on complexity and risk of the medical device, for each class of device
- defining the characteristics a product must have, and the risks that have to be dealt with, before the product can be put on the market ("essential principles/requirements")
- technical documentation required by the essential principles to support the marketing of medical devices

· reliance on international standards and the quality systems
approach, which provides assurances that a product is
designed and manufactured according to certain standards
and specifications regarding safety and performance
· formal product review or approval and clinical evaluation
for high risk devices
· product registration
· adverse incident reporting, investigation and an established
process for product withdrawal.

The current Australian medical device regulatory requirements do not include
all these common elements. Some of the current shortcomings include:

- **Limited pre-market evaluation of high risk medical device
  ("registrable").** Under the current system, only 12 types of
  medical devices are classified as "high risk" registrable and
  subject to detailed pre-market evaluation for quality, safety and
  efficacy. These comprise active implantables (pacemakers,
  defibrillators, deep brain stimulators), heart valves, intrauterine
  contraceptive devices, powered drug infusion pumps, intraocular
  lenses, intraocular viscoelastic fluids, breast implants, devices of
  human or animal origin (e.g., collagen implants), HIV and
  hepatitis C in vitro diagnostic test kits and instrument chemical
  disinfectants.

- **Limited assessment of other medical devices ("listable").** The
  remainder are approved for supply in Australia following a brief
  assessment of quality and safety, based on labelling and product
  information, and compliance with mandatory standards (for a
  limited number of devices: condoms, sutures, urethral catheters,
  dental restorative materials, and examination gloves). There are
  numerous examples of high risk technologies that are not subject
  to comprehensive pre-market assessment.

- **Inadequate classification.** Medical devices are presently
  classified as registrable or listable on a product by product basis.
  This classification is rigidly prescribed in Regulations, with lists
  of registrable and listable devices, exemptions and exclusions in
  Schedules. Consequently the Regulations cannot readily handle

technological change, as they have to be amended for each type of new device. Some new medical devices therefore are treated as listable regardless of their level of risk, until the legislation is amended to re-classify them as registrable. This means that many high risk devices based on insufficiently proven technology may enter the market having only undergone superficial scrutiny.

- **Limited use of standards.** For most medical devices there are no product specific standards under the therapeutic goods legislation. The default standard, the British Pharmacopoeia, has limited application to devices. In addition, the current legislation requires compliance with statutory Australian standards, referred to as Therapeutic Goods Orders (TGOs) which may impose compliance costs on the manufacturer.

- **Compliance with manufacturer quality systems.** Presently, compliance with quality systems standards is required for all registrable devices, for listable devices, which are implantable or sterile, and for a few selected non-sterile devices. However there are critical devices, such as surgical lasers and endoscopes, which are currently not required to be manufactured using a quality system standard.

- **Regulatory duplication.** Australia's medical device requirements differ from those of our major trading partners. Consequently Australian medical device importers and exporters have to comply with a number of different regulatory regimes with the attendant increase in compliance costs.

- **Limited emphasis on post-market surveillance of medical devices.** The importance of monitoring devices already on the market (post-market surveillance) to ensure continued quality, safety and efficacy is not always appreciated and is not explicit in the current legislation. It is a condition of placement of a medical device on the Australian Register of Therapeutic Goods (ARTG) that sponsors report device problems which have caused or may cause serious injury or death. However, it is estimated that only a small percentage of medical device problems are actually reported.

All active implantable medical devices, in vitro diagnostic goods and all other medical devices coming within the definition "medical device" would be regulated. The scope of medical devices would also include goods not included in the EC medical device legislation but covered under the current regulatory system. These goods would include:

> · devices incorporating material of human and animal origin
> · hospital grade and household/commercial grade disinfectants
> · menstrual tampons.

Medical devices would be classified under the following scheme:

- **Class I** ostomy pouches, cervical collars, compression hosiery, beds, wheelchairs, walking aids, spectacles, stethoscopes, external electrodes, gels, software for image processing, tubing for gravity drips, cotton wool, gauze dressings, dental impression materials, examination gloves, prostatic balloon dilatation catheters, scalpels, manual drills and saws, thermographic imagers, dental curing lights, removable dentures.

- **Class IIa** anaesthetic breathing circuits, devices for storage or transport of organs for transplantation, devices for long-term storage of corneas, sperm, embryos etc, hydrogel dressings, tracheal tubes, vaginal pessaries, fixed dental prostheses, suction catheters, single-use catheters, infusion cannulae, bridges, crowns, dental filling materials, TENS devices, external bone growth stimulators, cryosurgery equipment, dental drills, hearing aids, magnetic resonance equipment, gamma cameras, X-ray films, hospital and household / commercial grade disinfectants.

- **Class IIb** haemodialysers, cell separators, insulin pens, brachytherapy devices, surgical adhesives, stents, infusion ports, orthopaedic implants, peripheral vascular grafts, penile implants, non-absorbable sutures, lung ventilators, baby incubators, blood warmers, surgical, diathermy, external pacemakers, external defibrillators, surgical lasers, lithotripters, linear accelerators, radioactive therapy sources, diagnostic X-ray sources, intensive care monitoring systems, apnea monitors, ventilators, anaesthetic machines, blood pumps for heart-lung machines, condoms, contraceptive diaphragms, contact lens care products, viscoelastic products for eye surgery, sterilants and instrument grade disinfectants.

- **Class III** absorbable sutures, temporary pacing leads, neurological catheters, cortical electrodes, vascular prostheses, heart valves, vascular stents, heparin coated catheters, IUDs, condoms with spermicides, blood bags.
- **AIMD** implantable pulse generators, implantable electrodes and implantable drug infusion devices.

Under the proposed system registrable medical devices would be classified as follows:

- Active implantable medical devices, including implantable infusion systems — AIMD
- Cardiac pacemakers and accessories — AIMD
- Intrauterine contraceptive devices (not drug releasing) — Class III
- Prosthetic heart valve — Class III
- Intra ocular Fluids
  - If made from non-viable animal tissue — Class III
  - If synthetic and for transient use (< 60 minutes) — Class IIb
- Devices of animal origin — Class III
- Intra ocular lenses — Class IIb
- Powered drug infusion system, non-implantable — Class IIb
- Breast implants — Class IIb
- Barrier contraceptive devices — Class IIb
- Sterilents and instrument grade disinfectants — Class IIb
- Hospital, household / commercial grade disinfectants — Class IIa
- HIV/HCV *in vitro* diagnostics — IVD

The following products are specifically excluded by the EC directives and would not be regulated as medical devices under the proposed system:

- human tissues for direct donor to host transplantation
- medicinal products where device and drug form a single integral product which is intended exclusively for use in

the given combination and is not reusable e.g., a syringe
filled with a drug (but essential requirements still apply
to any device component)

- drug-device combinations where the principal intended
  purpose is reliant on the drug component e.g., IUD with
  hormone release
- cosmetic products and personal protective equipment.

Artificial tears, artificial saliva, preservatives for transplants/transport media
(other than for IVF) which are currently regulated as devices, would be
regulated as drugs. The conformity assessment procedure is detailed in Figure
7.1.

7.2   Japan

In Japan, compliance with mandatory regulations, if applicable to a
product, is required before a firm can sell its product or even display it in a
trade event -- this is true for all foreign and Japanese domestic firms. In some
instances, a product may be controlled by more than one law, or different laws
apply to products of the same group, since each law has its legislative objective.
Technical regulations are concerned not only with technical specifications of a
product itself, but also with packaging, marking or labeling requirements,
testing, transportation and storage, installation, etc. While "voluntary"
standards and "voluntary" quality marks are not mandatory in Japan, it is
strongly recommended that a firm try to comply with these requirements and
receive appropriate approval. Meeting Japanese standards or receiving a
Japanese quality mark is important for winning Japanese consumer acceptance.
Many Japanese consumers or end-users will only look for products meeting
these requirements.

A firm must determine if its product will be affected by Japanese
regulations and standards. Unfortunately, obtaining information in these areas
from outside of Japan can be difficult. In addition, Japanese approval
procedures are often slow and cumbersome and can be discouraging to those
unwilling to make a major commitment of their time, money, and energy.
However, significant progress has been made in specific product areas in the
last few years, and steps to simplify the system continue. It is absolutely

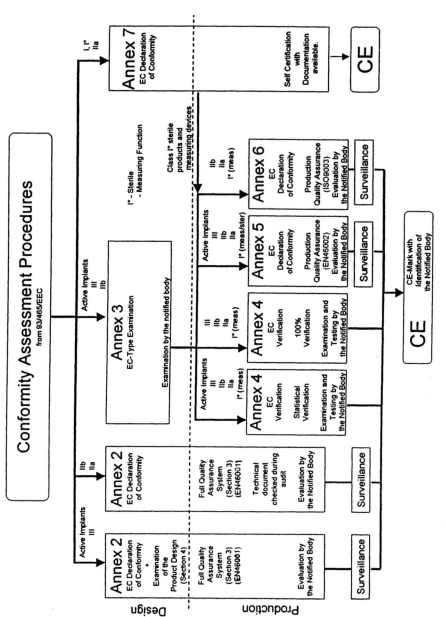

Figure 7-1 Australian conformity assessment procedure.   (From TGA, 1998.)

essential that a company work closely with its Japanese partner to ensure its product meets applicable regulations, standards, and quality marks. Even though some of this information is available here in the United States and is in English, much information on Japanese regulations and standards is only available through the appropriate Japanese governmental ministry and/or only exists in written form in the Japanese language. Therefore, it is often up to the firm's partner in Japan to supply it with information on regulations, standards, and quality marks. The partner will likely serve as the adviser on these matters and answer any questions. Moreover, a company should consider designating its partner as the point person in the company's dealings with the various Japanese Government agencies and ministries. It will be virtually impossible for the company to accomplish this work without someone knowledgeable about regulations, standards, and quality marks in Japan. A company will most likely have to provide detailed information on its product in Japanese and the firm or Japanese partner will have to know the appropriate contacts in the relevant Japanese Government ministry or ministries responsible for granting relevant product approvals.

The Japanese Industrial Standards (JIS) mark is widely used in Japan, and many diverse products are designated as eligible to bear this mark. The JIS are technical specifications which are applied to over 1,000 different products. These standards are comprised of three main elements:

- product standards relating to the function, configuration, and construction of the product
- production method standards which include the testing, analysis, performance criteria, and inspection of the product
- basic standards which relate to the terminology, units, series, and markings.

The JIS marking system is designed to promote quality standardization for individual product categories. There are about 8,600 JIS standards for all products covered under the JIS system. Presently, over 90 percent of these standards are available in English. Although the JIS mark is voluntary, compliance with these standards significantly enhances a product's image among Japanese consumers and is often essential for a product to sell in Japan. The Japanese consumer considers the JIS mark as a guarantee of a product's quality.

The JIS mark also ensures that a product is designed and produced in compliance with consumer safety concerns. Adherence to JIS is also an important determinant for companies competing on bids in the Japanese Government procurement process. Products that comply with these standards will be given preferential treatment in procurement decisions, as Japanese Government entities, in compliance with Article 26 of the Industrial Standardization Law, must give priority to products bearing the JIS mark when selecting winning procurement bids. JIS cover all industrial products except for those products regulated by specific national laws or for which other standard systems apply (i.e., Pharmaceutical Affairs Law and Japan Agricultural Standards). The American National Standards Institute (ANSI) can identify the particular JIS for specific products and provide a copy of these to companies for a fee.

In Japan various quality marks are affixed to products that are tested and approved. Some quality marks are mandatory, with the product approval process and application for the quality mark governed by specific national laws. Other quality marks are voluntary, but are often important for a product to be widely accepted by Japanese consumers. Mandatory quality marks and voluntary quality marks require both product type approval and factory inspections (these inspections are for quality control assessment) before a product can be affixed with the relevant quality mark. In instances where mandatory quality marks are applicable, it is important that the regulated products bear the appropriate mark when shipped to Japan. Japanese customs authorities will not allow imported goods that do not bear the appropriate mandatory quality mark.

7.2.1   Japanese Standards Association

The Japanese Standards Association was established as a public institution for the promotion of industrial standardization on December 6, 1945, under government authorization. JSA has no true performance standards, but tends to follow IEC 601-1. JSA does have a complicated approval process that can be very lengthy (up to 9 months). This process can delay distribution of products in Japan. JSA activities include:

- Standards and document publishing
- Seminars and consulting services
- Research on standardization
- National sales agent for foreign national standard bodies.

7.2.2   Other Japanese Standards Organizations

The unified national system of industrial standardization began to function by the setup of the Japanese Engineering Standards Committee (JESC) in 1921. This group undertook the establishment of national standards. In 1949, the Industrial Standardization Law was promulgated and the Japanese Industrial Standards Committee (JISC) was established under the law as an advisory organization of competent ministers in charge of the elaboration of Japanese Industrial Standards (JIS) and the designation of the JIS mark to products.

7.3   Russia

According to Russian law, all medical devices imported into Russia should be registered with the Ministry of Health of the Russian Federation. The registration certificate is issued by the State Inspectorate for Quality Control of Drugs and Medical equipment within the Ministry. Registration applications and forms may be obtained from the Department of Testing and Registration of New Foreign Medical Equipment in the State Inspectorate for Quality Control of Drugs and Medical Equipment. Completed forms and documents should be returned to the Department of Testing and Registration of New Foreign Medical Equipment.

Registration usually requires clinical trials. Registration fees depend on the type of medical device. Beginning October 1, 1995, imported medical devices must also be accompanied by a safety certificate. The main national testing and certification body of the Russian Federation is the Russian Federation State Committee on Standardization, Metrology and Certification (Gosstandart) which develops basic policies for certification and standards. Gosstandart does not issue certificates of conformity, but maintains lists of Russian national certification institutes.

Safety certificates requested by manufacturers of medical devices usually are issued for longer terms, up to three years. Certificates sought by distributors or trading companies are usually issued for shorter terms, up to one year. The testing company will require that the distributor or trading firm submit a contract with the manufacturer. Presenting a safety certificate issued by a foreign laboratory reduces the certification time to several days. Russian certification institutes accept certificates issued by foreign national certification institutes and testing laboratories in major European countries, Japan, the United States, Canada, Singapore, China, India, South Korea, and Israel. These institutes include TÜV (Germany) and UL Northbrook (United States). UL Northbrook is the only U.S. laboratory whose clinical tests results are accepted by Russian Testing Institutes.

7.4   China

7.4.1   Information Source

The China Information Institute of Technical Supervision was established through amalgamation of the former China Standards Information Center and China Information Service of Metrology, in January, 1990. It is affiliated with the State Bureau of Technical Supervision. It is a state professional information institution specializing in the collection, processing, research and servicing of information on standards, metrology, and the quality of products. The Institute provides the following services:

- access to standards documents
- text translations
- publishing standards catalogues and normative documents
- selling standards documents databases
- on-line standards documents retrieval
- consultation related to standards
- technical consultation on the database system
- consultation on quality certification.

7.4.2   Collective and Certification Marks

Procedures for the registration and administration of collective and certification marks have been formulated in accordance with the Trademark Law of the People's Republic of China and the Implementing Regulations under the Trademark Law. In these procedures, a collective mark refers to a goods mark or a service mark used by the members of an industrial or commercial group, association, or other collective organization for the purpose of indicating that the dealers in the goods or the providers of the services belong to the same organization. A certification mark refers to a goods mark or service mark controlled by an organization capable of testing and monitoring certain goods or services, but used by others for the purpose of certifying the place of origin, material, manufacturing process, quality, accuracy, or other specified characteristics of the goods or services.

The Trademark Office establishes a Collective Mark Register and a Certification Mark Register to list collective marks and certification marks. Such marks approved for registration by the Trademark Office are protected by law.

The party applying for the registration mark will submit to the Trademark Office an Application for Trademark Registration, copies of the reproduction of the mark, accompanied by a certificate of qualification. The application must also include a certifying document issued by the relevant competent department stating that the applicant is capable of testing and monitoring specified characteristics of their device. Once the party has fulfilled the conditions stipulated for administration of the certification mark, may use the mark on its goods or services.

References

Fries, Richard C., *Reliable Design of Medical Devices*. New York: Marcel Dekker, Inc., 1997.

Halverson, Fred S., "Global Harmonization and Mutual Recognition Efforts: Keeping Up The Pace," in *Medical Device and Diagnostic Industry,* April, 1999.

Information Institute of Technical Supervision, *China – Information Institute of Technical Supervision.* Chinanet Infotech & Service, Inc., 1998.

Japanese Regulations, Standards, Quality Marks, and Certification Systems. Japan, 1994.

Maksimova, Ludmila, *Registration and Certification of Medical Devices and Pharmaceuticals in Russia.* U.S. Foreign Commercial Service and U.S. Department of State, January, 1997.

Maksimova, Ludmila, An Update on *Registration and Certification of Medical Devices and Pharmaceuticals in Russia.* U.S. Foreign Commercial Service and U.S. Department of State, August, 1997.

Procedures for the Registration and Administration of Collective Marks and Certification Marks. State Administration for Industry and Commerce, December, 1994.

Sahota, Amarjit, "A Diagnosis for Southeast Asia," in *Medical Device and Diagnostic Industry.* March, 1999.

Therapeutic Goods Administration, *Background Information on the Proposed New Regulatory Requirements for Medical Devices.* Australia: Therapeutic Goods Administration, December, 1998.

Chapter 8

Overview of Software Standards

Nancy George – Software Quality Management, Inc.
Towson, Maryland

Up until the mid-19th century there were no national or international conventions as to how time should be measured or when the day would begin and end. Most towns or cities had a day made of 24 equal hours, with a primary fixed point in the day. The differences in local time did not really matter until the railway networks developed. Suddenly people could travel faster than the speed of the sun. With each town on the railway line following its own local time, the organization of the railway timetables became a nightmare. In October 1884, 41 delegates from 25 nations assembled in Washington, D.C., for the International Meridian Conference. In twenty-two days the delegates created and agreed on standard time and longitude.

Currently, we are experiencing related growth pains. Islands of software engineers all over the world are generating software products at ever-increasing rates. These products are being developed differently. Yet technology is bringing us closer together. We no longer just interact at a city-to-city level, dependent solely on a railway network. We now have a telecommunications network that bridges countries and continents. Daily, and on a global basis, we buy and sell these software-based products that result from these islands of development. Because of the uncertainty of the reliability and compatibility of these software-based products, many today are looking to national and international software standards to help. They are looking to them to help bring more consistent approaches to development, to help level the playing field worldwide as far as which islands are generating a good faith effort to develop reliable software, and to assist with pre-acquisition decisions.

Currently there are greater than 300 software standards and greater than 50 organizations developing software standards. Some estimate that the typical Institute of Electronic and Electrical Engineers (IEEE) standard takes 2 to 4 years to develop. Some estimates say that it costs (in labor and travel of volunteers) between $2,000 and $10,000 per page. Internationally, the development time is typically longer, generally greater than 7 years, with one standard taking 14 years. That is quite a difference from the 22 days taken in 1884 to create and agree on the standard for time and longitude.

Also the size of the actual standards have grown. The 1884 standard for time and longitude consisted of 7 bullets. The 1998 collection of IEEE standards was comprised of 2,300 pages. One international technical report, which is to become an international standard, is over 300 pages. The 7 bullets defined in 1884 have stood the test of time, but many of these current and in-process software standards have yet to stand the test of time regarding usability and usefulness.

Despite the relatively unproven nature of software standards, an entire infrastructure already exists, and grows each year, to support the use, implementation, conformance and competency based on the current and emerging software standards. Some contend that those fueling the standards development efforts are those positioning themselves to capitalize from their development. Others contend that standards development is necessary to enhance global trade and to bring harmonization and consistency to the software arena.

The Medical Device Industry has a goal of harmonization so that manufacturers can more easily sell worldwide. But this is not very easy when looking at the totality of software standards. The standards are not integrated, vary in detail, overlap and sometimes contradict. This lack of previous coordination of standards development efforts puts medical device manufacturers in a "difficult situation" because, as the adopters of these standards, they must themselves develop some mechanism to rationalize, explain, and relate the various standards chosen for implementation. Standards, and associated guidance, can be laborious to implement and turn into the standard operating procedures which are required in the regulated market.

Additionally, many software medical devices use cutting-edge technology. Technology that is rapidly changing. For instance, it took 30 years from initial concept until the radio was available to the average person. It took the web 4 years. Internet use is currently doubling every 100 days. Bandwidth is currently increasing 10 times faster than microprocessors, which are doubling every 18 months. The current and slow infrastructure that supports existing software standards development cannot keep pace with the rapidly changing technology. Yet the need to have consistent approaches to software development in order to reduce incompatibility problems is paramount to most medical device manufacturers. Because of this problem, some are inventing new ways to gain consensus for software technology standards, such as Object Management Group (OMG) which began a large standards making effort that included about 800 companies and which developed outside of the traditional standard making paths. After standards are developed, they have then requested that traditional standards making bodies accept their work efforts.

8.1   History

Following is a brief overview of the history of software standards, including Food and Drug Administration's (FDA) growing interest in standards:

- **1901** - The US National Bureau of Standards was formed. This was renamed the US National Institute of Standards and Technology (NIST) in 1988.
- **1966** – The NIST Computer Systems Laboratory (CSL) was formed to help resolve the problems associated with incompatible computer systems within the Federal

Government. The goal was to make computer system
procurement activities more uniform.

- **1974** – The US Navy began development of Mil-Std 1679,
  Weapons System Software Development.
- **1976** –The NIST Federal Information Processing Standards
  Publication (FIPS Pub.) *Guidelines for Documentation of
  Computer Programs and Automated Systems* was published.
  Ten documents were produced including: functional
  requirements, data requirements, system/subsystem
  specifications, program specifications, database
  specifications, user manual, operations manual, program
  maintenance manual, test plan, and test analysis report.
- **1976** – IEEE created the Software Engineering Standards
  Subcommittee (SESS).
- **1979** – IEEE Std. 730, Standard for a Quality Assurance Plan
  was approved for trial use.
- **1979** – FDA issued first notice of its intent to use consensus
  standards as part of the regulatory process.
- **1987** - International Organization for Standardization (ISO)
  and International Electrotechnical Committee (IEC) formed
  the a Joint Technical Committee 1 (JTC1) to address
  information technology (IT) and subcommittee 7 (SC7) was
  formed to focus on software engineering standards (ISO/IEC,
  JTC1/SC7).
- **1992** – Government Office of Management and Budget issued
  Circular A-119 encouraging government agencies to use the
  consensus process for procurement and such.
- **1995** - ISO/IEC, JTC1/SC7 finalized a standard for *Software
  Lifecycle Processes (ISO/IEC 12207)*.
- **1995** – Public law 104-113, the National Technology Transfer
  and Advancement Act codified and included paragraphs
  related to the use of standards by the agencies of the federal
  government for procurement, regulation, and other areas.
- **1996** – FDA outlined an intent to stretch the understanding of
  the use of standards by the adoption of consensus standards,
  particularly IEC 60601-1-4.
- **1997** – The Association for the Advancement of Medical
  Instrumentation (AAMI) began an effort to tailor *Software*

Lifecycle Processes (ISO/IEC 12207) for the software medical device community.

- **1998** – The FDA recognized the 1995 version of for *Software Lifecycle Processes (ISO/IEC 12207)* as its first and only consensus standard for software.

8.2   Major Standards Organizations

Standards making organizations can be classified as being international, national, professional in nature or sector specific. Some of the sector specific areas that have written software standards include: defense, financial, medical, nuclear, and transportation, etc. Some of the major software standards writing organizations that are often discussed include:

- AIAA – American Institute of Aeronautics and Astronauts
- ANS – American Nuclear Society
- ANSI – American National Standards Institute
- ASTM – American Society for Testing and Materials
- BSI – British Standards Institution
- CCITT – Telecommunication Standardization Bureau
- CEN - European Committee for Standardization
- CSA – Canadian Standards Association
- CSE – Communications Security Establishment
- DEF – British Defence Standards
- DIN - Drug Information Association
- DIN - Deutsches Institute für Normung e. Z.
- DoD – U.S. Department of Defense
- ISO – International Organization for Standardization
- IEC – International Electrotechnical Committee
- IEEE – Institute of Electronic and Electrical Engineers

8.3   The FDA's Interest in Standards

In an attempt to balance the need to ensure public safety in a time of shrinking resources, the FDA is now using standards in the regulatory review process. Some provisions of the FDA Modernization Act of 1997 allow manufacturers to submit a declaration of conformity to satisfy premarket review requirements. The FDA has issued a guidance on the recognition and use of consensus standards. This document describes how manufacturers may demonstrate substantial equivalence through special and abbreviated 510(k)s, in addition to traditional 510(k)s. Additionally, the FDA is interested in standards because they can help to serve as a common yardstick to assist with mutual recognition, based on the signed Mutual Recognition Agreement between the European Union and the United States. More than ever before, standards will have a more prominent role in the review of medical devices.

In the final legislation of the FDA Modernization Act of 1997, it is stated that the agency can withdraw recognition of a standard at any time if the standard changes in such a way that the FDA finds unacceptable.

8.4   ISO/IEC 12207 Information Technology - Software Life Cycle Process

In the 1980s it was determined that there was a need for an international process standard which could be a building block that would enhance trade and prevent artificial trade boundaries due to differences in national standards. Since software systems must sometimes be built with multinational participation, countries needed to agree on the key steps for developing software. The goal of this standard was for it to be an international framework that specified the best practices for software process. The development of this standard started in 1989. The standard was finalized and published in 1995. Seventeen countries played significant roles in developing this standard including Australia, Canada, France, Germany, Japan, the Netherlands, Spain, the United Kingdom, and the United States. The government agencies, industries and sectors providing active committee participation in this effort included the Army, Navy, Air Force, aeronautics, telecommunications, etc. Raghu Singh of the U.S. Department of Navy was the appointed project editor. James Roberts of Bellcore was the appointed U.S. convenor of the working group. Nancy George of SQM, Inc. represented the interests of the healthcare industry.

Because the goal of ISO/IEC 12207 was to make it the umbrella international standard for software life cycles, its impact could be significant to the healthcare industry, particularly the software medical device sector. But because of the large U.S. Department of Defense participation, there was a strong desire for this standard to be in line with the Department of Defense approaches to software development. These approaches differed fundamentally in some ways from those typically taken by software medical device manufacturers.

One difference was that the U.S. Department of Defense participants were currently relying on DoD Standards 2167A and Mil Standard 489 to define their software life cycle. Naturally, rather than changing directions, their desire was to keep ISO/IEC12207 in line with that standard. However, typically software medical device manufacturers do not use MIL Standard 498 as the basis for defining their software life cycle and their associated standard operating procedures (SOPs). Rather, they very often use IEEE standards as the basis for their software life cycle and standard operating procedures. MIL Standard 498 and IEEE Software Engineering Standards differ on two fundamental points: 1) the role of quality assurance in the process and 2) the role of validation and verification in the process. MIL Standard 498 defines the role of quality assurance as a supporting process that is basically called upon when needed. The IEEE Standards define quality assurance as an overriding process that is fully integrated in the development process. Similarly, MIL Standard 498 also defines validation and verification as being separate supporting processes that are also called upon when needed. The IEEE Standards define validation and verification as fully integrated into the development process, with a strong emphasis that there be an independent validation and verification function. For software medical device manufacturers, the 1987 Good Manufacturing Process Regulation defined quality assurance activities as fully integrated and independent. The concept of Preproduction Quality Assurance, which has fundamentally come to be known as Design Controls, was already out for discussion during the development of ISO/IEC12207. These concepts integrate validation and verification into the development life cycle.

Another fundamental difference was the concept of only using this proposed ISO/IEC international standard in two party contracts. Medical device manufactures are typically small development efforts where the manufacturer takes on both all of the development efforts and all of the responsibility for the product from cradle to grave. Rarely does one DOD company take product responsibility from cradle to grave. Additionally in the Department of Defense arena, the life cycle is very often segmented and contracted out. The DOD efforts are often very large projects that have a shelf life of up to about 25 years or longer. The shelf life of medical devices in not nearly that long. It was known at that time that despite the fact that ISO/IEC 9001 stated that it could only be used for two party contracts, a complete infrastructure was developing to certify companies to that standard. The concern was that if there were required certifications to ISO 12207, it could adversely impact the software medical device manufacturers. This was significant because if the FDA moved toward the approach of accepting certification to a standard without providing other options for compliance, or if the European Community added this requirement in order to sell in Europe as it had for ISO/IEC 9001, manufacturers could be in a difficult position. Because the Department of Defense was so well represented and there was such a small representation from the healthcare sector (one company) many positions that would be beneficial to the healthcare sector were overruled. However, one position was strongly lobbied for to protect the sector. In the end, the ISO/IEC committee in Geneva itself had to resolve the issue and ruled on the side of the free trade and the healthcare sector. The compromise was to include a clause in the Conformance section. This clause was so strongly lobbied for so that the healthcare sector, particularly the medical device sector, would not to be at the mercy of external certifications programs that might be imposed on them at great expense to manufacturers. The compromise clause states that "Any organization (for example, national, industrial association, company) imposing this International Standard, as a condition of trade, is responsible for specifying and making public the minimum set of required processes, activities, and tasks, which constitute suppliers' conformance with this International Standard" (ISO/IEC 12207 Section 1.4 - Conformance). This clause was also supported by Boeing. The clause is there because of the concern that the standard might be imposed on all products and that the software producer would not truly understand what was required because of the tailoring provision in the standard. This clause requires an organization to publicly define which software related tasks must be followed in order to be compliant to this standard.

8.5   The FDA Recognizes ISO/IEC 12207

ISO/IEC 12207 has been established as the FDA's baseline standard for software. It is the only standard currently on the FDA's list of recognized consensus standards for software. Additionally, the FDA has defined the inter-relationship between this standard and it's new software submission guidance, *Guidance for the Content of Premarket Submissions for Software Contained in Medical Devices* regarding what information companies must submit to the FDA. This means that manufacturers can claim conformance to this standard in lieu of submitting some of the defined documentation that should be forwarded to the FDA in a submission containing software.

Below will be found tables and lists that define:

- Table 8-1 Documentation in a Premarket Submission. The software documentation to be supplied to the FDA in a submission containing software. Table 8-2 FDA Recognition of ISO/IEC. The information that can be omitted if one states conformance to ISO/IEC 12207.

RECOGNITION LIST NUMBER: 002 EFFECTIVE DATE: August 14, 1998

Part B: SUPPLEMENTARY INFORMATION

Item: ISO/IEC 12207:1995 *Information technology - Software life cycle processes (Software)*

Address of Standards Organization:

International Organization for Standardization (ISO)*
International Electrotechnical Commission (IEC)*
1, rue de Varembe
Case Postale 56
CH 1211 Geneva 20
Switzerland

SOFTWARE DOCUMENTATION	MINOR CONCERN	MODERATE CONCERN	MAJOR CONCERN
Level of Concern	All levels of concern.		
Software Description	All levels of concern.		
Device Hazard Analysis	All levels of concern.		
Software Requirements Specification (SRS)	Software functional requirements from SRS.	SRS	
Architecture Design Chart	A chart depicting the partitioning of the software system into functional subsystems.	A chart depicting the partitioning of the software system into functional subsystems, listing of the functional modules and a description of how each fulfills the requirements.	
Design Specification	No documentation is necessary in the submission.	Software design specification document.	
Traceability Analysis	No documentation is necessary in the submission.	Traceability among requirements, identified hazards, and Verification and Validation testing.	

Table 8-1 Documentation for a Premarket Submission (From FDA, 1998.)

SOFTWARE DOCUMENTATION	MINOR CONCERN	MODERATE CONCERN	MAJOR CONCERN
Development	No documentation is necessary in the submission.	Summary of software life cycle development plan, including a summary of the configuration management and maintenance activities.	Summary of software life cycle development plan. Annotated list of control documents generated during the development process. Include the configuration management and maintenance plan documents.

Table 8-1 (continued)

SOFTWARE DOCUMENTATION	MINOR CONCERN	MODERATE CONCERN	MAJOR CONCERN
Validation, Verification, and Testing (VV&T)	Software functional test plan, pass/fail criteria, and results.	Description of VV&T activities at the unit, integration and system level. System level test protocol including pass/fail criteria, and tests results.	Description of VV&T activities at the unit, integration and system level. Unit, integration, and system level test protocols including pass/fail criteria, test report summary, and test results.
Revision Level History	No documentation is necessary in the submission.	Revision history log.	
Unresolved anomalies (bugs)	No documentation is necessary in the submission.	List of errors and bugs which remain in the device and an explanation how they were determined to not impact safety or effectiveness, including operator usage and human factors.	
Release Version Number	Version number and date for all levels of concern.		

Table 8-1 (continued)

CDRH Office(s) and Division(s) Associated with Recognized Standard:

Office of Device Evaluation
Office of Science and Technology

Devices Affected:
All medical devices containing software

Process(es) Impacted:
510(k), IDE, PMA, HDE

Type of Standard:
Horizontal, International

Extent of Recognition:
The following table defines the relationship between the standard ISO/IEC 12207 and the pre-market submission requirements for medical device software. The terms "SUBMIT" and "DON'T SUBMIT" are used to identify the applicability of the standard to individual pre-market submission requirements (as specified in "ODE Guidance for the Content of Premarket Submissions for Medical Devices Containing Software"). A "DON'T SUBMIT" indicates that compliance to ISO/IEC 12207 can be used in lieu of the specified submission requirement. A "SUBMIT" indicates that ISO/IEC 12207 cannot be substituted for the submission requirement. Whenever ISO/IEC 12207 is used, the medical device manufacturer must document all conformance declaration information in the pre-market submission. CDRH recognizes that no two medical devices are the same, and that it may be

appropriate for manufacturers to tailor a standard for their particular needs. However, if the standard is tailored, then the manufacturer is expected to submit a tailoring report in the pre-market submission. The tailoring report should identify specifically (section-by-section, and line-by- line if necessary) which parts of the standard have been modified or deleted. The tailoring report will be reviewed to establish that the manufacturer's application of the standard is adequate for the specific device under review. CDRH has the right to deny recognition to an improperly tailored standard.

Related CFR Citation(s) and Procode(s):
various

Relevant Guidance:
- ODE Guidance for the Content of Pre-market Submissions for Medical Devices Containing Software
- Guidance for Industry: General Principles of Software Validation (draft)
- Guidance for Off-the-Shelf Software Use in Medical Devices (draft)

FDA Technical Contact Person:
John F. Murray
FDA/CDRH/OST (HFZ-141)
12720 Twinbrook Parkway
Rockville, MD 20857
(301) 443-2536

- * In the United States, copies of this standard can be obtained from:

American National Standards Institute (ANSI)
11 West 42nd Street
New York, NY 10036.

- Table 8-3 Topics covered in ISO/IEC 12207. An overview of the topics in the ISO/IEC 12207 standard.
- List 8-1 Combining Tables 8-1, 8-2, and 8-3. Claiming conformance to ISO/IEC12207 in lieu of 510(k) documentation. The processes, activities and tasks that one must have in place if one states complete conformance to ISO/IEC 12207, as well as the remaining documentation that would need to be supplied to the FDA in a submission containing software. (From *Medical Software Weekly*, 1998)

8.6   Tailoring ISO/IEC 12207 for the Medical Device Business Sector

As mentioned before, ISO/IEC 12207 Section 1.4 (Conformance), states that "Any organization (for example, national, industrial associations or manufacturers} they have selected it as recognized consensus standards for software and therefore are allowing it as an option to manufacturers. However, based on the conformance clause above, ISO/IEC 12207 is being tailored (adapted for use) for the Medical Device Industry to define the minimum set of required processes, activities, and tasks, which constitute manufacturers' conformance with this Standard. The hope is that this Standard will provide a common framework and can be used by software practitioners. The Software Committee of the Association for the Advancement of Medical Instrumentation (AAMI) has taken on the task of drafting an adaptation of the 12207 standard for use in the medical device business sector.

This draft standard is [at the time of printing] still in development. The hope is that this standard can be used as the starting point for an International Standard on Medical Device Software to be developed through ISO and IEC. The Software Committee of the Association for the Advancement of Medical Instrumentation (AAMI) began its work in 1997. The co-chairs of this committee are John Murray, FDA and Sherman Eagles, (formerly Richard Fries) from Medtronic. The editor of the document is

(text continues on page 199)

Title: ISO/IEC 12207: 1995 Information technology - Software life cycle processes			
Software Documentation	Level of Concern		
	Minor	Moderate	Major
Software Description	SUBMIT	SUBMIT	SUBMIT
Device Hazard Analysis	SUBMIT	SUBMIT	SUBMIT
Software Requirements Specification	SUBMIT	SUBMIT	SUBMIT
Architectural Design	DON'T SUBMIT	DON'T SUBMIT	SUBMIT
Design Specification	DON'T SUBMIT	DON'T SUBMIT	SUBMIT
Traceability	DON'T SUBMIT	DON'T SUBMIT	SUBMIT
Development	DON'T SUBMIT	DON'T SUBMIT	DON'T SUBMIT
Validation, Verification and Testing (VV&T)	DON'T SUBMIT	DON'T SUBMIT	SUBMIT
Revision History	DON'T SUBMIT	DON'T SUBMIT	SUBMIT
Unresolved Anomalies	DON'T SUBMIT	DON'T SUBMIT	SUBMIT
Release Version Number	SUBMIT	SUBMIT	SUBMIT

Table 8-2   FDA Recognition of ISO/IEC 12207 (From FDA, 1998.)

Topics Covered	
Scope	Purpose
	Field of application
	Tailoring of this International Std
	Compliance
	Limitations
Normative references	
Definitions	
Application of this Int. Std.	Organization of this Int. Std.
	Life cycle processes
	Primary life cycle processes
	Supporting life cycle processes
	Organizational life cycle processes
	Tailoring process
	Relationship between the processes and organizations
Primary life cycle processes	Acquisition process
	Initiation
	Request-for-proposal preparation
	Contract preparation and update
	Supplier monitoring
	Acquisition and completion
Supply process	Initiation
	Preparation of response
	Contract
	Planning
	Execution and control
	Review and evaluation
	Delivery and completion
Development process	Process implementation
	System requirements analysis
	System architectural design
	Software requirements analysis
	Software architectural design
	Software detailed design

Table 8-3   Topics Covered in ISO/IEC 12207 (From Magee, 1988.)

Topics Covered	
Development process	Software coding and testing
	Software integration
	Software qualification testing
	System integration
	System qualification, installation, acceptance support
Operation process	Process implementation
	Operational testing
	System operation
	User support
Maintenance process	Process implementation
	Problem and modification analysis
	Modification implementation
	Maintenance review/acceptance
	Migration
	Software retirement
Supporting life cycle processes **Configuration management process**	Documentation process
	Process implementation
	Design and development
	Production
	Maintenance
	Process implementation
	Configuration identification
	Configuration control
	Configuration status accounting
	Configuration evaluation
	Release management and delivery

Table 8-3 (continued)

Topics Covered	
Quality assurance process	Process implementation
	Product assurance
	Process assurance
	Assurance of quality systems
	Verification process
	Process implementation
Verification	Contract verification
	Process verification
	Requirements verification
	Design verification
	Code verification
	Integration verification
	Documentation verification
Validation process	Process implementation
	Validation
Joint review process	Process implementation
	Project management reviews
	Technical reviews
Audit process	Process implementation
	Audit
	Problem resolution process
	Process implementation
	Problem resolution
Organizational life cycle processes	Management process
	Initiation and scope definition
	Planning
	Execution and control
	Review and evaluation
	Closure

Table 8-3 (continued)

Topics Covered	
Infrastructure process	Process implementation
	Establishment of infrastructure
	Maintenance of the infrastructure
	Improvement process
	Process establishment
	Process assessment
	Process improvement
Training process	Process implementation
	Training material development
	Training plan development
Tailoring process	Identifying project environment
	Soliciting inputs
	Selecting processes, activities, and tasks
	Documenting tailoring decisions and rationales
Guidance on tailoring	General tailoring guidance
Guidance on processes and organizations	Tailoring of the Development Process
	Tailoring of the evaluation-related activities
	Tailoring and application considerations
	Processes under key points of view
	Processes, organizations, and relationships
Bibliography	

Table 8-3 (continued)

Level of Concern
Minor, Moderate and Major Concern:
- Submit documentation to the FDA for all levels of concern

Software Description
Minor, Moderate and Major Concern:
- Submit documentation to the FDA for all levels of concern

Device Hazard Analysis
Minor, Moderate and Major Concern:
- Submit documentation to the FDA for all levels of concern

Software Requirements Specification (SRS)
Minor Concern:
- Submit documentation to the FDA detailing software functional requirements from SRS

Moderate and Major Concern:
- Submit documentation to the FDA detailing SRS

Architectural Design
Minor and Moderate Levels of Concern – In lieu of submitting documentation, state conformance to ISO/IEC 12207. The following concepts are listed in 12207 as being associated with "Architectural Design"
- Transform requirements into an architecture that describes top-level structure.
- Develop and document a top-level architecture of the system that identifies the elements and allocated requirements associated with them.
- Develop and document a top-level architecture of the software that identifies the major components and allocated requirements associated with them. Additionally, this shall be refined to facilitate detailed design.

List 8-1   Claiming Conformance to 12207 in Lieu of 510(k) Documentation. (From *Medical Software Weekly*, 1988.)

- Develop and document top-level design for software interfaces for both external and between components.
- Develop and document top-level design for software database.
- Develop and document top-level design for test requirements and software integration schedule.
- Review architectural design to evaluate system requirements
- Evaluate the architecture and requirements for traceability, consistency, appropriateness, and feasibility.
- Evaluate the architecture, interface, and database design for traceability, consistency, appropriateness, and feasibility.
- Perform technical reviews at the completion of the architectural design.

Major Level of Concern – Submit the following documentation:

- A chart depicting the partitioning of the software system into functional subsystems, listing of the functional modules and a description of how each fulfills the requirements.

Design Specification

Minor and Moderate Levels of Concern – In lieu of submitting documentation, state conformance to ISO/IEC 12207. The following concepts are listed in 12207 as being associated with "Design Specification"

- Develop and document design specification including functional capabilities of the system, safety, and security
- Develop and document detailed design for each software component
- Develop and document detailed design for internal and external software components

List 8-1 (continued)

- Develop and document detailed design for the database
- Evaluate feasibility of software design to appraise software requirements
- Evaluate the design based on traceability, consistency with architectural design and between components, design methods and standards, and operations and maintenance
- Evaluate the design based on test coverage, expected results, system integration and testing
- Establish a baseline for the design
- Verify design is correct, consistent and traceable to requirements
- Ensure that the design implements proper sequence of events
- Ensure selected design can be derived from the requirements
- Ensure design implements safety, security, and other critical requirements
- Ensure code can be derived from design
- Ensure critical code is traceable to design.

Major Level of Concern – Submit the following documentation:

- Software design specification document.

Traceability

Minor and Moderate Levels of Concern – In lieu of submitting documentation, state conformance to ISO/IEC 12207. The following concepts are listed in 12207 as being associated with "Traceability"

- Ensure backwards traceability from system requirements to the acquisition needs
- Ensure backwards traceability from system architecture, hardware and software requirements, and manual operations to the system requirements

List 8-1 (continued)

- Ensure backwards traceability from the software requirements to the system requirements and design
- Ensure backwards traceability from software architecture, interface and database design to the software requirements
- Ensure backwards traceability from software detailed design and test requirements to the software requirements
- Ensure backwards traceability from software code and test results to the software requirements and design
- Ensure critical code is traceable to design requirements
- Ensure backwards traceability from integration plan, design, code, tests, test results, and user's manuals to the system requirements
- Ensure traceability for each modification including reason and authorization
- Track problem reports.

Major Level of Concern – Submit the following documentation:

- Traceability among requirements, identified hazards, and Verification and Validation testing.

Development

Minor and Moderate Levels of Concern – In lieu of submitting documentation, state conformance to ISO/IEC 12207. The following concepts are listed in 12207 as being associated with "Development"

- Any life-cycle model is acceptable
- Develop plans for the development and qualification of all requirements
- Ensure development is conducted according to guidelines

List 8-1 (continued)

- [Perform the following] list of activities
  - Process implementation
  - System requirements analysis
  - System architectural design
  - Software requirements analysis
  - Software architectural design
  - Software detailed design
  - Software coding and testing
  - Software integration
  - Software qualification testing
  - System integration
  - System qualification testing
  - Software installation
  - Software acceptance support
  - Develop training material.

Major Level of Concern – Submit the following documentation:

- Summary of software life cycle development plan. Annotated list of control documents generated during development process. Include the configuration management and maintenance plan documents.

Validation, Verification and Testing (VV&T)

Minor and Moderate Levels of Concern – In lieu of submitting documentation, state conformance to ISO/IEC 12207. The following concepts are listed in 12207 as being associated with "Validation, Verification and Testing (VV&T)"

Verification

- Determine if the project warrants verification and if so, the degree of organizational independence necessary

List 8-1 (continued)

- Analyze the project requirements for criticality
- Determine if the project warrants verification and if so, implement a software verification process
- Determine if the project warrants independent verification and if so, select responsible organization
- Identify life-cycle activities and software products requiring verification based on criticality
- Define verification activities and tasks to be used for the life-cycle activities and software products
- Develop and document a verification plan including activities, products, resources, responsibilities, schedule, and procedures for forwarding reports to other organizations based on verification tasks
- Implement verification plan, resolve all problems and non-conformances, and provide results of verification activities to other organizations
- Evaluate contract verification based on supplier, requirements, procedures, and acceptance criteria
- Verify process by evaluating the project planning requirements, appropriateness, implementation, plan executed, compliance with contract, adequate standards, adequate procedures, adequate processes, and staff

List 8-1 (continued)

- Verify requirements by evaluating the system and software requirements for completeness, consistence, correctness, feasibility, and testable
- Verify requirements by evaluating the system requirements for appropriate allocation
- Verify requirements by evaluating the software requirements to ensure reflection of system requirements
- Verify requirements by evaluating the software requirements for safety, security, and criticality
- Verify design by evaluating correctness, and consistency and traceability to requirements
- Verify design by ensuring appropriateness
- Verify design by ensuring design can be derived from requirements
- Verify design by ensuring safety, security, and other critical requirements are implemented correctly
- Verify code by ensuring traceability to design and requirements, testability, correctness, and compliance to requirements and coding standards
- Verify code by ensuring appropriatness
- Verify code by ensuring code can be derived from requirements
- Verify code by ensuring safety, security, and other critical requirements are implemented correctly

List 8-1 (continued)

- Verify integration by ensuring all software components and units are completely and correctly incorporated into the software configuration items
- Verify integration by ensuring all system components are completely and correctly incorporated into the system
- Verify integration by ensuring all integration tasks have been performed according to plan
- Verify documentation for adequacy, completeness, and consistency
- Verify documentation is prepared in a timely manner
- Verify documentation follows configuration management procedures
- Coordinated effort with quality assurance
- Vary management control dependent on criticality.

Validation
- Validation is normally performed on the final product under defined operating conditions
- Multiple validations can be carried out if there are multiple intended uses
- Determine if the project warrants validation and if so, the degree of organizational independence necessary
- Verify code by ensuring code can be derived from requirements
- Determine if the project warrants independent validation and if so, select responsible organization

List 8-1 (continued)

- Develop a validation plan that includes items to be validated, tasks, resources, responsibilities, schedule, and procedures for forwarding reports
- Implement a validation plan, resolve all problems and non-conformances, and forward report
- Prepare validation requirements test cases, and test specifications for analyzing test results
- Ensure test requirements, test cases, and test specifications reflect requirements for intended use
- Conduct stress, boundary, and singular input tests
- Test software ability to minimize risk
- Validate that software meets specific criteria
- Validate that the software implements, safety, security, and other critical requirements appropriately
- Validate software in target environment
- Coordinated effort with quality assurance
- Vary management control dependent on criticality.

Testing

- Define and analyze testing standards and procedures
- Determine test cases, test data, test procedures and test environment
- Develop and document test procedures and data for each software unit and database
- Test each software unit to ensure it meets requirements and document results

List 8-1 (continued)

- Integrate test and document results
- Perform system qualification testing by testing each system requirement
- Test the software in its operational environment
- Test software in selected areas of target environment
- Conduct and document qualification testing - ensure all software requirements are tested for compliance
- Develop and document tests, test cases, and test procedures for conducting software qualification testing
- Conduct acceptance testing
- Perform operational testing for each software release
- Make testing reports available to acquirer
- Define and document test requirements and testing schedule
- Include stress testing in testing requirements
- Keep test requirements current
- Evaluate test requirements based on traceability, external and internal consistency, appropriateness, and feasibility
- Develop and document test procedures and data for each software unit and database
- Test each software unit to ensure it meets requirements and document results
- Evaluate test results based on traceability, external and internal consistency, test coverage, appropriateness, and feasibility

List 8-1 (continued)

- Evaluate tests and test results based on traceability, external and internal consistency, test coverage, appropriateness, and feasibility
- Evaluate software qualification tests and test results for test coverage, conformance, and feasibility
- Integrate test and document results
- Develop system qualification testing requirements for tests, test cases, and test procedures
- Evaluate integrated system based on test coverage, test methods, conformance, qualification testing and feasibility
- Ensure critical code is testable
- Prepare test requirements, test cases, test specifications for analyzing test results
- Ensure test requirements, test cases, and test specification match requirements for the specific intended use
- Test software for its ability to reduce risk
- Ensure software successfully tested to meet specifications
- Ensure test data meets specifications
- Vary management control dependent on criticality.

Major Level of Concern – Submit the following documentation:

- Description of VV&T activities at the unit, integration and system level. Unit, integration and system level test protocols including pass/fail criteria, test report, summary, and test results.

List 8-1 (continued)

Revision History
Minor and Moderate Levels of Concern – In lieu of
submitting documentation, state conformance to
ISO/IEC 12207. The following concepts are listed in
12207 as being associated with "Revision History"
- Maintain management records and status reports
  including the status and history with baseline of
  controlled items
- Collect historical, technical and evaluation data
  to analyze the quality of the process.

Major Level of Concern – Submit the following
documentation:
  - Revision History Log.

Unresolved Anomalies
Minor and Moderate Levels of Concern – In lieu of
submitting documentation, state conformance to
ISO/IEC 12207. The following concepts are listed in
12207 as being associated with "Unresolved
Anomalies"
- Document problems using the
  problem/modification request
- Record and enter all problems into the problem
  resolution process
- Analyze all problem reports
- Where possible eliminate all detected problems
- All problems must be replicated or verified
- Problem resolution process is a closed loop
  process
- All problems and non-conformances shall be
  resolved
- Document all problems and their resolutions.

Major Level of Concern – Submit the following
documentation:
  - List of errors and bugs which remain in
    the device and an explanation [of] how
    they were determined to not impact
    safety or effectiveness, including
    operator usage and human factors.

List 8-1 (continued)

Release Version Number
Minor, Moderate and Major concern:
- Version number and date for all levels of concern.

Additionally, ISO/IEC 12207 lists six standards as normative references. In order to state conformance to ISO/IEC 12207, an organization must also conform to the normative references listed below:

ISO/IEC/AFNOR: Dictionary of Computer Science

ISO/IEC 8402: Quality Management and Quality Assurance; Vocabulary

ISO/IEC 2382/1: Data Processing – Vocabulary – Section 01: Fundamental terms

ISO/IEC 2382-20: Information Technology – Vocabulary; Part 20: System Development

ISO/IEC 9126: Information Technology – Software Product Evaluation – Quality Characteristics and Guidelines for their Use

ISO/IEC 9001: Quality Systems – Models for Quality Assurance in Design/Development, Production, Installation and Servicing

List 8-1(continued)

Sherman Eagles. The Secretary of this committee is Nancy George, SQM, Inc. There is an Executive Board for this committee that includes: John Murray, FDA; Sherman Eagles, Medtronic; Ed Antonio, Shared Medical Systems; Bryan Fitzgerald, Underwriter's Laboratory ; Richard Fries, Datex-Ohmeda; Nancy George, SQM, Inc., Alan Kusinitz, Expertech Associates; Bernie Liebler, HIMA; Donna-Bea Tillman, FDA; and Nick Tongson, AAMI. The goal of this Executive Board was to generate the first draft, which is to be submitted for review in the first quarter, 1999, as well as to drive the effort to successful completion.

8.7   Summary

Standards, both international and national, are increasing in use as the manufacturers develop and sell in the global economy. We have moved from the need to standardize the time zones so that railway time schedules could to developed to standardizing the necessary information needed to develop, buy or sell software products without trade barriers.

References

FDA, Appendix A, *FDA Recognized Consensus Standards*. October, 1998.

FDA, *Guidance for the Content of Premarket Submissions for Software Contained in Medical Devices*. May, 1998.

FDA, *Guidance for Industry: General Principles of Software Validation*, (draft). June 1997.

FDA, *Guidance for Off-the-Shelf Software Use in Medical Devices*, (draft). August, 1998.

Instrumentation & Technology. Volume 32, Number 5, September/October, 1998.

Magee, Stan and Leondard Tripp, *Guide to Software Engineering Standards and Specifications*. Boston, Massachusetts, Artech House, 1997.

Magee, Stan, "ISO/IEC Software Life Cycle Standard 12207," *Datapro Management of Applications Software*. February, 1995.

Moore, James W., *Software Engineering Standards: A User's Road Map*. Los Alamitos, California: IEEE Computer Society, 1998.

Rechen, E. and D. Barth and D. Marlowe and L. Kroger, "FDA Use of International Standards in the Premarket Review Process," *Biomedical* SQM, Inc., "Claiming Conformance to 12207 in lieu of 510(k) Documentation," *Medical Software Weekly*, Volume 2, Issue 35. August, 1998.

Section 2

Determining and Documenting Requirements

Chapter 9

Defining the Device

Richard C. Fries, PE, CRE – Datex-Ohmeda, Inc.
Madison, Wisconsin

New product ideas are not simply born. New product ideas come from examining the needs of hospitals, nurses, respiratory therapists, physicians and other medical professionals, as well as from sales and marketing personnel. It is also important to talk with physicians and nurses and determine what their problems are and how they can be addressed. These problems generally represent product opportunities. A successful new product demands that it meet the end user's needs. It must have the features and provide the benefits the customer expects.

The multiphased process of defining a product involves the customer, the company, potential vendors, and current technologies (Figure 9-1). The result is a clear definition of what the product is, and is expected to do, included in a Business Proposal. The first inputs to the process are the needs of the customer and the needs of the company.

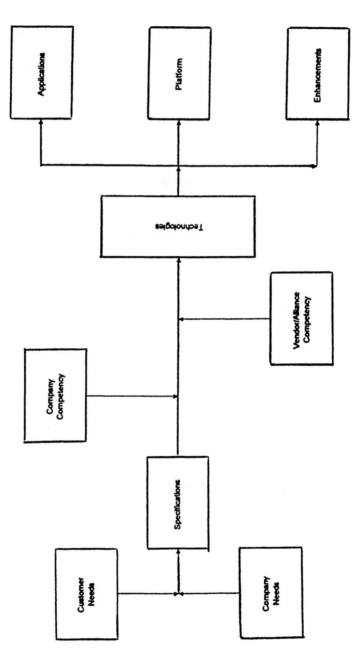

Figure 9-1   The product definition process. (From Fries, 1997.)

The customer's needs and expectations are the primary source of information when defining a device. If the new product does not meet the customer's needs or expectations, there is no market for the device. In addition, the needs of the company are important in defining the device. Issues such as market need, product niche, etc., must be considered in the definition process.

The company's competencies must be taken into consideration. What are they, how do they match the customer's and company's needs, what is required outside of the company's competencies, and is it easily available? In addition, the competencies of potential vendors or other companies in alliance or partnership with the original company must be considered.

Once a rough idea of the potential device is taking shape, the next consideration is technologies. What technologies are appropriate for the proposed device, how available are they, are they within the company's competency, are resources readily available?

Finally, the type of proposed device must be decided. Is it a new application for older devices, is it a new platform, or is it an enhancement to an older device?

Establishing answers in these areas leads to the definition of a device which leads to the development of a product specification. Let's look at each area in more detail.

9.1   The Product Definition Process

Numerous methods of obtaining new product information exist. They include various ways of collecting data, such as internal sources, industry analysis, and technology analysis. Then the information is screened and a business analysis is conducted. Regardless of the method of obtaining the information, there are certain key questions:

Where are we in the market now?
Where do we want to go?
How big is the potential market?
What does the customer really want?

How feasible is technical development?
How do we get where we want to go?
What are the chances of success?

9.1.1   Surveying the Customer

The customer survey is an important tool in changing an idea into a product. The criticality of the survey is exhibited by an estimate that, on the average, it takes 58 initial ideas to get one commercially successful new product to market. It is therefore necessary to talk with various leaders in potential markets to build a credible database of product ideas.

The goal of the customer survey is to match the needs of the customer with the product concept. Quality has been defined as meeting the customer needs. So a quality product is one that does what the customer wants it to do. The objective of consumer analysis is to identify segments or groups within a population with similar needs so that marketing efforts can be directly targeted to them. Several important questions must be asked to find that market which will unlock untold marketing riches:

What is the *need* category?
Who is buying and who is using the product?
What is the *buying* process?
Is what I'm selling a high- or low-involvement product?
How can the market be segmented?

9.1.2   Defining the Company's Needs

While segmentation analysis focuses on consumers as individuals, market analysis takes a broader view of potential consumers to include market sizes and trends. Market analysis also includes a review of the competitive and regulatory environment. Three questions are important in evaluating a market:

What is the *relevant* market?
Where is the product in its product life cycle?
What are the key *competitive* factors in the industry?

9.1.3 What Are the Company's Competencies?

Once a market segment has been chosen, a plan to beat the competition must be chosen. To accomplish this, a company must look at itself with the same level of objectivity it looks at its competitors. Important questions to assist in this analysis include:

> What are our core competencies?
> What are our weaknesses?
> How can we capitalize on our strengths?
> How can we exploit the weaknesses of our competitors?
> Who are we in the marketplace?
> How does my product map against the competition?

9.1.4 What Are the Outside Competencies?

Once a company has objectively looked at itself, it must then look at others in the marketplace:

> What are the strengths of the competition?
> What are their weaknesses?
> What are the resources of the competition?
> What are the market shares of the industry players?

9.1.5 Completing the Product Definition

There are many other questions that need to be answered in order to complete the product definition. In addition to those mentioned above, an organization needs to determine:

> How does the potential product fit with our other products?
> Do our current technologies match the potential product?
> How will we differentiate the new product?
> How does the product life cycle affect our plans?

It is also important to consider the marketing mix of products, distribution networks, pricing structure, and the overall economics of the product plan. These are all important pieces of the overall product plan as developed in a Business Proposal. However, the needs and wants of the customer remain the most important information to be collected. One method of obtaining the required customer requirements is Quality Function Deployment.

9.2   Overview of Quality Function Deployment

Quality Function Deployment (QFD) is a process in which the "voice of the customer" is first heard and then deployed through an orderly, four-phase process in which a product is planned, designed, made and then made consistently. It is a well-defined process which begins with customer requirements and keeps them evident throughout the four phases. The process is analytical enough to provide a means of prioritizing design trade-offs, to track product features against competitive products, and to select the best manufacturing process to optimize product features. Moreover, once in production, the process affords a means of working backwards to determine what a prospective change in the manufacturing process or in the product's components may do to the overall product attributes.

The fundamental insight of QFD from an engineering perspective is that customer wants and technical solutions do not exist in a one-to-one correspondence. Though this sounds simplistic, the implications are profound. It means that product "features" are not what customers want; instead, they want the "benefits" provided by those features. To make this distinction clear, QFD explicitly distinguishes between customer attributes that the product may have and technical characteristics which may provide some of the attributes the customer is looking for. Taking a pacemaker as an example, the customer attribute might be that the patient wants to extend their life, while the technical characteristic is that the pacemaker reduces arrhythmia's.

9.3   The QFD Process

The QFD process begins with the wants of the customer, since meeting these is essential to the success of the product. Product features should not be defined by what the developers think their customers want. For clear product definition that will lead to market acceptance, manufacturers must spend both time and money learning about their customer's environments, their constraints, and the obstacles they face in using the product. By fully understanding these influencers, a manufacturer can develop products that are not obvious to its customers or competitors at the outset, but will have high customer appeal.

Quality Function Deployment should be viewed from a very global perspective as a methodology that will link a company with its customers and assist the organization in its planning processes. Often, an organization's introduction to QFD takes the form of building matrices. A common result is that building the matrix becomes the main objective of the process. The purpose of QFD is to get in touch with the customer and use this knowledge to develop products which satisfy the customer, not to build matrices.

QFD uses a matrix format to capture a number of issues pertinent and vital to the planning process. The matrix represents these issues in an outline form which permits the organization to examine the information in a multidimensional manner. This encourages effective decisions based on a team's examination and integration of the pertinent data.

The QFD matrix has two principal parts. The horizontal portion of the matrix contains information relative to the customer (Figure 9-2). The vertical portion of the matrix contains technical information that responds to the customer inputs (Figure 9-3).

9.3.1   The Voice of the Customer

The voice of the customer is the basic input required to begin a QFD project. The customer's importance rating is a measure of the relative importance that customers assign to each of the voices. The customer's competitive evaluation of the company's products or services permits a company to observe how its customers rate its products or services on a numerical scale. Any complaints that customers have personally registered with the company serve as an indication of dissatisfaction.

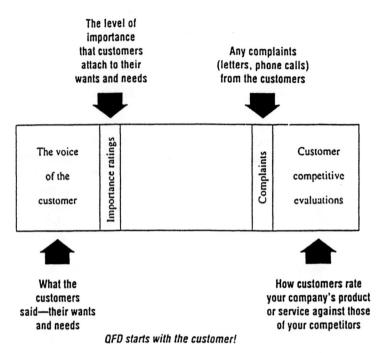

Figure 9-2   The customer information portion of the matrix.
(From Fries, 1997.)

9.3.2   The Technical Portion of the Matrix

The first step in developing the technical portion of the matrix is to determine how the company will respond to each voice. The technical or design requirements that the company will use to describe and measure each customer's voice are placed across the top of the matrix. For example, if the voice of the customer stated "want the control to be easy to operate," the technical requirement might be "operating effort." The technical requirements represent how the company will respond to its customers' wants and needs.

The center of the matrix, where the customer and technical portion intersect, provides an opportunity to record the presence and strength of relationships between these inputs and action items. Symbols may be used to indicate the strength of these relationships. The information in the matrix can

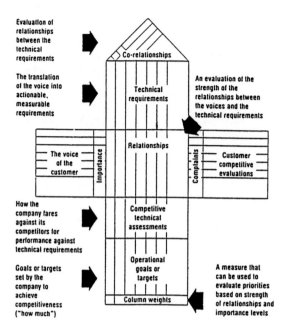

Figure 9-3   The technical portion of the matrix.. (From Fries, 1997.)

be examined and weighed by the appropriate team. Goals or targets can be established for each technical requirement.

Tradeoffs can be examined and recorded in the triangular matrix at the top of Figure 9-3. This is accomplished by comparing each technical requirement against the other technical requirements. Each relationship is examined to determine the net result that changing one requirement has on the others.

9.3.3   Overview of the QFD Process

The Quality Function Deployment process is a 9-step process consisting of:

- determining the voice of the customer

- customer surveys for importance ratings and competitive evaluation
- developing the customer portion of the matrix
- developing the technical portion of the matrix
- analyzing the matrix and choosing priority items
- comparing proposed design concepts and synthesizing the best
- developing a part planning matrix for priority design requirements
- developing a process planning matrix for priority process requirements
- developing a manufacturing planning chart.

In planning a new project or revisions to an old one, organizations need to be in touch with the people who buy and use their products and services. This is vital for hard issues, such as a product whose sales are dependent on the customers' evaluation of how well their needs and wants are satisfied. It is equally crucial for softer issues, such as site selection and business planning.

Once the customers' wants and needs are known, the organization can obtain other pertinent customer information. Through surveys, it can establish how its customers feel about the relative importance of the various wants and needs. It can also sample a number of customers who use its products and competitors' products. This provides the customers evaluation of both the organization's performance and that of its chief competitors.

Records can be examined to determine the presence of any customer complaint issues. This can be the result of letters of complaint, phone complaints, reports to the FDA, or other inquiries and comments.

Once this information is available, it can be organized and placed in the horizontal customer information portion of the QFD matrix. The voices of the customers represent their wants and needs: their requirements. These are the inputs to the matrix, along with importance ratings, competitive evaluations, and complaints.

The appropriate team can then begin developing the technical information portion of the matrix. The customers' voices must be translated into items that are measurable and actionable within the organization. Companies use a variety of names to describe these measurable items, such as design requirements, technical requirements, product characteristics, and product criteria.

The relationship between the inputs and the actionable items can then be examined. Each technical requirement is analyzed to determine if action on the item will affect the customer's requirements. A typical question may be: "Would the organization work on this technical requirement to respond favorably to the customers' requirements?"

For those items in which a relationship is determined to exist, the team then must decide on the strength of the relationship. Symbols are normally used to denote a strong, moderate, or weak relationship. Some of the symbols commonly used are a double circle, single circle, and a triangle, respectively. The symbols provide a quick visual impression of the overall relationship strengths of the technical requirements and the customers' wants and needs.

The team must instigate testing to develop technical data showing the performance of the parent company and its competitors for each of the technical requirements. Once this information is available, the team can begin a study to determine the target value that should be established for each technical requirement. The objective is to ensure that the next-generation product will be truly competitive and satisfy its customers' wants and needs. A comparison of the customers' competitive ranges and the competitive technical assessments helps the organization determine these targets.

Additional information can be added to the matrix depending on the team's judgement of value. Significant internal and regulatory requirements may be added. Measure of organizational difficulty can be added. Column weights can be calculated. These can serve as an index for highlighting those technical requirements that have the largest relative effect on the product.

Once this matrix is complete, the analysis stage begins. The chief focus should be on the customer portion of the matrix. It should be examined to determine which customer requirements need the most attention. This is an integrated decision involving the customers' competitive evaluation, their importance ratings, and their complaint histories. The number of priority items selected will be a balance between their importance and the resources available within the company.

Items selected for action can be treated as a special project or can be handled by use of the QFD matrix at the next level of detail. Any items so selected can become the input to the new matrix. Whereas the first matrix was a planning matrix for the complete product, this new matrix is at a lower level. It concerns the subsystem or assembly that affects the requirement.

The challenge in the second-level matrix (Figure 9-4) is to determine the concept that best satisfies the deployed requirement. This requires evaluation of some design concept alternatives. Several techniques are available for this type of comparative review. The criteria or requirements for the product or service are listed at the left of the matrix. Concept alternatives are listed across the top. The results of the evaluation of each concept versus the criteria can be entered in the center portion.

Once the best concept alternative is selected, a QFD part planning matrix can be generated for the component level (Figure 9-5). The development of this matrix follows the same sequence as that of the prior matrix. Generally, less competitive information is available at this level and the matrix is simpler. The technical requirements from the prior matrix are the inputs. Each component in the selected design concept is examined to determine its critical part requirements. These are listed in the upper portion. Relationships are examined and symbols are entered in the center portion. The specifications are then entered for these selected critical part requirements in the lower portion of the matrix.

The part planning matrix should then be examined. Experience with similar parts and assemblies should be a major factor in this review. The analysis should involve the issue of which of the critical part requirements listed are the most difficult to control or ensure continually. This review will likely lead to the selection of certain critical part requirements that the team believes deserve specific follow-up attention.

If a team believes the selected critical part characteristics are best handled through the QFD process, a matrix should be developed (Figure 9-6)

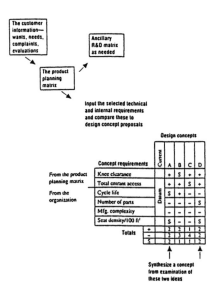

Figure 9-4   Second level matrix. (From Fries, 1997.)

for process planning. The critical part concerns from the Part Planning matrix
should be used as inputs in the left area of the matrix. The critical process
requirements are listed across the top. Relationships are developed and
examined in the central area. The specification for operating levels for each
process requirement are recorded in the lower area of the matrix. For example,
if a critical part requirement was spot-weld strength, one critical process
parameter would be weld current. The amount of current would be a
critical process parameter to ensure proper spot weld strength. The
specification for this critical process requirement would be the amperes of
current required to ensure the weld strength.

Upon completion of the planning at the part and process levels, the
key concerns should be deployed to the manufacturing level. Most
organizations have detailed planning at this level and have developed
spreadsheets and forms for recording their planning decisions. The
determinations from the prior matrices should become inputs to these
documents. Often, the primary document at this level is a basic planning chart
(Figure 9-7). Items of concern are entered in the area farthest left. The risk

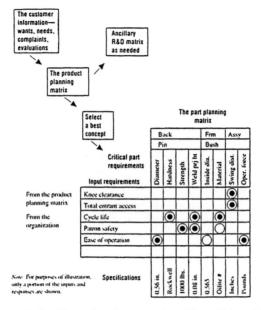

Figure 9-5   Part planning matrix. (From Fries, 1997.)

associated with these items is assessed and recorded in the next column. In typical risk assessments, the level of the concern and the probability of its occurrence are listed, as are the severity of any developing problems and the probability of detection. These items, along with other concerns, can be used to develop an index to highlight items of significant concern. Other areas in the chart can be use to indicate issues such as the general types of controls, frequency of checking, measuring devices, responsibility, and timing.

9.4   Summary of QFD

The input to the QFD Planning Matrix is the voice of the customer. The matrix cannot be started until the customers' requirements are known This applies to internal planning projects as well as products and services that will be sold to marketplace customers. Use of the QFD process leads an organization to develop a vital customer focus.

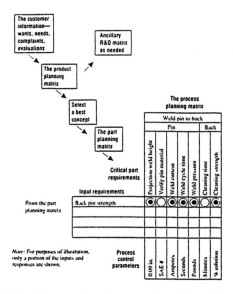

Figure 9-6   Process planning matrix. (From Day, 1993.)

The initial matrix is usually the planning matrix. The customers'
requirements are inputs. Subsequent matrices may be used to deploy or flow
down selected requirements from the product planning matrix for part planning
and process planning. Some forms of a manufacturing chart or matrix can be
used to enter critical product and process requirements from prior matrices.

The principal objective of the QFD process is to help a company
organize and analyze all the pertinent information associated with a project and
to use the process to help it select the items demanding priority attention. All
companies do many things right. The QFD process will help them focus on the
areas that need special attention.

9.5   The Business Proposal

The purpose of the Business Proposal is to identify and document
market needs, market potential, the proposed product and product alternatives,
risks and unknowns, and potential financial benefits. The Business Proposal

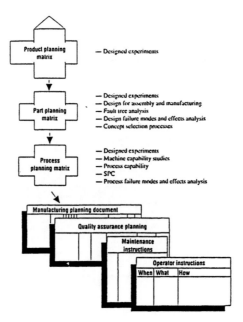

Figure 9-7   Manufacturing planning chart. (From Day, 1993.)

also contains a proposal for further research into risks and unknowns, estimated project costs, schedule, and a request to form a core team to carry out needed research, to define the product and to prepare the project plan.

The Business Proposal usually contains:

- Project Overview, Objectives, Major Milestones, Schedule
- Market Need and Market Potential
- Product Proposal
- Strategic Fit
- Risk Analysis and Research Plan
- Economic Analysis
- Recommendation to Form a Core Project Team
- Supporting Documentation.

9.5.1 Project Overview, Objectives, Major Milestones, and Schedule

This portion of the Business Proposal contains a statement of overall project objectives and major milestones to be achieved. The objectives clearly define the project scope and provide specific direction to the project team.

The Major Milestones and Schedule follows the statement of objectives. The schedule anticipates key decision points and completion of the primary deliverables throughout all phases of development and implementation. The schedule contains target completion dates, however, it must be stressed that these dates are tentative and carry an element of risk. Events contingent upon achievement of the estimated dates should be clearly stated. Examples of milestones include:

- design feasibility
- patent search completed
- product specification verified by customers
- design concept verified through completion of sub-system functional model completed
- process validation completed
- regulatory approval obtained
- successful launch into Territory A
- project assessment complete, project transferred to manufacturing and sustaining engineering.

9.5.2 Market Need and Market Potential

This section of the Business Proposal defines the customer and clinical need for the product or service and, identifies the potential territories to be served. Specific issues which are to be addressed include, but should not be limited, to the following:

- What is the market need for this product, i.e., what is the problem to be solved?
- What clinical value will be delivered?
- What incremental clinical value will be added over existing company or competitive offerings?
- What trends are occurring that predict this need?

- In which markets are these trends occurring?
- What markets are being considered, what is the size of the market and what are the competitive shares?
- What is the market size and the estimated growth rate for each territory to be served?
- What are the typical selling prices and margins for similar products?
- When must the product be launched to capture the market opportunity?
- If competitors plan to launch similar products, what is our assessment of their launch date?
- Have competitors announced a launch date?
- What other similar products compose the market?
- Will the same product fit in all markets served? If not, what are the anticipated gross differences and why? What modifications will be required?
- Is the target market broad-based and multifaceted or a focused niche?
- What are the regulatory requirements, standards and local practices which may impact the product design for every market to be served?

9.5.3   Product Proposal

The Product Proposal section proposes the product idea that fulfills the market need sufficiently well to differentiate its features and explain how user and/or clinical value will be derived. The product specification is not written nor does design commence during this phase. It may be necessary to perform some initial feasibility studies, construct non-working models, perform simulations and conduct research in order to have a reasonable assurance that the product can be designed, manufactured, and serviced. Additionally, models, simulations, and product descriptions will be useful to verify the idea with customers. It is also recommended that several alternative product ideas be evaluated against the "base case" idea. Such evaluation will compare risks, development timelines, costs and success probabilities.

9.5.4   Strategic Fit

This section discusses how the proposed product conforms with (or departs from) stated strategy with respect to product, market, clinical setting, technology, design, manufacturing and service.

9.5.5   Risk Analysis and Research Plan

This section contains an assessment of risks and unknowns, an estimate of the resources needed to reduce the risks to a level whereby the product can be designed, manufactured, and serviced with a reasonable high level of confidence. The personnel resource requirement should be accompanied by the plan and timetable for addressing, researching and reducing the risks.

The following categories of risks and unknowns should be addressed. Not all of these categories apply for every project. Select those which could have a significant impact on achieving project objectives.

- Technical
  Feasibility (proven, unknown, or unfamiliar?)
  New technology
  Design
  Manufacturing process
  Accessibility to technologies
  Congruence with core competencies
  Manufacturing process capability
  Cost constraints
  Component and system reliability
  Interface compatibility

- Market
  Perception of need in market place
  Window of opportunity; competitive race
  Pricing
  Competitive positioning and reaction

Cannibalization of existing products
Customer acceptance

- Financial
    Margins
    Cost to develop
    Investment required

- Regulatory
    Filings and approvals (IDE, PMA, 510k,
    CE, TUV, etc.)
    Compliance with international standards
    Clinical studies; clinical trials
    Clinical utility and factors, unknowns

- Intellectual property
    Patents
    Licensing agreements
    Software copyrights

- Requisite skill sets available to design and
  develop
    Electrical
    Mechanical
    Software
    Industrial Design
    Reliability

- Manpower availability

- Vendor selection
    Quality system
    Documentation controls
    Process capability
    Component reliability
    Business stability

- Schedule
    Critical path
    Early or fixed completion date
    Resource availability

- Budget.

9.5.6   Economic Analysis

This section includes a rough estimate of the costs and personnel required to specify, design, develop, and launch each product variant into the market place.

9.5.7   Core Project Team

This section discusses the formation of a core project team to perform the research required to reduce risks and unknowns to a manageable level, to develop and verify the User Specification. and to prepare the project plan

The requisite skills of the proposed team members should also be outlined. To the extent possible, the following functions should be involved in research, preparation of the User Specification, and the preparation of the project plan.

- Marketing
- Engineering
- Manufacturing
- Service
- Regulatory
- Quality Assurance
- Finance.

The approximate amount of time required of each participant as well as incremental expenses should also be estimated. Some examples of incremental expenses include: model development, simulation software, travel for customer verification activities, laboratory supplies, market research, and project status reviews.

References

Brodie, Christina Hepner and Gary Burchill, *Voices Into Choices – Acting on the Voice of the Customer*. Madison: Joiner Associates, Inc., 1997.

Day, Ronald G., *Quality Function Deployment - Linking a Company with Its Customers*. Milwaukee, WI: ASQC Quality Press, 1993.

Fries, Richard C., *Reliable Design of Medical Devices*. New York: Marcel Dekker, Inc., 1997.

Gause, Donald C. and Gerald M. Weinberg, *Exploring Requirements: Quality Before Design*. New York: Dorset House Publishing, 1989.

Guinta, Lawrence R. and Nancy C. Praizler, *The QFD Bool: The Team Approach to Solving Problems and Satisfying Customers Through Quality Function Deployment*. New York: AMACOM Books, 1993.

Kriewall, Timothy J. and Gregory P. Widin, "An Application of Quality Function Deployment to Medical Device Development," in *Case Studies in Medical Instrument Design*. New York: The Institute of Electrical and Electronics Engineers, Inc., 1991.

Potts, Colin, Kenji Takahashi, and Annie I. Anton, "Inquiry-Based Requirements Analysis," in *IEEE Software*, Volume 11, Number 2, March, 1994.

Silbiger, Steven, *The Ten Day MBA*. New York: William Morrow and Company, Inc., 1993.

Taylor, J. W. *Planning Profitable New Product Strategies*. Radnor, PA: Chilton Book Company, 1984.

Chapter 10

Documenting Product Requirements

Richard C. Fries, PE, CRE – Datex-Ohmeda, Inc.
Madison, Wisconsin

A widely shared piece of conventional wisdom states that requirements constitute a complete statement of what the system will do without referring to how it will do it. The resiliency of this view is indeed surprising since researchers have long argued against this simple distinction.

Clearly, requirements and design are interdependent, as practitioners surely realize. Perhaps the continuing prevalence of the "what vs how" distinction is due to the well meaning desire on the part of requirements engineers to avoid over-constraining implementers.

10.1   Requirements, Design, Verification, and Validation

As medical products encompass more features and technology, they will grow in complexity and sophistication. The hardware and software for these products will be driven by necessity to become highly synergistic and intricate which will in turn dictate tightly coupled designs. The dilemma is whether to tolerate longer development schedules in order to achieve the features and technology, or to pursue shorter development schedules. There really is no choice given the competitive situation of the marketplace. Fortunately, there are several possible solutions to this difficulty. One solution that viably achieves shorter development schedules is a reduction of the quantity of requirements that represent the desired feature set to be implemented. By documenting requirements in a simpler way, the development effort can be reduced by lowering the overall product development complexity. This would reduce the overall hardware and software requirements which in turn reduces the overall verification and validation time.

The issue is how to reduce the number of documented requirements without sacrificing feature descriptions. This can be achieved by limiting the number of product requirements, being more judicious about how the specified requirements are defined, or by recognizing that some requirements are really design specifications. A large part of requirements definition should be geared toward providing a means to delay making decisions about product feature requirements that are not understood until further investigation is carried out.

As stated above, verification and validation must test the product to assure that the requirements have been met and that the specified design has been implemented. At worst, every requirement will necessitate at least one test to demonstrate that it has been satisfied. At best, several requirements might be grouped such that at least one test will be required to demonstrate that they all have been satisfied. The goal for the design engineer is to specify the requirements in such a manner as to achieve as few requirements as are absolutely necessary and still allow the desired feature set to be implemented. Several methods for achieving this goal are refinement of requirements, assimilation of requirements and requirements versus design.

10.1.1   Refinement of Requirements

As an example, suppose a mythical device has the requirement "the output of the analog to digital converter (ADC) must be accurate to within plus or minus 5%." Although conceptually this appears to be a straight forward requirement, to the software engineer performing the testing to demonstrate satisfaction of this requirement, it is not as simple as it looks. As stated, this requirement will necessitate at least three independent tests and most likely five tests. One test will have to establish that the ADC is outputting the specified nominal value. The second and third tests will be needed to confirm that the output is within the plus or minus 5% range. Being a good software engineer, the 5% limit is not as arbitrary as it may seem due to the round off error of the percent calculation with the ADC output units. Consequently, the fourth and fifth test will be made to ascertain the sensitivity of the round off calculation.

A better way to specify this requirement is to state "the output of the analog to digital converter (ADC) must be between X and Y," where X and Y values correspond to the original requirement of "plus or minus 5%." This is a better requirement statement because it simplifies the testing that occurs. In this case, only two tests are required to demonstrate satisfaction of this requirement. Test one is for the X value and test two is for the Y value. The requirement statements are equivalent but the latter is more effective because it has reduced the test set size, resulting in less testing time and consequently a potential for the product to reach the market earlier.

10.1.2   Assimilation of Requirements

Consider the situation where several requirements can be condensed into a single equivalent requirement. In this instance, the total test set can be reduced through careful analysis and an insightful design. Suppose that the user interface of a product is required to display several fields of information that indicate various parameters, states and values. It is also required that the user be able to interactively edit the fields, and that key system critical fields must flash or blink so that the user knows that a system critical field is being edited. Further assume that the software requirements document specifies that "all displayed fields can be edited. The rate field shall flash while being edited. The exposure time shall flash while being edited. The volume delivered field shall flash while being edited."

These statements are viable and suitable for the requirements specification but they may not be optimum from an implementation and test point of view. There are three possible implementation strategies for these requirements. First, a "monolithic" editor routine can be designed and implemented that handles all aspects of the field editing, including the flash function. Second, a generic field editor can be designed which is passed a parameter that indicates whether or not the field should flash during field editing. Third, an editor executive could be designed such that it selects either a non-flashing or flashing field editor routine depending on whether the field was critical or not. Conceptually, based on these requirements statements, the validation team would ensure that 1) only the correct fields can be displayed, 2) the displayed fields can be edited, 3) critical fields blink when edited, and 4) each explicitly named field blinks.

The first "monolithic" design option potentially presents the severest test case load and should be avoided. Since it is monolithic in structure and performs all editing functions, all validation tests must be performed within a single routine in order to determine whether the requirements are met. The validation testing would consist of the four test scenarios presented above.

The second design option represents an improvement over the first design. Because the flash/no flash flag is passed as a parameter into the routine, the testing internally to the routine is reduced because part of the testing burden has been shifted to the interface between the calling and called routines. This is easier to test because the flash/no flash discrimination is made at a higher level. It is an inherent part of the calling sequence of the routine and therefore can be visually verified without formal tests. The validation testing would consist of test situations 1, 2, and 4 as presented above.

The third design option represents the optimum from a test stand point because the majority of the validation testing can be accomplished with visual inspections. This is possible because the flash/no flash discrimination is also implemented at a higher level and the result of the differentiation is a flashing field or a non-flashing field. The validation testing would consist of test situations 2 and 4 as presented above.

Based on the design options, the requirements could be rewritten in order to simplify testing even further. Assume that the third design option in fact requires less testing time and is easier to test. The requirement statements can then be written in order to facilitate this situation even more. The following requirements statements are equivalent to those above and in fact tends to drive the design in the direction of the third design option. "All displayed fields can be edited. All critical items being edited shall flash to inform the user that editing is in progress." In this instance, the third design can be augmented by creating a list or look-up table of the fields required to be edited and a flag can be associated with each that indicates whether the field should flash or not. this approach allows a completely visual inspection to replace the testing because the field is either in the edit list or it is not, and if it is, then it either flashes or it does not. testing within the routine is still required, but it now is associated with debug testing during development and not with formal validation testing after implementation.

10.1.3   Requirements versus Design

There is agreement that there is a lot of overlap between requirements and design, yet the division between these two is not a hard line. Design can itself be considered a requirement. Many individuals, however, do not appreciate that the distinction between them can be used to simplify testing and consequently shorten overall software development times. Requirements and their specification concentrates on the functions that are needed by the system or product and the users. Requirements need to be discussed in terms of what has to be done, and not how it is to be done.

The requirement "hardcopy strip chart analysis shall be available" is a functional requirement. The requirement "hardcopy strip chart analysis shall be from a pull down menu" has design requirements mixed with the functional requirements. Consequently, there may be times when requirements specifications will contain information that can be construed as design. When developing a requirements specification, resist placing the "how to" design requirements in the system requirements specification and concentrate on the underlying "what" requirements.

As more "how" requirements creep into the requirements specification, more testing must occur on principally two levels. First, there is more detail to test for and second, but strategically more important, there is more validation than verification that needs to be done. Since verification is qualitative in nature and ascertains that the process and design were met, low-key activities have been transferred from the visual and inspection methods into validation testing which is more rigorous and requires formal proof of requirements fulfillment. The distinction of design versus requirements is difficult, but a careful discrimination of what goes where is of profound benefit. As a rule of thumb, if it looks like a description of "what" needs to be implemented, then it belongs in the requirements specification. If it looks like a "how to" description, if a feature can be implemented in two or more ways and one way is preferred over another, or if it is indeterminate as to whether it is a requirement or design, then it belongs in the design specification.

There is another distinct advantage to moving as many "how" requirements to design as possible. The use of computer aided software engineering (CASE) tools has greatly automated the generation of code from design. If a feature or function can be delayed until the design phase, it can then be implemented in an automated fashion. This simplifies the verification of the design because the automation tool has been previously verified and validated so that the demonstration that the design was implemented is simple.

10.2   The Product Specification

The product specification is the first step in the process of transforming product ideas into approved product development efforts. It details the results of the customer survey and subsequent interface between the Marketing, Design Engineering, Reliability Assurance and Regulatory Affairs personnel. It specifies what the product will do, how it will do it and how reliable it will be. To be effective, it must be as precise as possible.

The product specification should be a controlled document, that is, subject to revision level control, so that any changes that arise are subjected to review and approval prior to implementation. It prevents the all too typical habit of making verbal changes to the specification, without all concerned personnel informed. This often leads to total confusion in later stages of development, as the current specification is only a figment of someone's imagination or a pile of handwritten papers in someone's desk.

The specification should also have joint ownership. It should only be written after all concerned departments have discussed the concept and its alternatives and have agreed on the feasibility of the design. Agreement should come from Marketing, Design Engineering, Manufacturing, Customer Service, Reliability Assurance and Regulatory Affairs.

The specification is a detailed review of the proposed product and includes:

- the type of product
- the market it addresses
- the function of the product
- the product parameters necessary to function effectively
- accuracy requirements
- tolerances necessary for function
- the anticipated environment for the device
- cautions for anticipated misuse
- safety issues
- human factors issues
- the anticipated life of the product
- the reliability goal
- requirements from applicable domestic or international standards.

Each requirement should be identified with some form of notation, such as brackets and a number. For traceability purposes, each numbered subsection of the specification should start numbering its requirements with the number 1. For example:

5.3.1   Analog to Digital Converter

The output of the analog to digital converter must be between X and Y [1].

In parsing the requirements, this particular one would be referred to as 5.3.1-1. Subsequent requirements in this paragraph would be numbered in consecutive order. Requirements in the next paragraph would restart the numbering with #1.

Software programs are available to assist in the parsing process. The software establishes a database of requirements for which a set of attributes are developed that help trace each requirement. Some attributes which might be established include:

- Paragraph number

- Requirement number

- Author of the requirement

- System or subsystem responsible for the requirement

- Type of verification or validation test

The database might appear as shown in Table 10-1.

10.3   Specification Review

Once the marketing survey is complete, the reliability goal
established and the product specification drafted, a review of the specification is
held. The review is attended by Marketing, Design Engineering, Manufacturing,
Customer Service, Reliability Engineering and Regulatory Affairs. The draft of
the specification is reviewed in detail. Discussion and appropriate action items
are documented. Once the specification is approved, it is placed under revision
level control.

With the successful completion of the review, the development process
moves into the design phase, where the Design Specification is produced from
the Product Specification.

10.4   The Design Specification

The Design Specification is a document that is derived from the
Product Specification. The requirements found in the Product Specification are
partitioned and distilled down into specific design requirements for each
subassembly. The Design Specification should address the following areas for
each subsystem:

Total Requirement #	Requirement	Paragraph #	Req #	Author	Requirement Responsibility	Test Type
1221	The machine shall contain no burrs or sharp edges	3.1	1	Smith	System	Visual
1222	The maximum height of the machine shall be 175 cm	3.1	2	Smith	System	Validation
1223	The maximum height of the shipping package shall be 185 cm	3.1	3	Smith	System	Validation
1224	The power supply shall have a maximum inrush current of 7.3 volts	3.2	1	Jones	Subsystem B	Verification
1225	The power supply shall provide currents of +5V, +15V, and −15V	3.2	2	Jones	Subsystem B	Verification
1226	The check valve shall withstand a pressure of 150 psi	3.3	1	Thomas	Subsystem C	Verification

Table 10-1   Example of a Parsing Database (Fries, 1997.)

- the reliability budget
- service strategy
- manufacturing strategy
- hazard consideration
- environmental constraints
- safety
- cost budgets
- standards requirements
- size and packaging
- the power budget
- the heat generation budget

- industrial design/human factors
- controls/adjustments
- material compatibility.

In addition, all electrical and mechanical inputs and outputs and their corresponding limits under all operating modes must be defined.

Each performance specification should be listed with nominal and worst case requirements under all environmental conditions. Typical performance parameters to be considered include:

- gain
- span
- linearity
- drift
- offset
- noise
- power dissipation
- frequency response
- leakage
- burst pressure
- vibration
- long term stability
- operation forces/torques.

As in the Product Specification, the requirements in the Design Specification should be identified by a notation such as a bracket and numbers. The parsing tool works well for focusing on these requirements.

10.5   The Software Quality Assurance Plan

The term *Software Quality Assurance* is defined as a planned and systematic pattern of activities performed to assure the procedures, tools and techniques used during software development and modification are adequate to provide the desired level of confidence in the final product. The purpose of a Software Quality Assurance program is to assure the software is of such quality that it does not reduce the reliability of the device. Assurance that a product works reliably has been classically provided by a test of the product at the end of its development period. However, because of the nature of software, no test appears sufficiently comprehensive to adequately test all aspects of the program. Software Quality Assurance has thus taken the form of directing and documenting the development process itself, including checks and balances.

Specifying the software is the first step in the development process. It is a detailed summary of what the software is to do and how it will do it. The specification may consist of several documents, including the Software Quality Assurance Plan, the Software Requirements Specification and the Software Design Specification. These documents serve not only to define the software package, but are the main source for requirements to be used for software verification and validation. A typical Software Quality Assurance Plan (SQAP) includes the following sections.

10.5.1 Purpose

This section delineates the specific purpose and scope of the particular SQAP. It lists the names of the software items covered by the SQAP and the intended use of the software. It states the portion of the software life cycle covered by the SQAP for each software item specified.

10.5.2 Reference Documents

This section provides a complete list of documents referenced elsewhere in the text of the SQAP.

10.5.3 Management

This section describes the organizational structure that influences and controls the quality of the software. It also describes that portion of the software life cycle covered by the SQAP, the tasks to be performed with special emphasis on software quality assurance activities, and the relationships between these tasks and the planned major checkpoints. The sequence of the tasks shall be indicated as well as the specific organizational elements responsible for each task.

10. 5.4   Documentation

This section identifies the documentation governing the development, verification and validation, use, and maintenance of the software. It also states how the documents are to be checked for adequacy.

10.5.5   Standards, Practices, Conventions, and Metrics

This section identifies the standards, practices, conventions and metrics to be applied as well as how compliance with these items is to be monitored and assured.

10.5.6   Review and Audits

This section defines the technical and managerial reviews and audits to be conducted, states how the reviews and audits are to be accomplished, and states what further actions are required and how they are to be implemented and verified.

10.5.7   Test

This section identifies all the tests not included in the Software Verification and Validation Plan and states how the tests are to be implemented.

10.5.8   Problem Reporting and Corrective Action

This section describes the practices and procedures to be followed for reporting, tracking, and resolving problems identified in software items and the software development and maintenance processes. It also states the specific organizational responsibilities.

10.5.9 Tools, Techniques, and Methodologies

This section identifies the special software tools, techniques, and methodologies that support SQA, states their purpose, and describes their use.

10.5.10 Code Control

This section defines the methods and facilities used to maintain, store, secure and document controlled versions of the identified software during all phases of the software life cycle.

10.5.11 Media Control

This section states the methods and facilities used to identify the media for each computer product and the documentation required to store the media and protect computer program physical media from unauthorized access or inadvertent damage or degradation during all phases of the software life cycle.

10.5.12 Supplier Control

This section states the provisions for assuring that software provided by suppliers meets established requirements. It also states the methods that will be used to assure that the software supplier receives adequate and complete requirements.

10.5.13 Records Collection, Maintenance and Retention

This section identifies the SQA documentation to be retained, states the methods and facilities to be used to assemble, safeguard, and maintain this documentation, and designates the retention period.

10.5.14 Training

This section identifies the training activities necessary to meet the needs of the SQAP.

10.5.15 Risk Management

This section specifies the methods and procedures employed to identify, assess, monitor, and control areas of risk arising during the portion of the software life cycle covered by the SQAP.

10.5.16 Additional Sections as Required

Some material may appear in other documents. Reference to these documents should be made in the body of the SQAP. The contents of each section of the plan shall be specified either directly or by reference to another document.

10.6   Software Requirements Specification

The Software Requirements Specification (SRS) is a specification for a particular software product, program, or set of programs that perform certain functions. The SRS must correctly define all of the software requirements, but no more. It should not describe any design, verification, or project management details, except for required design constraints. A good SRS is unambiguous, complete, verifiable, consistent, modifiable, traceable, and usable during the Operation and Maintenance phase.

Each software requirement in an SRS is a statement of some essential capability of the software to be developed. Requirements can be expressed in a number of ways:

- through input/output specifications
- by use of a set of representative examples
  by the specification of models.

A typical Software Requirements Specification includes the following sections.

10.6.1 Purpose

This section should delineate the purpose of the particular SRS and specify the intended audience.

10.6.2 Scope

This section should identify the software product to be produced by name, explain what the software product will do, and if necessary, will not do, and describe the application of the software being specified.

10.6.3 Definitions, Acronyms, and Abbreviations

This section provides the definitions of all terms, acronyms, and abbreviations required to properly interpret the SRS.

10.6.4 References

This section should provide a complete list of all documents referenced elsewhere in the SRS or in a separate specified document. Each document should be identified by title, report number if applicable, date, and publishing organization. It is also helpful to specify the sources from which the references can be obtained.

10.6.5 Overview

This section should describe what the rest of the SRS contains and explain how the SRS is organized.

10.6.6   Product Perspective

This section puts the product into perspective with other related products. If the product is independent and totally self-contained, it should be stated here. If the SRS defines a product that is a component of a larger system, then this section should describe the functions of each subcomponent of the system, identify internal interfaces, and identify the principal external interfaces of the software product.

10.6.7   Product Functions

This section provides a summary of the functions that the software will perform. The functions should be organized in a way that makes the list of functions understandable to the customer or to anyone else reading the document for the first time. Block diagrams showing the different functions and their relationships can be helpful. This section should not be used to state specific requirements.

10.6.8   User Characteristics

This section describes those general characteristics of the eventual users of the product that will affect the specific requirements. Certain characteristics of these people, such as educational level, experience, and technical expertise, impose important constraints on the system's operating environment. This section should not be used to state specific requirements or to impose specific design constraints on the solution.

10.6.9   General Constraints

This section provides a general description of any other items that will limit the developer's options for designing the system. These can include regulatory policies, hardware limitations, interfaces to other applications, parallel operation, control functions, higher-order language requirements, criticality of the application, or safety and security considerations.

10.6.10 Assumptions and Dependencies

This section lists each of the factors that affect the requirements stated in the SRS. These factors are not design constraints on the software, but are any changes to them that can affect the requirements.

10.6.11 Specific Requirements

This section contains all the details the software developer needs to create a design. The details should be defined as individual specific requirements. Background should be provided by cross referencing each specific requirement to any related discussion in other sections. Each requirement should be organized in a logical and readable fashion. Each requirement should be stated such that its achievement can be objectively verified by a prescribed method.

The specific requirements may be classified to aid in their logical organization. One method of classification would include:

- functional requirements
- performance requirements
- design constraints
- attributes
- external interface requirements.

This section is typically the largest section within the SRS.

10.7   The Software Design Description

A software design description is a representation of a software system that is used as a medium for communicating software design information. The Software Design Description (SDD) is a document that specifies the necessary information content and recommended organization for a software design description. The SDD shows how the software system will be structured to satisfy the requirements identified in the software requirements specification. It is a translation of requirements into a description of the software structure, software components, interfaces, and data necessary for the implementation phase. In essence, the SDD becomes a detailed blueprint for the implementation activity. In a complete SDD, each requirement must be traceable to one or more design entities.

The SDD should contain the following information:

- Introduction
- References
- Decomposition description
- Dependency description
- Interface description
- Detailed design.

10.7.1   Decomposition Description

The decomposition description records the division of the software system into design entities. It describes the way the system has been structured and the purpose and function of each entity. For each entity, it provides a reference to the detailed description via the identification attribute.

The decomposition description can be used by designers and maintainers to identify the major design entities of the system for purposes such as determining which entity is responsible for performing specific functions and tracing requirements to design entities. Design entities can be grouped into major classes to assist in locating a particular type of information and to assist in reviewing the decomposition for completeness. In addition, the information in the decomposition description can be used for planning, monitoring and control of a software project.

10.7.2   Dependency Description

The dependency description specifies the relationships among entities. It identifies the dependent entities, describes their coupling, and identifies the required resources. This design view defines the strategies for interactions among design entities and provides the information needed to easily perceive how, why, where, and at what level system actions occur. It specifies the type of relationships that exist among the entities.

The dependency description provides an overall picture of how the system works in order to assess the impact of requirements and design changes. It can help maintenance personnel to isolate entities causing system failures or resource bottlenecks. It can aid in producing the system integration plan by identifying the entities that are needed by other entities and that must be developed first. This description can also be used by integration testing to aid in the production of integration test cases.

10.7.3   Interface Description

The entity interface description provides everything designers, programmers, and testers need to know to correctly use the functions provided by an entity. This description includes the details of external and internal interfaces not provided in the Software Requirements Specification.

The interface description serves as a binding contract among designers, programmers, customers, and testers. It provides them with an agreement needed before proceeding with the detailed design of entities. In addition, the interface description may be used by technical writers to produce customer documentation or may be used directly by customers.

10.7.4   Detailed Design Description

The detailed design description contains the internal details of each design entity. These details include the attribute descriptions for identification, processing, and data.

The description contains the details needed by programmers prior to implementation. The detailed design description can also be used to aid in producing unit test plans.

References

ANSI/IEEE Standard 730, *IEEE Standard for Software Quality Assurance Plans*. New York: The Institute of Electrical and Electronics Engineers, Inc., 1989.

ANSI/IEEE Standard 830, *IEEE Guide to Software Requirements Specifications*. New York: The Institute of Electrical and Electronics Engineers, Inc., 1984.

ANSI IEEE Standard 1016, *IEEE Recommended Practice for Software Design Descriptions*. New York: The Institute of Electrical and Electronics Engineers, Inc., 1987.

Chevlin, David H. and Joseph Jorgens III, "Medical Device Software Requirements: Definition and Specification," *Medical Instrumentation* Volume 30, Number 2, March/April, 1996.

Davis, Alan M. and Pei Hsia, "Giving Voice to Requirements Engineering," in *IEEE Software*. Volume 11, Number 2, March, 1994.

Fairly, Richard E., *Software Engineering Concepts*. New York: McGraw-Hill Book Company, 1985.

Fries, Richard C., *Reliable Design of Medical Products*. New York: Marcel Dekker, Inc., 1997.

Fries, Richard C., *Reliability Assurance for Medical Devices, Equipment and Software*. Buffalo Grove, IL: Interpharm Press, 1991.

Gause, Donald C. and Gerald M. Weinberg, *Exploring Requirements: Quality Before Design*. New York: Dorset House Publishing, 1989.

Keller, Marilyn and Ken Shumate, *Software Specification and Design: A Disciplined Approach for Real-Time Systems*. New York: John Wiley & Sons, Inc., 1992.

Potts, Colin, Kenji Takahashi, and Annie I. Anton, "Inquiry-Based Requirements Analysis," in *IEEE Software*. Volume 11, Number 2, March, 1994.

Pressman, Roger S., *Software Engineering: A Practitioner's Approach*. New York: McGraw-Hill Book Company, 1987.

Siddiqi, Jawed and M. Chandra Shekaran, "Requirements Engineering: The Emerging Wisdom," in *Software*. Volume 13, Number 2, March, 1996.

Chapter 11

Medical Device Records

Richard C. Fries, PE, CRE – Datex-Ohmeda, Inc.
Madison, Wisconsin

All records required by the Quality System Regulation and the Medical Device Directives must be maintained at the manufacturing establishment or other location that is reasonably accessible to responsible officials of the manufacturer and to auditors. The records must be legible and stored so as to minimize deterioration and to prevent loss. Those records stored in computer systems must be backed up.

Records deemed confidential by the manufacturer may be marked in order to aid the auditor in determining whether information may be disclosed. All records must be retained for a period of time equivalent to the design and expected life of the device, but not less than two years from the date of release of the product by the manufacturer.

There are four primary types of records that must be kept by every medical device manufacturer. These types are:

- Design History File (DHF)
- Device Master Record (DMR)
- Device History Record (DHR)
- Technical Documentation File (TDF).

Each type of record is discussed in the following sections.

11.1   The Design History File

The Design History File (DHF) is a compilation of records that describes the design history of a finished device. It covers the design activities used to develop the device, accessories, major components, labeling, packaging and production processes.

The Design History File contains or references the records necessary to demonstrate that the design was developed in accordance with the approved design plans and the requirements of the Quality System (QS) regulation.

The design controls in CFR 21 820.30(j) require that each manufacturer establish and maintain a DHF for each type of device. Each type of device means a device or family of devices that are manufactured according to one DMR. That is, if the variations in the family of devices are simple enough that they can be handled by minor variations on the drawings, then only one DMR exists. It is common practice to identify device variations on drawings by dash numbers. For this case, only one DHF could exist because only one set of related design documentation exists. Documents are never created just to go into the DHF.

The QS regulation also requires that the DHF shall contain or reference the records necessary to demonstrate that the design was developed in accordance with the approved design plan and the requirements of this part. As noted, this requirement cannot be met unless the manufacturer develops and maintains plans that meet the design control requirements. The plans and subsequent updates should be part of the DHF. In addition, the QS regulation specifically requires that:

- the results of a design review, including identification of the design, the date, and the individual(s) performing the review, shall be documented in the DHF
- design verification shall confirm that the design output meets the design input requirements. The results of the design verification, including identification of the design, method(s), the date, and the individual(s) performing the verification, shall be documented in the DHF.

Typical documents that may be in, or referenced in, a DHF include:

- design plans
- design review meeting information
- sketches
- drawings
- procedures
- photos
- engineering notebooks
- component qualification information
- biocompatibility (verification) protocols and data
- design review notes
- verification protocols and data for evaluating prototypes
- validation protocols and data for initial finished devices
- contractor/consultants information
- parts of design output/DMR documents that show plans were followed
- parts of design output/DMR documents that show specifications were met.

The DHF contains documents such as the design plans and input requirements, preliminary input specs, validation data and preliminary versions of key DMR documents. These are needed to show that plans were created, followed and specifications were met. The DHF is not required to contain all design documents or to contain the DMR, however, it will contain historical versions of key DMR documents that show how the design evolved.

The DHF also has value for the manufacturer. When problems occur during re-design and for new designs, the DHF has the "institutional" memory of previous design activities. The DHF also contains valuable verification and validation protocols that are not in DMR. This information may be very valuable in helping to solve a problem; pointing to the correct direction to solve a problem; or, most important, preventing the manufacturer from repeating an already tried and found-to-be-useless design.

11.2   The Device Master Record

The Device Master Record (DMR) is a compilation of those records containing the specifications and procedures for a finished device. It is set up to contain or reference the procedures and specifications that are current on the manufacturing floor. The Device Master Record for each type of device should include or refer to the location of the following information:

- device specifications including appropriate drawings, composition, formulation, component specifications, and software specifications
- production process specifications including the appropriate equipment specifications, production methods, production procedures, and production environment specifications
- quality assurance procedures and specifications including acceptance criteria and the quality assurance equipment used
- packaging and labeling specifications, including methods and processed used
- installation, maintenance, and servicing procedures and methods.

It is more important to construct a document structure that is workable and traceable than to worry about whether something is contained in one file or another.

11.3   The Device History Record

The Device History Record (DHR) is the actual production records for a particular device. It should be able to show the processes, tests, rework, etc. that the device went through from the beginning of its manufacture through distribution. The Device History Record should include or refer to the location of the following information:

- the dates of manufacture
- the quantity manufactured
- the quantity released for distribution
- the acceptance records which demonstrate the device is manufactured in accordance with the Device Master Record
- the primary identification label and labeling used for each production unit
- any device identification and control numbers used.

11.4   The Technical Documentation File

The Technical Documentation File (TDF) contains all the relevant design data by means of which the product can be demonstrated to satisfy the essential safety requirements which are formulated in the Medical Device Directives. In the case of liability proceedings or a control procedure, it must be possible to turn over the relevant portion of this file. For this reason, the file must be compiled in a proper manner and must be kept for a period of 10 years after the production of the last product.

The Technical Documentation File must allow assessment of the conformity of the product with the requirements of the Medical Device Directives. It must include:

- a general description of the product, including any planned variants
- design drawings, methods of manufacture envisaged and diagrams of components, sub-assemblies, circuits, etc.

- the descriptions and explanations necessary to understand the above mentioned drawings and diagrams and the operations of the product

- the results of the risk analysis and a list of applicable standards applied in full or in part, and descriptions of the solutions adopted to meet the Essential Requirements of the Directives if the standards have not been applied in full

- in the case of products placed on the market in a sterile condition, a description of the methods used

- the results of the design calculations and of the inspections carried out. If the device is to be connected to other device(s) in order to operate as intended, proof must be provided that it conforms to the Essential Requirements when connected to any such device(s) having the characteristics specified by the manufacturer

- the test reports and, where appropriate, clinical data

- labels and instructions for use.

The manufacturer must keep copies of EC type-examination certificates and/or the supplements thereto in the Technical Documentation File. These copies must be kept for a period ending at least five years after the last device has been manufactured.

11.5   A Comparison of the Medical Device Records

A manufacturer will accumulate a large amount of documentation during the typical product development process. The primary question then becomes which documentation is kept and where is it kept? Table 11-1 is an attempt to summarize the typical types of documentation and where they are kept. This is not an exclusive list, but serves only as guidance.

Record	Inclusion			
	DHF	DMR	DHR	TF
Agency submittals		X		X
Assembly inspection records		X	X	
Bills of material		X		
Calibration instructions/records		X		
Certificate of vendor compliance			X	
Certificates of compliance	X			X
Check sheets			X	
Clinical trial information	X			X
Combined product analysis				X
Component specifications		X		
Declarations of Conformity				X
Design review records	X			
Design specification	X	X		
Design test protocols	X			
Design test results	X			X
Design validation plans	X			
Design validation protocols	X			
Design validation results	X	X		
Design verification plans	X			
Design verification protocols	X			
Design verification results	X			X
Engineering drawings	X	X		
Essential Requirements checklists				X
Evaluations of potential vendors	X			
Evaluations of contractors	X			
Evaluations of consultants	X			
Field action reports			X	
Field service reports			X	
Final inspection instructions		X		
Incoming material quality records		X		
Inspection instructions		X		
Inspection plans		X		

Table 11-1   Comparison of Record Storage

Record	Inclusion			
	DHF	DMR	DHR	TF
Installation instructions		X		
Labeling requirements	X	X		X
Lab notebooks	X	X		
Letters of transmittal		X		
Listings of applicable standards				X
Machining inspection records			X	
Maintenance procedures		X		
Maintenance service reports			X	
MDD design specifications				X
Medical Device Reports (MDRs)			X	
Medical device vigilance reports			X	
Nonconforming material reports			X	
Packaging instructions		X		
Packaging specifications		X		
Post-release design control change records		X		
Pre-release design control change records	X			
Primary inspection records		X		
Process change control records		X		
Process validation records		X		
Product complaints			X	
Product descriptions		X		X
Product environmental specs		X		
Product manuals		X		
Product routings		X		
Product specifications	X	X		
Product test specifications	X	X		
Production release documentation		X		
Project plans	X			
Project team minutes	X			
Promotional materials		X		
Purchase orders			X	

Table 11-1 (continued)

Record	Inclusion			
	DHF	DMR	DHR	TF
Quality inspection audit reports		X		
Quality problem reporting sheets			X	
Quality memorandums		X		
Rationale for deviation from standards/regulations				X
Receipt vouchers			X	
Regulatory submittals		X		
Rework plans	X			
Risk analysis	X			X
Sales order reports			X	
Service specifications		X		
Shipping orders			X	
Software source code	X	X		
Tooling specs/revision log		X		
Work orders			X	

Table 11-1 (continued)

References

Fries, Richard C., *Reliable Design of Medical Devices*. New York: Marcel Dekker, Inc., 1997.

Higson, Gordon R., *The Medical Devices Directives – A Manufacturer's Handbook*. Brussles: Medical Technology Consultants Europe Ltd., 1993.

Schoenmakers, C.C.W., *CE Marking for Medical Devices*. New York: The Institute of Electrical and Electronic Engineers, 1997.

21 CFR §820. Washington DC: Food and Drug Administration, 1996.

Trautman, Kimberly A., *The FDA and Worldwide Quality System Requirements Guidebook for Medical Devices.* Milwaukee: American Society for Quality Press, 1997.

Section 3

The Design Phase

Chapter 12

Hazard and Risk Analysis

Markus Weber – System Safety, Inc.
San Diego, California

Hazard and risk analysis is a methodical approach to assist in designing safe and efficient medical devices. Safety critical industries like nuclear, aerospace or chemical industries have used various approaches to assess hazards and minimize the risk potential of their installation or products for years. The earliest approaches have been to identify hazards after the basic design decisions have been made and successively mitigate or change the design to address potentially hazardous failure modes. Techniques like FTA and FMEA have been used extensively to achieve this goal. However the techniques employed during a hazard analysis try to accomplish this at an even earlier time during the development process, thus allowing a more economical and speedier development process by developing valuable design information before the design process is initiated.

The hazard and risk analysis builds the foundation on which all other safety-related activities are based upon. The specification of safety requirements, the evaluation of hazard mitigating measures and the verification and validation of safety-related functions of a device solely depend on the completeness and correctness of the hazard and risk analysis. Any hazard, which is not identified, will not be addressed by safety measures and will not be detected during testing. It is crucial to be aware of this vulnerability, because it requires paying close attention to detail and completeness of the hazard analysis.

The hazard and risk analysis will have to consider the entire system including necessary or optional accessories and sub-systems. The analysis for a TMR laser system should therefore include, the laser itself, the delivery catheter and the ECG monitor used to gate the beam delivery. If necessary certain parts of the system hazard analysis can be detailed in subsequent subsystem hazard analyses, however to only perform a sub-system hazard analysis like a software criticality analysis will result in an incomplete or incorrect assessment and is to be considered potentially dangerous.

Keep in mind:

SAFETY is a SYSTEM PROPERTY.

12.1   Hazards, Risks, and Mitigation

Casually the terms hazard and risk are often used synonymously. The definition used in this text will closely differentiate between the two terms:

Hazard is a potentially dangerous condition, which is triggered by an event. This event is often called the cause of the hazards. A hazard will not necessarily cause harm, because any hazard will have to be existent for a period of time before it will become dangerous. This time is often called hazard latency time. Examples are radiation or exposure hazards, which need to exceed a specific dose in order to become dangerous. The hazard latency time is an important property of each individual hazard and determining this time should be part of the hazard identification process. A second important hazard property is the observability and detectability. These factors are also hazard specific and will provide important information for the design of risk mitigation measures.

Risk is a hazard that is associated with a severity and a probability of occurrence. This definition is intuitive; if a hazard is occurring more often or the result is more severe, the risk will be increased. In determining the risk, it is often considered difficult to identify the unmitigated risk because the design engineers often think ahead and are already considering the implementation of a mitigation or control measure. For reasons discussed later it is advantageous to determine the unmitigated risk before the reduced mitigated risk is determined.

A risk can be so low that no action is necessary to reduce the severity or occurrence probability. Many risks however are considered severe enough that measures have to be implemented to reduce the risk. The measures are usually avoidance, mitigation or organizational measures like user information.

The activities of hazard analysis, risk analysis and risk reduction are consecutive, closely interrelated steps that will be addressed in detail. The overall interaction of these activities is shown in Figure 12-1.

Every device follows certain steps during its useful life. Various lifecycle models have been developed to identify these steps. The hazard analysis is part of the 'safety lifecycle' of a device. Figure 12-2 illustrates how the safety lifecycle integrates into the design device lifecycle and has impact on almost every activity during the design process.

12.1.1   The Safety Life Cycle

Software Engineering has long used lifecycle models to describe the activities and deliverable during the design, validation and decommissioning of software systems. Modern development technologies applied this model to the entire development process. Adopting a lifecycle model allows to better identify the relation of process steps and the relevant process step in- and outputs. The safety part of the device development cycle should also follow the adopted lifecycle model. The most commonly used (and apparently most practicable) model is the so-called V-model. It defines a detailed succession of steps, is scalable (meaning is can be applied to the entire system as well as to sub or sub-sub systems) and is sufficiently generic to be implemented without

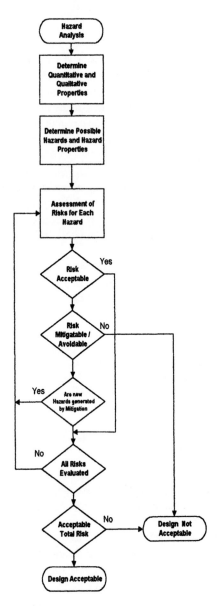

Figure 12-1   Hazard and risk analysis flow.

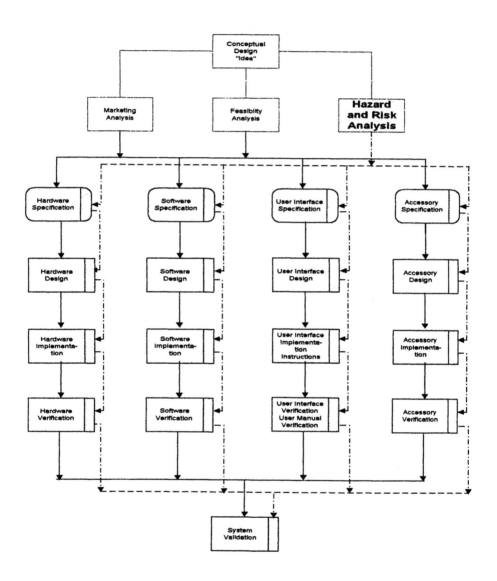

Figure 12-2   Hazard analysis as part of the development process.

conflicting too much with already established policies and procedures. The hazard analysis is the cornerstone of any lifecycle model and its placement within the overall V- lifecycle model is depicted in Figure 12-3.

12.2   Hazard Analysis

12.2.1   Purpose

The purpose of a hazard and risk analysis is to identify all possible hazards potentially created by a device, process or application. It is very important to try to identify all possible hazards and not omit potential hazards because their occurrence probability at the time of the analysis seems to be too remote. A hazard analysis should give a complete unbiased picture of all potential hazards and show how these are avoided, mitigated or controlled. It is often difficult to know where to draw the line and determine which hazards to list and omit. The appropriate approach is to include even remotely possible hazards in the analysis. It is a commonly made mistake to neglect 'obviously' less likely hazards from the analysis. If the hazard analysis is ever to be scrutinized during a quality system audit, GMP inspection, or during legal proceedings, it will be difficult to explain, why certain hazards are not addressed. The determination that these 'unlikely' hazards are unrealistic or improbable is a task performed during the risk assessment, not during the hazard analysis and it is important to document that these hazards have been considered. The hazard analysis is the cornerstone of the 'safety lifecycle' of a device and puts down the basis for safety requirements, safety verification and safety validation of a device.

12.2.2   Scope and Exclusions

The hazard analysis, like a marketing analysis and a feasibility study, is an activity that should be performed before the actual design of a device begins. The analysis determines basic design parameters and generates considerable input information for the design process. It is imperative to define the exact scope of the analysis to make clear which parts of the system or procedure are considered and which are excluded. The scope of the analysis

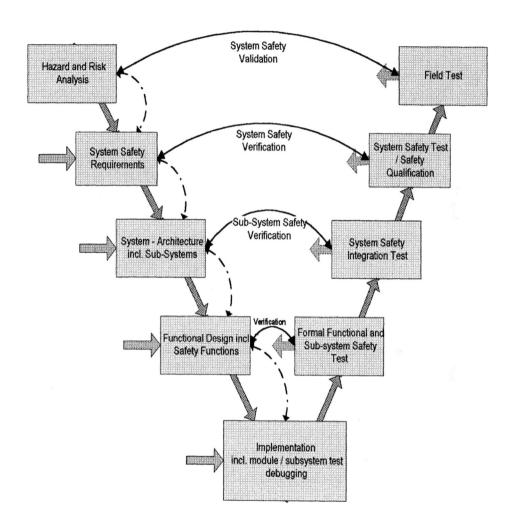

Figure 12-3   The V-model lifecycle.

should contain the intended use and environment of the device but should also include foreseeable unintended use or environmental impact. If exclusions in scope are made these exclusions should be clearly identified. Criminal use, sabotage or use by untrained personnel, are some exclusions that should be considered. A clear and concise definition of the scope of the analysis is one predetermination that should be carefully considered and will in part determine the labeling of the device.

12.2.2.1 Intended Use

The definition of the intended use should be either part of the hazard analysis or specified in separate documents. The intended use is essential to identify one of the scope boundaries of the hazard analysis. However the hazard analysis should go beyond this boundary and evaluate:

- Intended use of the device
- Foreseeable misuse of the device
- Under normal operation conditions
- Under or beyond marginal operating conditions
- Under fault conditions.

Additionally it should be defined which kind of operators and patients are assumed intended users of the device. This will give a clearer indication which use-environment the device is targeted for. The operator could be:

- Specially trained, licensed professional
- Professional
- Untrained medical personnel
- Patient.

In addition, the patient treated or diagnosed by the device could be categorized as:

- Healthy unaffected (donor)
- Healthy affected (patient)
- Fragile, elderly or slightly ill
- Heavily or critically ill
- Life-sustained, terminally ill

This incomplete list shows that the definition of intended use is necessary information to determine a hazard potential. It also allows better evaluation of to risk/benefit trade-offs that are necessary to determine the level of risk reduction and acceptable risk level during the risk analysis. A specially trained professional is less likely to use the device incorrectly, and a healthy patient is less likely to be sensitive to certain hazards.

12.2.3   Sources for Hazard Identification

As many sources as possible should be used to develop the list of potential hazards and their properties. Incident reports from similar devices, scientific literature, the body of applicable or related standards and the wealth of knowledge of professionals are all resources that can be utilized. It should not be underestimated that different professional groups have widely differing views on what could be considered hazardous. The design engineers often have a different understanding of a medical procedure and the associated hazards than a clinician who performs the procedure. A research scientist has a different perspective that a biomedical technician. These different views are parts of the puzzle, which once put together display the picture of a complete hazard analysis. It is very valuable to make the development of the hazard list not an exercise solely performed by design engineers and marketing.

Very sound sources to identify potential hazards are procedure or device specific safety standards. Even though standards define requirements, these requirements very often have their origin in potential hazards and are actually prescribing implementations to mitigate these hazards. Standards are generally consensus documents and their content summarizes the collective knowledge of many experts in a specific field. The requirements imposed in a standard often point to the most likely hazards occurring. If a standard for instance prescribes that the air sensor of an infusion pump has to be fail safe, it is a strong indication that the addressed hazard (in infusion) is very severe. The body of standards, even certain standards not directly applicable to the application investigated, are an excellent source of hazard information if they are read 'backwards', deriving potential hazard from implementation requirements. Compliance with recognized standards often is considered sufficient mitigation for specific hazards as compliance to UL 2601 and IEC 601-1 is considered sufficient to prove appropriate mitigation of electrical and mechanical device hazards if these hazards coincide with the hazards addresses in these standards. The last disclaimer however is very important – it is an important task of any hazard analysis to establish whether the requirements of a standard are sufficient to cover all possible hazards of the device. Standards often lag behind current state-of-the-art technology and may not cover all potential hazards for a given high-tech device. However the importance and legal impact of consensus documents should never be estimated. A comprehensive identification of applicable standards requirements and a strong rationale, if and why a requirement is not applicable, is advised.

The first step of the hazard analysis should consist of a comprehensive collection of potential hazards and is primarily a cause-effects analysis. This list may be refined as the implementation of the device becomes more defined, but should be free from implementation details. All hazards should be collected taking various factors into account. The following list can assist in identifying these hazards, but it should be cautioned that usually not all hazards are identified immediately. Specifically long-term hazards, secondary hazards or 'cloaked hazards' are not easily identifiable, because the direct cause-effect relationship may not be obvious. A hazard analysis should therefore be periodically reviewed and updated. At this stage the detailed factors that are involved in the hazard (software, hardware, control systems, accessory, etc.) should not be evaluated in detail to ensure that the general scope of the identification is maintained. However as many interactions of the device in different states of the device including the fault-free and faulty state with the environment are possible and should be identified. Figure 12-4 illustrates how the device becomes part of multiple interactions with its environment depending on internal states.

12.2.4   Commonly Known Hazard Sources

The following list attempts to categorize the most commonly known sources for hazards as outlined in EN 1441 and ISO 14971. The list of categories however is not complete and must be amended depending on the specific device envisioned.

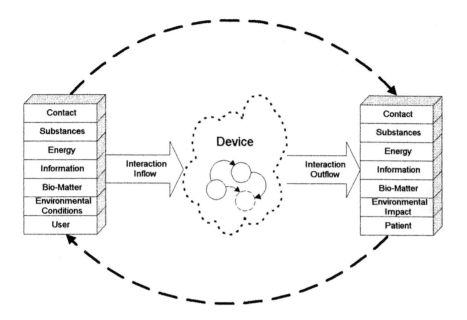

Figure 12-4   Device properties and interactions.

Energy Hazards

- Electricity
- Heat
- Ionizing Radiation
- Non-Ionizing Radiation
- Electromagnetic Fields
- Moving Parts
- Suspended Masses
- Patient Support Device Failure
- Pressure (Vessel Rupture)
- Acoustic Pressure
- Vibration
- Magnetic Fields (MRI).

Biological Hazards

- Bio-Burden
- Bio-Contamination
- Bio-Incompatibility
- Incorrect Output Of Substances / Energy
- Toxicity
- (Cross-) Infection Or Contamination
- Pyrogenicity
- Inability To Maintain Hygienic Safety
- Degradation.

Environmental Hazards

- Electromagnetic Interference
- Inadequate Supply Of Coolant
- Restriction Of Cooling (Air-Flow)
- Likelihood Of Operation Outside Prescribed Environmental Conditions
- Incompatibility With Other Devices
- Accidental Mechanical Damage To The Device
- Contamination Due To Waste Products and/or Device Disposal.

Hazards Related to the Use of the Device

- Inadequate Labeling
- Inadequate Operating Instructions
- Inadequate Specification Of Pre-Use Checks
- Inadequate Specification Of Accessories
- Over–Complicated User Instructions
- Unavailable Or Separated User Instructions
- Use By Unskilled/Untrained Personnel
- Reasonably Foreseeable Misuse
- Insufficient Warning Of Side Effects
- Inadequate Warning Of Hazards Likely With Re-Use Of Single Use Devices
- Incorrect Measurement And Other Methodical Aspects

- Incorrect Diagnosis
- Erroneous Data Transfer
- Mispresentation Of Results
- Incompatibility With Consumables / Accessories / Other Devices.

Hazards Due to Functional Failure, Maintenance and Aging

- Inadequacy Of Performance Characteristics For The Intended Use
- Lack Of, Or Inadequate Specification For Maintenance, Including Post Maintenance Functional Checks
- Inadequate Maintenance
- Lack Of Adequate Determination Of End Of Device Life
- Inadequate Packaging (Contamination Or Deterioration)
- Improper Re-Use.

The following addresses the most common concerns identified in the above list.

12.2.4.1 Patient / Person Contact

Devices that contact a patient directly or are invasive usually have a higher hazard potential than devices, which are isolated from the human body. An evaluation of the kind and duration of all physical contact with humans should be evaluated such as:

- Surface contact points
- Invasive contact / Contact through bodily orifices
- Implantable contact.

The kind and duration of the contact will allow identifying hazards propagating through these contact points.

12.2.4.2 Materials

The materials used in the design have a direct impact on potential hazards. This applies not only to human contact materials and the resulting sterility and biohazards but also to materials used in the construction of the device. Materials that could generate hazardous by-products under normal operating conditions (ozone) or under environmental extremes like fire / heat (poisonous fumes) may not be suitable for use in a device.

12.2.4.3 Energy

Energy delivered or extracted is one of the predominant hazards. Incorrect energy levels, energy delivery or extraction can lead to life-threatening situations (laser, hypothermia equipment, RF surgery devices). In general the potential of a device to emit or absorb energy should be evaluated not only in respect to the patient, but also the operator and other medical personnel should be taken into account, specifically for long term exposure effects (x-ray devices, nuclear medicine devices). The physical and physiological properties of the primary energy transfer on humans should be identified. Additionally secondary energy generated by the primary energy source through energy transformation should be evaluated like the transformation of light energy into thermal energy in laser surgery.

12.2.4.4 Delivery of Substances

Another prime hazard is the delivery of drugs or other substances to the patient. Absolute dose and rate (dose/time) are potential hazards if the delivery is unintended or an intended delivery does not occur. It will be difficult to specify an absolute dose or rate at which a hazard will develop because this will depend on multiple factors like the potency of the drug, the patient weight, interacting substances, pharmacokinetics, etc. However it should be a defined design goal to meet a self-imposed rate/dose accuracy limit as well as a maximum limit under fault conditions. Also the effects of non-delivery should be investigated.

12.2.4.5 Information

Even though information will not directly generate a hazard, incorrect information has hazard potential if used to control or direct a potential hazard source. This is immediately obvious in closed loop systems (control of drug delivery by a physiological parameter like blood pressure) but even if in incorrect path for treating a patient is selected based on incorrect information presented to the physician, the incorrect information is the primary cause of the hazard. The point in time during which information becomes available may also be critical.

Not only correctness and proper timing of information are potentially critical but also the absence of information may be hazardous. This applies specifically for critical alarms like the apnea alarm of a ventilator.

12.2.4.6 Bio-Matter

If the device processes biological materials biohazards may result in its operation. Extracorporeal processing of bodily fluids like blood processing or dialysis may generate hazards for the patient or the operator. This concern also applies to in vitro diagnosis or processing devices. Haemolysis, viral infections, and bacterial or chemical contamination are some of these biohazards.

12.2.4.7 Time Delayed Dose/Effects

Time and dose are important properties of potential hazards. Usually there are limits to when the hazard becomes negligible. Determining these limits is important for the design of a device since they decide how the implementation will control the hazard. The duration of exposure to a hazard source before the hazard manifests itself is also an important variable. This time allows evaluating accumulative or time-delayed hazards like exposure to low frequency electromagnetic fields or iodine accumulation in the thyroid gland.

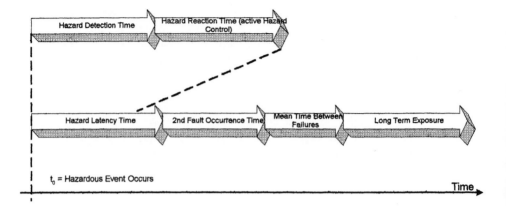

Figure 12-5   Safety critical times.

12.2.4.8 Environment

A device can affect or be affected by the environment in which it is used. It may alter the patient environment (pressure, temperature, humidity) but it will also be influenced by the environment (electromagnetic susceptibility, temperature). Both factors should be investigated in terms of their hazard potential.

12.2.4.9 User Interface

To determine possible intentional or foreseeable unintentional use of the device that could cause a hazard, the user interface is an important part of the device's safety system. Incorrect parameter input, misinterpretation of information presented by the device or ambiguous user interfaces can be hazardous. An evaluation of the parts of the user/device interface that could be the cause of a hazard should be part of the hazard identification.

12.2.4.10 Miscellaneous Factors

Miscellaneous factors may have to be addressed during the hazard identification, such as:

- Calibration
- Sterility
- Storage environment
- Ergonomic considerations
- Influence of accessory devices.

It is important to be aware that the hazard identification is a multi-faceted approach that should not involve a single person. Input from multiple areas like physiological, pharmacological, chemical, electrical sciences, etc. will be necessary to ensure a comprehensive and complete as possible identification of hazards. If a device uses a programmable system the software will not directly factor into the hazard identification process because implementation details will not change the hazard potential of a device. It will however have great influence on potential of functional risk, hazard control and mitigation.

A valuable tool during the analysis are group sessions in which as many disciplines as possible should be involved. A tool to facilitate the free flow of ideas, the scenario approach is often used, in which all participants mentally execute many 'what-if' situations.

12.2.4.11 Qualitative and Quantitative Properties of the Device

To better structure the areas, which should be investigated regarding a potential hazard, it is useful to identify the qualitative and quantitative properties of the proposed device. The standards EN1441 and ISO 14971 use a series of questions to guide the though process. These questions relate to the following areas:

- What is the intended use and how is the device to be used?
- Is the device intended to contact the patient or other persons?
- What materials and/or are incorporated in the device or are used?

- Is energy delivered or extracted from the patient?
- Are substances delivered or extracted from the patient?
- Does the device for subsequent use process biological materials?
- Is the device supplied sterile or intended to be sterilized by the user or are other microbiological controls applicable?
- Is the device intended to modify the patient environment?
- Are measurements made?
- Is the device interpretive?
- Is the device intended to control or interact with other devices or drugs?
- Are there unwanted outputs of energy or substances?
- Is the device susceptible to environmental influences?
- Are essential consumables or accessories associated with the device?
- Is routine maintenance and calibration necessary?
- Does the device contain software?
- Does the device have a restricted shelf life?
- Are there possible delayed and long-term effects?
- To what mechanical forces will the device be subjected?
- What determines the lifetime of the device?
- Is the device intended for single / multiple use?

It has been proven a helpful activity to formally answer these questions in the hazard analysis document. Annex C of the standards also give the above mentioned categories of hazards and sources, each of which should be addressed in detail by either finding a rationale, if a category is not applicable, or by identifying hazards that are related to the category.

Additionally it is helpful to consider if a hazard is likely to cause to a 'secondary hazard'. Very often a hazard source does not only generate a single hazard but additional secondary hazards, like optical energy (a laser beam) causing eye damage, tissue damage and an explosion hazard or thermal energy caused by an overheating component causing tissue damage, a fire hazard and the generation of toxic fumes.

12.2.4.12 Hazards Induced by Hazards Mitigation

One hazard category will not be evaluated during the initial hazard analysis but carries significant importance during any subsequent review of the initial, often call preliminary, hazard analysis. This category contains all hazards induced by avoidance or mitigation of any hazard identified during the first pass of the hazard analysis. Examples are the exposure to biohazards if an operator intervenes and exposing him/herself to blood or the decrease in availability of device function if a mitigation safety component malfunctions and shuts down a life-sustaining device like a lung ventilator.

12.2.5 Hazards Identification Matrix

To manage the number of identified hazards efficiently and establish the root for hazard, risk and mitigation traceability the identified hazards are often summarized in a hazards identification matrix. Such a matrix is shown in Table 12-1.

The biggest problem during the hazard identification is the inadequacy of the generated list. Any hazard that has not been identified will not be addressed in the consecutive steps of the analysis and design of the device. The omission may result in a hazardous device carrying a high risk of injury or death. Therefore the hazard list should not omit hazards because they seem to be unlikely or because historical precedence is missing. These factors are already part of the analysis and should not be considered during the identification phase.

12.3 Risk Analysis

The next step after the collection of potential hazards is the interpretation and analysis of the risk for each identified hazard. Risk in this context is the probability and severity of the hazard becoming reality. These two factors require a judgment to be made on the occurrence probability of the uncontrolled hazard and the severity of the unmitigated occurrence. Additionally it must be identified how a risk can be avoided, controlled or mitigated to reduce the risk to an acceptable level. Very often it is useful not to

Hazard ID	Hazard Description	Cause	Secondary Hazards	Hazard Source	Hazard Latency Time/Dose	Observability
Physiological Hazards / Procedure Hazards						
1 (Infusion pump)	Air embolism	Infusion of air into the patient	NA	Infusion bag empty	15 ml air / hour	No
				Leak in upstream infusion set	15 ml air / hour	No
Energy Hazards						
2 (Surgical laser)	Retinal damage	Exposure to laser light	Minor tissue damage	Focused invisible laser beam	< 100ms	No
3 (Defibrillator)	Ventricular Fibrillations	Over-energy delivered to patient	Tissue burns	Overcharged capacitors	< 100ms	No
4 (ESU)	?					
Bio-Hazard						
5 (Sterile Package)	Exposure to bodily fluids	Sharp punctures sterile package	Patient infection	Sterile package exposed to mechanical stress	< 10 ms	Eventually (visual inspection of package)

Table 12-1   Hazards identification matrix.

intermingle the assessment of 'raw' hazards with the investigation of 'risk-reduced' hazards. During the risk assessment it is often tempting to identify the already mitigated risk. For example the unmitigated risk of electrocution is very high (due to high severity and high probability) if fundamental isolation requirements are not implemented. These requirements appear to any engineer, as being so natural that proper isolation is already assumed and the risk of the unmitigated hazards is down-rated.

The identification of the unmitigated risk is however essential to identify the safety integrity of the mitigation. The safety integrity is understood as the probability of a mitigator to perform its function. In other terms, the more risk reduction is burdened upon a mitigation measure the higher the required safety integrity for that measure. To determine the 'spread' between unmitigated and mitigated risk it is therefore necessary to determine the unmitigated risk. This 'spread' is directly related to the safety integrity of the measure and signify the actual risk reduction achieve by this measure.

Hazards with a high severity rating should be paid special attention to regardless of the occurrence probability and risk-reduction measures because a misjudgment in the two later factors can cloak potentially severe hazards by assuming either incorrect probability or a higher safety integrity of the mitigator. For example if a hazard is identified to be lethal to a patient, however it was determined that the probability of the hazardous event is unlikely, this hazard will still need close attention. For example if the probability of the lethal event is determined to 10^{-9}/hour (one billion hours or more than 100,000 years between lethal events), this low probability seems to make the event sufficiently unlikely to cause this hazard not be mitigated. However, if it is expected that 10,000 units be sold, the incident occurrence probability goes down to 10^{-5}/hour. This will cause a lethal accident every 100,000 operation-hours or every 11 years. This may be well within the expected life of the device.

A second factor aggregates the above example. Normally probability numbers are considered a statistical average of a set of data. The probability does not imply that every 10^{-9}/hours the lethal event will happen, but that within every 10^9 hour window the event will statistically happen once. Two issues arise from that fact:

1. It is not determined when the event will happen. The reasoning that a device will never reach the number of operating hours is not a valid argument. The lethal event can happen within the first hour of operation. Additionally the occurrence of the first event does not imply that the next 10^9 hours will be free of incidents.
2. The confidence that one can have in this data is very low. The probabilities are usually assumed or derived based on a very limited set of data. This will make the statistical base very unreliable. Safety engineering is the art of working with very little data in hoping of not generating more.

Furthermore it should be identified if the hazard can occur under fault-free, single fault or multiple fault conditions. Severe hazards should not be acceptable under normal and single fault conditions.

12.3.1   Qualitative versus Quantitative

Two different methodologies can be used to determine the risk of each hazard: quantitative and qualitative assessment. Both have pros and cons and whichever method is chosen one should be aware of its strengths and weaknesses. The previous sections touched on some technical problems using the quantitative risk assessment. One should also be aware that identifying a quantitative risk could imply the acceptance of a certain number of incidents (like killing a patent every million hours), which could be a potential legal issue. Very few legal requirements worldwide are in fact identifying quantitative risks that are deemed acceptable. Therefore the burden of proof in case of an incident lies with the manufacturer. The quantitative approach is widely considered to be more vulnerable to legal challenge than the less defined qualitative approach.

The quantitative method uses occurrence probabilities combined with a severity rating. These probabilities can be derived using statistical methods. Severe hazards should be assessed independent as in the qualitative method. The weakness of this method, as explained above, is that sound statistical data may not be available and that using questionable data may falsely assume a high level of accuracy.

The qualitative method assigns certain discreet levels to the severity and probability of a hazard. The granularity of the levels can range from minor, moderate and major to more detailed levels (1-10). The assignment of these levels may be used to determine the risk. If a severity scale of 1-10 and the product of the probability scale of 1-10 is used the resulting risk scale will be 1-100. It is obvious that a low severity combined with a high probability will generate the same risk rating as a high severity and low probability. Since a severe hazard resulting in death or irreversible injury should be avoided at all cost, this method has to evaluate not only the risk rating but must also address all hazards with a high severity rating separately. The weakness of this method is that the assignment of levels may be arbitrary without underlying detail knowledge. Whichever method is used the reason for the risk parameter selection should be documented including the rating schema data sources used.

To increase the confidence in the risk evaluation various methods can be used like technical discussion, examples from industries with related safety issues like aerospace, chemical process or nuclear industries. Additionally a 'blind voting' of all risk assignment team members can be used during which each member assigns the risk parameters individually and secretly. The results are then openly review and compared. The author has experienced a group convergence on certain hazards and a wide swing of parameters on others. The items with wide divergence were than further investigated until a near consensus of the blind 'votes' was achieved.

12.3.2   Risk Reduction

The next step is to identify measures implemented into a device to avoid, control or mitigate a hazard in order to achieve a risk reduction. These measures may involve the operator, additional equipment, self-testing and other ways that result in reducing the risks. These measures however shall not introduce new hazards unless these hazards are also addressed in the hazard analysis. A review and amendment of the hazard analysis will be necessary after all mitigators have been defined.

The order of measures to reduce the risk of a hazard should be ranked in the following order (in fact the European Medical Device Directive legally requires this order):

1.   Risk Avoidance
2.   Risk Mitigation down to a level 'as low as reasonably possible'
3.   User intervention, labeling, training.

Additionally only observable hazards or hazards made observable through technical means, which have a sufficiently long hazard latency time, can be mitigated by user intervention.

12.3.2.1 Risk Avoidance

If a hazard is identified to be above the risk acceptance level, the device is to be considered unsafe. However a different implementation can sometimes be employed to avoid the hazard entirely. This may result in a new design approach or in substituting components responsible for the hazard like substituting chemical agents or changing from a DC motor to a stepper. If such a general design change is made, the new design has to be evaluated by performing a separate hazard analysis.

Avoiding a hazard all together is the best of all possible methods. Avoidance can be achieved by using different technology (electrical, optical, pneumatic), different agents (less hazardous chemicals) and different materials (less flammable, higher thermal insulation). Unfortunately using these methods is not always possible or will itself generate an entire new set of hazards. However it is a useful exercise during a hazard analysis to evaluate if avoidance is possible and to document if this approach is not feasible. Avoidance is the prime method in handling systematic errors in software. Since fault detection and control mechanisms are difficult to implement or limited in their effectiveness, avoiding programming and design failures is extremely important. A software development process controlled by effective software quality assurance measures can ensure a high level of 'bug' avoidance.

12.3.2.2 Rick Control

Means to control hazards can be of an active or a passive nature. Passive means do not require an active reaction to a hazardous event. Examples are safety goggles to protect against laser light or double or reinforced isolation to prevent electric shock hazards. Active controls require the detection of a potentially hazardous event and an appropriate reaction to avoid or mitigate the developing hazard. Active controls need a definition of the 'safe state' of the device. The 'safe state' is the state into which the control has to place the device before the hazard becomes critical. A single device may have multiple safe states like alarm, shutdown, user notification, activation of a backup device, etc. If active controls are used each hazard should to be assigned the appropriate safe state or combination of safe states.

The time and dose properties of a hazard require the active control mechanism to detect and react to the event causing the hazard before time or dose limits are exceeded. These requirements may preclude certain measures such as self-testing or operator intervention.

12.3.2.2.1 Passive Mitigation

Passive mitigation is the next best level to manage a potential hazard. The goal of the mitigating measures should be to lower the severity (not the occurrence probability) sufficiently to meet the risk acceptance level. Shielding, encapsulation, antidotes, etc., can achieve passive mitigation. Lead aprons, laser goggles and protective clothing are examples of passive mitigating measures. The reaction time of mitigation to a hazardous event is instantaneous and can therefore be used to deal with 'fast' developing hazards like laser exposure, ex- or implosive events, etc., and usually does not require energy to be effective.

12.3.2.2.2 Active Mitigation

Active mitigation like testing and corrective action is a measure consisting of two parts, hazard detection (testing) and hazard control (corrective action). This method usually requires energy to be effective and the reaction time is limited by the sum of the detection plus the reaction time. The timing requirements of the hazards will determine the necessary test cycle time, which can range from microseconds (hardware implementation) to minutes or hours (software implementation). Testing and corrective action usually require additional resources like sensors, hardware circuits and software, which themselves can induce new hazards to the device.

12.3.2.3 User Intervention and Labeling

Only observable hazards or hazards made observable through technical means, which have a sufficiently long hazard latency time, can be mitigated by user intervention. Because the user intervention is considered the least reliable means reducing risk (which relates to having a low safety integrity level) it is to be considered the last possible action. The human interface is of utmost importance. Consider how a nurse taking the correct action within an ICU, while 20 different devices are blaring out alarms of varying importance, is prone to mistake.

There is very little guidance on human-device interfaces for critical devices and especially in integrated environments as described above. The safety and reliable implementation of human interaction may be a challenge.

The reluctance to consider user interaction should not be interpreted as a reluctance to implement user interaction to control or eventually override certain device functions. There is a substantial difference in a physician discharging a defibrillator even if the device cannot achieve the necessary charge level for a given Joule setting and a nurse having to bag a ventilated patient due to a ventilator malfunction.

In certain environments like surgery, human interaction can be utilized to achieve hazard control. Especially if the measures necessary to control a hazard are not easily quantifiable, or depend on multiple parameters not accessible by the device, human intervention may be the only appropriate means to mitigate a hazard.

As stated earlier user intervention as a risk reduction method should be used very carefully and will require detailed user instructions and training. In many cases however, it may be the only reasonable way to reduce a specific device risk.

12.3.2.3.1 Residual Risk

Whichever mitigation measures or combination of measures are implemented there always will be residual risks with any potentially hazardous device. This is partly due to the limited level of risk reduction achieved. It is also influenced by the limited safety integrity of the measures implemented. It is important to identify these risks by identifying the remaining risk after mitigation.

12.3.3   Risk Acceptance Level and Risk Reduction

The acceptable level of risk reduction is a complex issue. It has not only technical but also ethical and liability implications. Basically it has to answer the question "How much safety is sufficient and how much risk do I accept?" One difficult factor will be the risk/benefit determination that will allow accepting higher risk levels if the benefits far outweigh the risks (i.e., defibrillator). There is no regulation available on how to quantify the acceptable risk, but the minimal acceptable level should prevent irreversible injury or death under single fault conditions. Any medical device should never exceed this acceptance level. Different hazards may be linked to different acceptance levels depending on their severity and possible external counteracting measures, i.e., antidotes. Figure 12-6 illustrates the risk-reduction using more that one measure enabling the actual risk to be below the risk acceptance level.

Depending on the methodology used the risk acceptance level will either be a probability figure or a classification of an acceptable risk rating. One suggestion for the classifications of risk parameters can be found in an IEC document that establishes four risk classes with proposed acceptance criteria:

Risk Class	Interpretation
Class I	Intolerable risk
Class II	Undesirable risk and tolerable only if risk reduction is impracticable or if the costs are grossly disproportionate to the improvements gained
Class III	Tolerable risk if the cost of risk reduction would exceed the improvement gained
Class IV	Negligible risk

These risk classes are then linked to occurrence probability and the consequence of the event:

Frequency	Consequence			
	Catastrophic	Critical	Marginal	Negligible
Frequent	I	I	I	II
Probable	I	I	II	III
Occasional	I	II	III	III
Remote	II	III	III	IV
Improbable	III	III	IV	IV
Incredible	IV	IV	IV	IV

Another approach is using the concept of safety integrity levels. This concept can be utilized for both the quantitative and qualitative approach. The quantitative method can briefly be described as:

$$R = F * C$$

where R is the unmitigated risk, F the occurrence frequency and C the consequence. If the resulting risk R is greater than the acceptable risk R_a, a reduction of the risk by reducing F to achieve a reduction by $\Delta R = R - R_a$.

The parameter F is composed of three factors:

- Exposure to the hazard
- Probability of avoiding the hazardous event
- Probability of occurrence.

12.3.3.1 Safety Integrity

Safety integrity is defined as the probability of a safety function to perform on demand. In other words the criticality of a function is directly related to the necessary safety integrity. For example if the only device preventing a nuclear

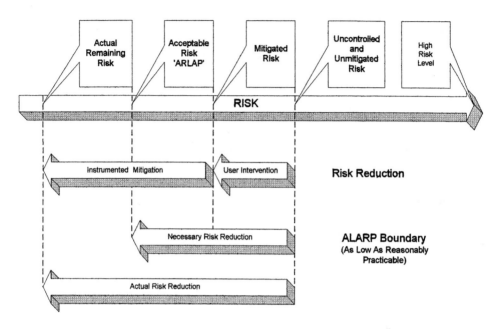

Figure 12-6   Risk, acceptable risk, and risk reduction.

reactor from becoming critical would rest upon a PC based system with software written under object oriented methodology, it is highly questionable that such a system is fit for the desired purpose. In other terms – the safety integrity of the system is too low for the necessary risk reduction.

It is often helpful to think of 'safety integrity' in terms of 'safety burden' placed onto a function. The safety integrity if human interaction may be considered low and not sufficient if a high amount of risk reduction must be achieved.

An important aspect of the safety integrity approach however is the scalability of risk reduction though combined measures of different safety integrity. If multiple means are used to independently mitigate the same risk, the individual means may not provide sufficient safety integrity individually. However the combined use of multiple means may achieve the necessary risk reduction.

12.3.3.2 Fault Tree Analysis

The fault tree analysis (FTA) is a methodology that can be used to trace hazards to possible component failures. It identifies components that are involved in the hazard generation and the combination and conditions of these components that will lead to a hazard in a structured manner. FTA originally was used to investigate possible critical as well a non-critical faults, but is also an excellent method to use as a tool for a structured hazard analysis approach. FTA however does not account for parts of the hazard analysis like risk-level determination, risk reduction evaluation, etc. FTA is also an excellent method to verify a hazard analysis that used a matrix approach.

FTA is call a top-down methodology because the starting point of each branch is a system level event, which is than decomposed into more detailed branches and sub-branches.

FTA methodology can be used to evaluate the sufficient mitigation of each hazard by identifying the causal relationship of events and trace them down to system component failures. It however does not replace the hazard and Risk Analysis because the list of potential hazards is needed as input information into the FTA tree in which each hazard constitutes one root event for the hazards analysis. If event probabilities are used, the FTA can give an excellent overview of combined mitigation and helps to identify critical components or subsystems.

12.3.3.3 Failure Mode Effects and Criticality Analysis

Failure Mode Effects and Criticality Analysis (FMECA) is a modification of the well known Failure Mode and Effects Analysis (FMEA). It uses the bottom-up approach of the FMEA on a system level to investigate known failure modes of system parts in their capability to create a hazard. The advantage of FMECA is the fact, that every component of the system becomes part of the evaluation. This is not necessarily the case using FTA.

FMECA is often considered a hazard analysis. This belief is however incorrect. The hazard analysis generates a set of hazards and their associated mitigators, whereas the FMECA uses the known hazards of the hazard analysis to identify if a given implementation causes any of these hazards if a component fails. Here is a list of the substantial differences between hazards analysis and FMECA.

The FMEC(D)A is an amplification of the FMECA that not only identifies the criticality of a failure mode but also determines to which degree the failure mode is detected and can be actively mitigated.

However, the significant differences between a Hazard and Risk Analysis and a FMEA are illustrated in Table 12-2. Prerequisite to FMECA and FMEC(D)A is a modularized design and sufficient knowledge of all failure modes of a component as well as the identified hazards.

12.4   Risk Analysis Matrix

The hazard analysis is usually summarized in table format listing the various components attached to a hazard. The resulting risk analysis most likely will follow a similar approach. It is useful to number each line to be able to refer and back-trace to each hazard. The matrix format is independent of the methodology used during the actual analysis, but presents the results in an easy-to-read form. It is important to mention that the matrix is not the only component of a hazard and risk analysis documentation because it usually does not sufficiently cover other parts like scope identification, assumptions and exclusions, and the conclusion.

Additionally the table format has limited capabilities if it is used in complex systems, which usually deal with many hazards and mitigation

	Hazard and Risk Analysis	**FMECA**
When performed	Before the design begins	After the design is determined
Information generated	List of potential hazards and risks List of mitigation measures	Failure modes of a device Criticality and detectability of the failure
	Safety requirements for design	Analysis whether the design meets the requirements
Information used	Literature, scenarios, expert opinions	Component failure modes and rates Hazard Analysis Results
Impact on design if unmitigated hazard is detected	Proactive prevention of hazards by appropriate design	Redesign of existing device

Table 12-2   Hazard anlaysis and FMEA.

combinations. In these cases the application of a hazard and risk database can be more appropriate, especially since the data storage will allow multiple views into the data such as:

- Which hazards are mitigated by measure A?
- Are all hazards mitigated?
- What is the average/minimum/maximum safety integrity level?

Tables 12-3 and 12-4 give an example of a quantitative and qualitative Risk Analysis Matrix. The columns identify the hazard as earlier identified during the Hazard Analysis, the occurrence probabilities and estimated severities for the unmitigated and mitigated hazard. The hazards latency time and the observability of the hazards are repeated to easier identify and assess possible mitigations. The hazard control is the key column of the table. It identifies the implementation of a measure to mitigate the risk down to an acceptable level. Each row of to table is clearly identified by a unique identifier (mitigator number). There may be more mitigators than hazards, but each mitigator will be back-traceable to the associated hazard by the hazard number.

Each mitigator will later be verified regarding effectiveness and completeness as well as for proper implementation regarding the requirements derived from the risk analysis. It can be helpful to include forward references (hazard number $\Rightarrow$ mitigating measure $\Rightarrow$ requirements $\Rightarrow$ verification and

Mitigation Number	Hazard Number	Hazard Description	Hazard Latency Time	Possible Cause	Probability	Severity	Uncontrolled Risk	Method of Control	Risk Reduction	Controlled Risk	Req. Reference
1	1	Inadvertent Radiation (LASER)	100 ms	Shutter failure	8	9	72	Shutter position sense	4	36	
2	1		100 ms	Control system failure	8	9	72	Second processor			
3		Overdose (IV)	Depending on drug	Motor runaway	10	10	60	Motor monitoring	2	80	
4		Ventilator Stops	5 sec	Power loss	7	10	70	Power loss alarm	5	50	
			5 sec	CPU failure	5	10	50	Watchdog	2	20	

Table 12-3 Quantitative Hazard Analysis

Mitigation Number	Hazard Number	Hazard Description	Hazard Latency Time	Possible Cause	Probability	Severity	Uncontrolled Risk	Method of Control	Risk Reduction	Controlled Risk	Req. Reference
1	1	Inadvertent Radiation (LASER)	100 ms	Shutter failure	10^{-8}	10^{2}	10^{-6}	Shutter position sense	10^{-3}	10^{-9}	2.3.1
2	1		100 ms	Control system failure	10^{-6}	10^{2}	10^{-4}	Second processor	10^{-4}	10^{-8}	4.5.2
3	2	Overdose (IV)	Depending on drug	Motor runaway	10^{-3}	10^{3}	10^{-3}	Motor monitoring	10^{-3}	10^{-6}	SSR15
4	3	Ventilator Stops	5 sec	Power loss	10^{-6}	10^{4}	10^{-2}	Power loss alarm	10^{-3}	10^{-5}	
			5 sec	CPU failure	10^{-7}	10^{4}	10^{-3}	Watchdog	10^{-3}	10^{-6}	

Table 12-4 Qualitative Hazard Analysis

validation tests) as well as backward references (mitigating measure $\Rightarrow$ hazards number, etc.) in each table. This will allow easier referencing between the related items and will establish traceability between them. Ultimately it will have to be proven at the end of the device design, that each of the identified hazards is sufficiently mitigated. analysis.

Table 12-5 shows one possible structure of a hazard analysis matrix that can be used as a template for qualitative evaluations. Table 12-6 shows one possible structure of a hazard analysis matrix that can be used as a template for qualitative evaluations. The values assumed are for illustration purposes only and do not resemble realistic data.

12.5   Software Hazard Analysis

If the hazard analysis shows that software is a critical component special care will have to be taken while designing and implementing the software system. Failure in software can be divided into the following main categories:

- Random failure of hardware that the software system runs on
- Systematic faults of hardware that the software runs on
- Systematic faults in the software itself.

The first two failures are not 'classical' software failures known as bugs, but the complexity of today's computer components blurs the border between failures and faults and any malfunction of these components will have a direct impact on the behavior of the software system. Both fault types have inherent different characteristics:

Random faults are spontaneous faults of a component within a single physical system. It is generally known that they occur and they have underlying physical fault characteristics. These faults can be diagnosed but never entirely avoided and they can be found in the hardware that the software runs on. Examples for random faults are component failures like a loose contact but also incorrect operation of the device by the operator.

Systematic faults are errors in design or implementation that are hidden in every system. These faults and their characterization are generally unknown. Once they are detected they can be eliminated entirely. Systematic faults can be hidden in hard- and software and they can be found by extensive testing. An incorrect instruction in a users manual can also be considered a systematic fault since users will be performing the same incorrect action every time they refer to the instructions for use. A widely published incarnation of a systematic fault was the 'Year 2000 Problem'.

The characteristics of a systematic fault make it very difficult to assign an occurrence probability to these faults and as of today no methodology has been developed to measure the degree of fault-freeness of a system, even though some methods exist that try to derive a metric out of various factors like complexity, testing time, etc. A quantitative hazard analysis of software systems should therefore be viewed with caution.

To deal with the unknown number and severity of systematic faults in software the overall criticality of the entire software system has to be considered within the scope of the device. Any hazard that could be induced by software malfunction has to be addressed. However only the severity can be assigned to the hazard since the probability is unknown. Conservatively the occurrence probability should be considered 1. The mitigation strategies for software dependent hazards are slightly different than the hardware or procedure related approaches.

12.5.1   Risk Avoidance

The software risk can altogether be avoided if software is not used or only used in non safety-related functions. However this approach is often not practical due to design constrains like flexibility, complexity and user interaction. Additionally the probability of software faults is closely linked to the controls and rigor of the software design process. The employment of current software engineering principles, the adherence to a well defined software lifecycle, requirements based software testing, strict configuration control, etc. are all measure targeted at avoiding the induction of systematic faults into software.

If software is potentially harmful, as many design controls as possible should be used. The analysis of safety requirements in terms of correctness and completeness as well as the capture of all software related mitigation measures defined in the Hazard and Risk Analysis is essential. The modularization of the software system into manageable and separately testable units with known interfaces should be used to reduce the complexity. The more complex a system is, the more it is prone to systematic faults.

At the end of the software development cycle the software should be thoroughly tested to prove that all hazards are mitigated and all requirements are correctly and completely implemented. Stress and challenge testing of the device is also highly recommended to detect a potentially missing requirement.

To coordinate all these activities the application of a lifecycle model ensures to proper steps are taken at an appropriate time. The V-model is most widely used to show activities and their relations during a development lifecycle. This model has several advantages over others like Waterfall or Spiral because it is scalable (meaning various V-model lifecycles can be nested for subsystems) and is universally applicable system level, hardware and software development.

12.5.2   Risk Control

Risk control or active mitigation is difficult to achieve in software systems. This is mainly due to the fact that the manifestation of the fault is unknown (if we knew where the bug is, we would fix it). Therefore a limited toolbox is available to implement risk control. Two main technologies have proven practical.

12.5.2.1 Diverse Redundancy

Diverse redundancy processes critical data twice in different ways and compares the results. For safety purposes it is often not necessary to perform both processing paths with the same accuracy or even on separate hardware processors. Important is that different algorithms are used. Redundancy is often used in hardware systems to increase the availability of a critical function (think of the dual hydraulic brake system in your car), it is however not sufficient to address systematic faults of the system (like water in your brake fluid that will influence both brake circuits at the same time). Diverse redundancy relies on the notion that it is less likely that you make the same mistake twice.

Diverse redundancy can be effectively employed without increasing the device significantly. Two implementations are most common.

12.5.2.1.1 Backward Calculation

Backward calculation is software that runs on the same processor but tries to revalidate a set-parameter by reverse calculation of the control parameter to the set-parameter. For instance if an infusion rate of 100 ml/hour results in a motor speed between 5 and 8 RPM (depending on certain correction factors like temperature) a motor speed of 10 RPM can never be correct for an infusion rate of 80 ml/hour. Reverse calculation of the infusion rate based on the motor RPM will detect if the algorithm has a fault.

12.5.2.1.2 Control – Monitoring System

Since the critical parameters can usually be reduced to a few, it is not necessary that the diverse safety system has the same processing and complexity requirements as the control system. Usually the safety of a device depends on very few parameters. An independent monitoring system is therefore often used to minimize possible systematic faults. Examples for these monitoring systems may be a second small processor (like a PIC) monitoring critical parameters of the device. In an infusion pump it may be sufficient to monitor the motor speed, direction and an air-senor. It is important however to provide the monitoring system with independent data like sensor reading or user-set parameters to achieve true independence and systematic fault protection. Often it is not necessary to monitor all critical parameters independently, but restrain the monitoring system to the most critical (in terms of software hazard potential) properties. Also an already existing second processor, like a micro controller handling the display or keyboard, can often be used to provide these safety functions without unduly increasing hardware cost.

It is important however that any independent system, may it be an secondary software monitoring device or a hardware safety device such as a watchdog, are independently capable to put the device into it's safe state. It does not help if it is detected that the primary control is defective and the very same primary system is then used to assert the safe state. (If the controlling FET of an infusion pump motor is shorted there must be other means to stop the pump from killing the patient).

It may be noted at this point that the suggested control-monitoring architecture also provides protection against certain potential hardware faults and it is recommended to seriously consider architectural solutions to potential hazards that mitigate effectively multiple hazards at the same time.

12.5.2.1.3 Assertions and Plausability Checks

Assertions and plausibility checks are another means to detect systematic faults. Plausibility checks assume certain reasonable value ranges for clinical or device parameters. The definition of these checks and their implementation in (often considered "useless") code requires creative thinking and in-depth knowledge of the application of the device.

Checks can be introduced into the software system as safeguards against systematic faults, such as:

- Is it reasonable that an adult ventilator ventilates at 240 Bpm?

- Should the blood pump really draw blood from the patient during prime?

- Is an infusion rate of 100ml/hour reasonable if the VTBI is only 2 ml?

Each of these questions will be initially considered to be irrational until a systematic fault manifests itself and potentially induces a hazard. If such checks would have been implemented accidents like the Therac-20 incidents could have been avoided.

Assertions follow the same principle but address the inner workings of the software. Checking parameters like stack size, pointer validity, array indices, etc. are means to avoid commonly known programming errors like memory leaks, garbage collection problems or just plain algorithmic errors such as division by zero errors.

Assertions and plausibility checks follow the same notion of assuming the software does not what it is supposed to do (or what the programmed thinks it should do). Therefore the programmers often consider these software checks plain 'nuts'. They appear to check something that is already implemented – so everybody thinks. However software bugs are about the things that nobody considered.

It is, however, very difficult to determine the effectiveness of these assertions, but this just goes along the lines of not being able to determine the 'software failure rate'.

12.5.3   Software System Boundaries

In analyzing the hazard potential of the software system one has to be aware of the interaction boundaries between the various software modules. A software system on a single processor usually consists of critical and non-critical modules if only the functionality of these modules is evaluated. However both types of modules share many resources like memory, busses, the CPU etc. An apparently non-critical module can easily change data of a critical module (except if 100% data hiding is implemented). A software system or software module can therefore only be declared non-critical if no negative interference with critical modules is possible. This boundary can more easily be drawn in multiprocessor systems, where critical and non-critical software systems may co-exist. In a single processor system that mixes both types of software the entire software system should be considered critical. Modern programming techniques like object oriented programming help substantially to minimize the interference between modules (objects), if the methodological approach is consequently implemented. Lower level modules that access hardware directly however very often break the paradigm and are implemented in a low level language.

The translation / compilation process of a software system should also be taken into account if the attempt is made to separate critical and non-critical modules. The fact that the high level language suggests that a decoupling has been achieved often proves incorrect. The actual binary code may still contain coupling point, i.e., the stack, library routines, memory allocation, operating systems, etc. To avoid extensive analysis the approach to treat the entire software system as critical, once it performs a single critical function, is often the most viable and surely the safer one.

The dynamic nature of real-time applications make it very difficult to correctly evaluate software hazards caused in real-time environment. Especially in event driven systems the number of possible combinations is almost infinite, making the hazard assessment even more difficult.

The following are some key questions that should be answered during the software hazard analysis. Will a hazard occur if:

- Software is executed using incorrect data (bad sensor)?
- Software is executed in an incorrect order (program flow)?
- Software is not executed (stalled processor)?
- Software is not or incorrectly responding to external or internal events?

If any of these questions can be answered YES a corrective action executed by an entity independent from the software system may be necessary. In other terms the software should be evaluated in terms of incorrect behavior in four separate domains:

- **The Data Domain** – Which hazards can arise if the software if the software is provided with incorrect data (sensors, users inputs or data provided from other software functions).
- **The Program Domain** - Which hazards can arise if the software is executed through the wrong processing paths or algorithms (incorrect if/case statements, incorrect algorithms, infinite or incorrect looping, etc.)?
- **The Time Domain** - Which hazards can arise if certain program parts are executed at an inappropriate time (too early, too late, not at all or too often)?

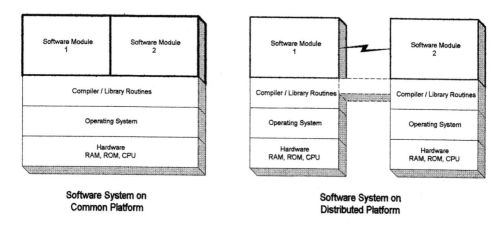

Figure 12-7   Software boundaries and coupling points.

- **The Event and State Domain** - Which hazards can arise if the
  software is correctly responding to real-time events of does not
  reflect the state of the 'real word" (state mismatch, interrupt overload or stacking, task inversion, etc.).

12.6   Safety Requirements Specification

The results of the hazard analysis should find their way into the
documentation defining the requirements necessary to ensure the safety of the
proposed device. The safety requirements should be traceable to the identified
hazard and will be an important set within all requirements, which needs to be
carefully implemented and thoroughly tested, verified and validated through the
device development process. The verification and validation procedures should
emphasize the importance of these requirements.

Safety requirements can be part of a specific safety requirements
document or can be integrated in various requirement documents. If the later

approach is taken the requirements should be clearly identifiable as safety requirements. This can be achieved by introducing a separate chapter for these requirements throughout the document trail. The specified safety requirements should be evaluated to confirm they cover all identified hazards sufficiently.

12.7   Hazard Analysis and Quality Control

Documentation developed during the hazard analysis is an essential part of the device file and should therefore be controlled by policies and procedures. The Hazard and Risk Analysis is the first step of a risk management lifecycle. This lifecycle and all activities and work products produce there under should be governed by a risk management procedure. It is important to understand that quality control and the strict adherence to a quality process are the most potent weapons to avoid systematic faults. Since the importance of software in critical system functions steadily increases the avoidance of systematic faults becomes more and more important.

Is obvious that the documents need to be under a document control system. The quality control system should ensure that all issues that surface during the analysis process are adequately addressed and should provide procedures to co-ordinate the involvement of all persons that participate in the hazard analysis process. As stated earlier the analysis is an effort that should involve multiple persons with different fields of expertise to ensure sufficient coverage of all concerns. Performing the analysis under a structured procedure will allow a clear definition of assignments and responsibilities and will ensure closure of all addressed issues.

As mentioned earlier quality control and a well-defined development process are not only a regulatory requirement, but also are one of the very few means to avoid systematic faults. Historically systematic faults and the related accidents have increased almost exponentially over the last twenty years. This can partly attributed to the increasing complexity of modern medical devices and the predominance of software functionality. More and more people die due to the omission of proper thinking rather than due to the random failure of a component. Quality control and diligent software engineering is essential to reduce these risks and should never be considered an unnecessary burden, even if their success can hardly be measured (such as advertising success can not be scientifically measured or proven either).

12.8 Conclusion

Hazard and Risk Analysis are state-of-the art tools to minimize the risk to human life and health as well as environmental impact of any technological implementation. For medical devices they become more and more legally or regulatory required activities, since these devices carry a significant public health risk. Even though it is difficult to ultimately statistically prove that these methodologies achieve their goals, it is commonly believed that these methods work sufficiently well to make them mandatory. Their use has been proven over and over again (who has not leaned about a new aspect of a device application during a thorough hazard analysis?). Even if the use of these methods would not be mandatory, engineering ethics would have to call for their implementation.

Many questions will have to remain unanswered in this chapter, like: How many hazards do I have to identify, or the most important one: How much risk is acceptable? There is not a single global requirement or standard that will provide this answer. This is only partly due to the fact that everybody is reluctant to put a figure on human life or suffering. The nature of safety engineering also calls for assuming hazards that may (hopefully) never happen and think of ways to prevent them from ever happening. Safety is only an exact science as long as it deals with known facts like accidents happened in the past, but is a highly speculative endeavor as far as the prediction and assumption of not yet known hazards is concerned. This fact, however, does not justify the omission of safety engineering. The ultimate answer to the open questions in this chapter lies beyond the scope of this chapter and this book.

References

Functional safety of electrical/electronic/programmable electronic safety-related systems, IEC 61508 Part 1: General requirements Part 4: Definitions and abbreviations Part 5: Examples of methods for the determination of safety integrity levels. Bureau Central dl la Commission Electrotechnique Internationale (IEC), 3 rue de Varembre, Geneve, Switzerland, 1998.

Medical Devices - Risk Analysis, EN 1441, CEN - European committee for Standardization, Rue de Stassart 36, Bruxelles. Belgium, B-1050, 1997.

Medical Devices - Risk Management, ISO/IEC 14971-1, International Organization for Standardization, Case Postale 56, Geneva, Switzerland, CH-1211.

Medical electrical equipment - Part 1: General requirements for safety - 4 Collateral Standard, Programmable electrical medical systems, IEC 60601-1-4, 1st. ed., Geneva, Switzerland, International Electrotechnical Commission, 1996.

Guidance for the Content of Premarket Submissions for Software Contained in Medical Devices, Rockville, MD, FDA, Center for Devices and Radiological Health, May 29, 1998.

William M Goble, *Evaluating Control Systems Reliability*, Instrument Society of America, 1992.

Chapter 13

Hardware Design

Richard C. Fries – Datex-Ohmeda, Inc.
Madison, Wisconsin

Design input provides the foundation for product development. The objective of the design input process is to establish and document the design input requirements for the device. The design input document is as comprehensive and precise as possible. It contains the information necessary to direct the remainder of the design process. It includes design constraints, but does not impose design solutions.

Once the documentation describing the design and the organized approach to the design is complete, the actual design work begins. As the design activity proceeds, there are several failure-free or failure tolerant principles that must be considered to make the design more reliable. Each is important and has its own place in the design process.

13.1   Block Diagram

The first step in an organized design is the development of a block diagram of the device (see Figure 13-1). The block diagram is basically a flow chart of the signal movement within the device and is an aid to organizing the design. Individual blocks within the block diagram can be approached for component design, making the task more organized and less tedious. Once all blocks have been designed, their connections are all that remain.

13.2   Redundancy

One method of addressing the high failure rate of certain components is the use of redundancy, that is, the use of more than one component for the same purpose in the circuit. The philosophy behind redundancy is if one component fails, another will take its place and the operation will continue. An example would be the inclusion of two reed switches in parallel where if one fails because the reeds have stuck together, the other is available to continue the operation.

Redundancy may be of two types:

- Active
- Standby.

13.2.1   Active Redundancy

Active redundancy occurs when two or more components are placed in parallel, with all components being operational. Satisfactory operation occurs if at least one of the components functions. If one component fails, the remaining parts will function to sustain the operation. Active redundancy is important in improving the reliability of a device. Placing components redundantly increases the MTBF of the circuit, thus improving reliability. Consider the following example.

Figure 13-2 shows a circuit for an amplifier. Let's use the component U1 as our candidate for redundancy. The failure rate for the component in MIL-HDBK-217 gives a value for our intended use of 0.320

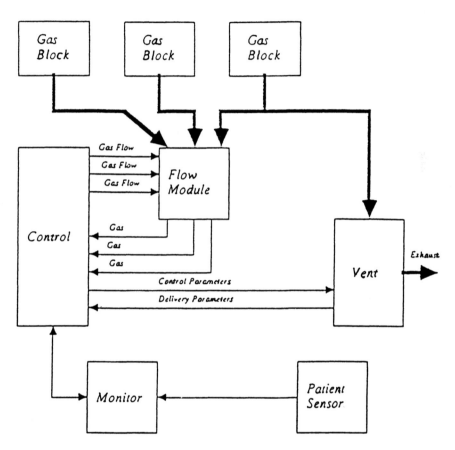

Figure 13-1   Block diagram. (From Fries, 1997.)

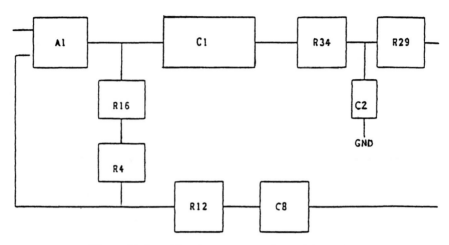

Figure 13-2   Circuit example. (From Fries, 1997.)

failures/million hours. The failure rate assumption is that the component was
in its useful life period. Therefore, the reciprocal of the failure rate is the
Mean Time Between Failure (MTBF). When calculating the MTBF, the failure
rate must be specified in failures per hour. Therefore, the failure rate,
as listed in the handbook or in vendor literature must be divided by one million.

$$MTBF = 1/\lambda$$

$$= 1/0.00000032$$
$$= 3{,}125{,}000 \text{ hours}$$

Let's assume for our particular application, this MTBF value is not
acceptable. Therefore, we decide to put two components in parallel
(Figure 13-3). Again, we assume the useful life period of the component. For
this case:

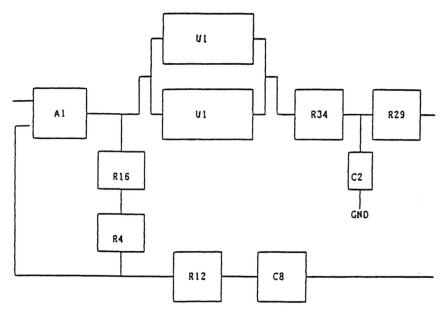

Figure 13-3   Active redundancy. (From Fries, 1997.)

$$MTBF = 3/2\lambda$$
$$= 3/2(0.00000032)$$
$$= 3/0.00000064$$
$$= 4,687,500 \text{ hours}$$

By putting two components in active redundancy, the MTBF of the circuit has increased by 50%.

13.2.2   Standby Redundancy

Standby redundancy occurs when two or more components are placed in parallel, but only one component is active. The remaining components are in standby mode.

Returning to our previous example, we have decided to use standby redundancy to increase our reliability (Figure 13-4). Again assuming the useful life period and ignoring the failure rate of the switch,

$$MTBF = 2/\lambda$$
$$= 2/0.00000032$$
$$= 6,250,000 \text{ hours}$$

By using standby redundancy, the MTBF has increased by 100% over the use of the single component and by 33% over active redundancy.

Obviously, the use of redundancy is dependent upon the circuit and the failure rates of the individual components in the circuit. However, the use of redundancy definitely increases the reliability of the circuit. What type of redundancy is used again depends on the individual circuit and its intended application.

13.3   Component Selection

As certain portions of the design become firm, the job of selecting the proper components becomes a primary concern, especially where there are long lead times for orders. How are the vendors for these components chosen? If one is honest in looking back at previous design developments and honest in listing the three main criteria for choosing a component vendor, they would be:

>Lowest cost
>Lowest cost
>Lowest cost.

The only other parameter which may play a part in choosing a vendor is loyalty to a particular vendor, no matter what his incoming quality may be. Obviously, these are not the most desirable parameters to consider if the design is to be reliable. The parameters of choice include:

- Fitness for use
- Criticality vs non-criticality

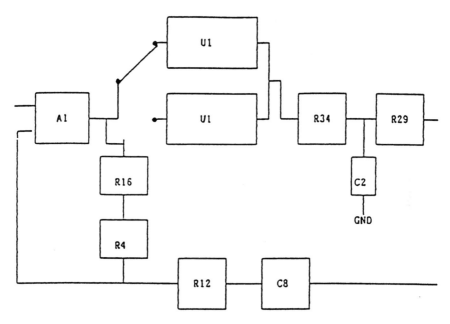

Figure 13-4   Standby redundancy. (From Fries, 1997.)

- Reliability
- History
- Safety.

13.3.1   Component Fitness for Use

Fitness for use includes analyzing a component for the purpose to which it was designed. Many vendors list common applications for their components and tolerances for those applications. Where the desired application is different than that listed, the component must be analyzed and verified in that application. This includes specifying parameters particular to its intended use, specifying tolerances, inclusion of a safety margin and a review of the history of that part in other applications.

For components being used for the first time in a particular application and for which no history or vendor data is available, testing in the desired application should be conducted. There is more about this in the chapter on validation.

13.3.2   Component Reliability

The process of assuring the reliability of a component is a multi-step procedure, including:

> Initial vendor assessment
> Vendor audit
> Vendor evaluation
> Vendor qualification.

The initial vendor assessment should be a review of any past history of parts delivery, including on time deliveries, incoming rejection rate, willingness of the vendor to work with the company and handling of rejected components. The vendor should also be questioned as to the nature of his acceptance criteria, what type of reliability tests were performed and what the results of the tests were. It is also important to determine whether the nature of the test performed was similar to the environment the component will experience in your device.

Once the initial vendor assessment is satisfactorily completed, an audit of the vendor's facility is in order. The vendor's processes should be reviewed, the production capabilities assessed, rejection rates and failure analysis discussed. Sometimes the appearance of the facility provides a clue as to what type of vendor you are dealing with. A facility that is unorganized or dirty may tell you about the quality of the work performed.

Once components are shipped, you need to ensure that the quality of the incoming product is what you expect. A typical approach to the evaluation would be to do 100% inspection on the first several lots to check for consistent quality. Once you have an idea of the incoming quality and you are satisfied with it, components can be randomly inspected or inspected on a skip-lot basis.

Many companies have established a system of qualified vendors to determine what components will be used and the extent of incoming inspection. Some vendors qualify through a rigorous testing scheme that determines the incoming components meet the specification. Other companies have based qualification on a certain number of deliveries with no failures at incoming. Only components from qualified vendors should be used in any medical device. This is especially important when dealing with critical components.

13.3.3   Component History

Component history is an important tool in deciding what components to use in a design. It is important to review the use of the component in previous products, whether similar or not. When looking at previous products, the incoming rejection history, performance of the component in field use and failure rate history need to be analyzed.

A helpful tool in looking at component history is the use of available data banks of component information. One such data bank is MIL-HDBK-217. This military standard lists component failure rates based upon the environment in which they are used. The information has been accumulated from the use of military hardware. Some environments are similar to that seen by medical devices and the data is applicable. MIL-HDBK-217 is discussed in greater detail later in this chapter.

Another component data bank is a government program named GIDEP. The only cost for joining this group is a report listing failure rates of components in your applications. You receive reports listing summaries of other reports the group has received. It is a good way to get a history on components you intend to use. More information may be obtained by writing to:

GIDEP Operations Center
Department of the Navy
Naval Weapons Station
Seal Beach, Corona Annex
Corona, CA   91720

A good source for both mechanical and electrical component failure rates is the books produced by the Reliability Analysis Center. They may be contacted at:

> Reliability Analysis Center
> P. O. Box 4700
> Rome, NY   13442-4700
> Telephone: +1+800+526-4802

13.3.4   Component Safety

The safety of each component in your application must be analyzed. Do this by performing a fault tree analysis, where possible failures are traced back to the components causing them. This is discussed later in this chapter.

A failure mode analysis can be performed that looks at the results of single point failures of components. Unlike the fault tree, which works from the failure back to the component, failure mode analysis works from the component to the resultant failure. This is also discussed in more detail later in the chapter.

13.4   Component Derating

Component failure in a given application is determined by the interaction between the strength and the stress level. When the operational stress levels of a component exceed the rated strength of the

component, the failure rate increases. When the operational stress level falls below the rated strength, the failure rate decreases.

With the various ways for improving the reliability of products, derating of components is an often-used method to guarantee the good performance as well as the extended life of a product. Derating is the practice of limiting the stresses, which may be applied to a component, to levels below the specified maximum.

Derating enhances reliability by:

- reducing the likelihood that marginal components will fail during the life of the system
- reducing the effects of parameter variations
- reducing the long-term drift in parameter values
- providing allowance for uncertainty in stress calculations
- providing some protection against transient stresses, such as voltage spikes.

An example of component derating is the use of a 2 watt resistor in a 1 watt application. It has been shown that derating a component to 50% of its operating value generally decreases its failure rate by a factor greater than 30%. As the failure rate is decreased, the reliability is increased.

Components are derated with respect to those stresses to which the component is most sensitive. These stresses fall into two categories, operational stresses and application stresses. Operational stresses include:

- temperature
- humidity
- atmospheric pressure.

Application stresses include:

- voltage
- current
- friction
- vibration.

These latter stresses are particularly applicable to mechanical components.

Electrical-stress usage rating values are expressed as ratios of Maximum Applied Stress to the Component's Stress Rating. The equation for table guidelines is:

Usage Ratio = Maximum Applied Stress/Component Stress Rating

For most electronic components, the usage ratio varies between 0.5 and 0.9.

Thermal derating is expressed as a maximum temperature value allowed or as a ratio of "actual junction temperature" to "maximum allowed junction temperature" of the device. The standard expression for temperature measurement is the Celsius scale.

Derating guidelines should be considered to minimize the degradation effect on reliability. In examining the results from a derating analysis, one often finds that a design needs less than 25 components aggressively derated to greatly improve its reliability. And, depending on the design of the product, these components often relate to an increase in capacitance voltage rating, a change of propagation speed, an increase in the wattage capacity of a selected few power resistors, etc.

13.5   Safety Margin

Components or assemblies will fail when the applied load exceeds the strength at the time of application. The consideration of the load should take into account combined loads, such as voltage and temperature or humidity and friction. Combined loads can have effects that are out of proportion to their separate contributions, both in terms of instantaneous effects and strength degradation effects.

Establishing tolerances is an essential element of assuring adequate safety margins. Establishing tolerances, with appropriate controls on manufacturing provides control over the resulting strength distributions. Analysis should be based on worst case strength or distributional analysis, rather than on an anticipated strength distribution.

Safety margin is calculated as follows:

$$\text{Safety Margin} = (\text{Mean safety factor}) - 1$$
$$= (\text{Mean strength/mean stress}) - 1$$

An example illustrates the concept:

> A structure is required to withstand a pressure of 20,000 psi. A safety margin of 0.5 is to be designed into the device. What is the strength that must be designed in?

$$\text{Safety Margin} = (\text{strength/stress}) - 1$$
$$0.5 = (\text{strength}/20{,}000) - 1$$
$$1.5 = \text{strength}/20{,}000$$
$$(20{,}000 \times 1.5) = \text{strength}$$
$$30{,}000 \text{ psi} = \text{strength}$$

Most handbooks list a safety margin of 2.0 as the minimum required for high reliability devices. In some cases, this may result in an over-design. The safety margin must be evaluated according to device function, the importance of its application and the safety requirements. For most medical applications, a minimum safety margin of 0.5 is adequate.

13.6   Load Protection

Protection against extreme loads should be considered whenever practicable. In many cases, extreme loading situations can occur and must be protected against. When overload protection is provided, the reliability analysis should be performed on the basis of the maximum load which can be anticipated, bearing in mind the tolerances of the protection system.

13.7   Environmental Protection

Medical devices should be designed to withstand the worst case environmental conditions in the product specification, with a safety margin included. Some typical environmental ranges that the device may experience include:

operating temperature	0 to +55 degrees centigrade
storage temperature	-40 to +65 degrees centigrade
humidity	95% RH at 40 degrees centigrade

mechanical vibration   5 to 300 Hz at 2 Gs
mechanical shock 24" to 48" drop
mechanical impact   10 Gs at a 50 msec pulse width
electrostatic discharge   up to 50,000 volts

Electromagnetic compatibility becomes an issue in an environment, like an operating room. Each medical device should be protected from interference from other equipment, such as electrocautery and should be designed to eliminate radiation to other equipment.

13.8   Product Misuse

An area of design concern that was briefly addressed earlier in this chapter is the subject of product misuse. Whether through failure to properly read the operation manual or through improper training, medical devices are going to be misused and even abused. There are many stories of product misuse, such as the hand held monitor that was dropped into the toilet bowl, the user who used a hammer to pound a 9-volt battery into a monitor backwards or the user who spilled a can of soda on and into a device. Practically, it is impossible to make a device completely misuse-proof. But it is highly desirable to design around the ones that can be anticipated.

Some common examples of product misuse include:

- excess application of cleaning solutions
- physical abuse
- spills
- excess weight applied to certain parts
- excess torque applied to controls or screws
- improper voltages, frequencies or pressures
- improper or interchangeable electrical or pneumatic connections.

Product misuse should be discussed with Marketing to define as many possible misuse situations as can be anticipated. The designer must then design around these situations, including a safety margin, which will serve to increase the reliability of the device. Where design restrictions limit the degree of protection against misuse and abuse, the device should alarm or should malfunction in a manner that is obvious to the user.

13.9   Design for Variation

During design, one may need to deal with the problem of assessing the combined effects of multiple variables on a measurable output or other characteristic of a product, by means of experiments. This is not a problem that is important in all designs, particularly when there are fairly large margins between capability and required performance, or for design involving negligible risk or uncertainty, or when only one or a few items are to be manufactured. However, when designs have to be optimized in relation to variations in parameter values, processes, and environmental conditions, particularly if these variations can have combined effects, it is necessary to use methods that can evaluate the effects of the simultaneous variations.

Statistical methods of experimentation have been developed which enable the effects of variation to be evaluated in these types of situation. They are applicable whenever the effects cannot be theoretically evaluated, particularly when there is a large component of random variation or interactions between variables. For multivariable problems, the methods are much more economical than traditional experiments, in which the effect of one variable is evaluated at a time. The traditional approach also does not enable interactions to be analyzed, when these are not known empirically.

13.10   Design of Experiments

The statistical approach to design of experiments is a very elegant, economical, and powerful method for determining the s-significant effects and interactions in multivariable situations.

13.10.1 The Taguchi Method

Genichi Taguchi developed a framework for statistical design of experiments adapted to the particular requirements of engineering design.

Taguchi suggested that the design process consists of three phases: system
design, parameter design, and tolerance design. In the system design phase, the
basic concept is decided, using theoretical knowledge and experience to
calculate the basic parameter values to provide the performance required.
Parameter design involves refining the values so that the performance is
optimized in relation to factors and variation which are not under the effective
control of the designer, so that the design is robust in relation to these.
Tolerance design is the final stage, in which the effects of random variation of
manufacturing processes and environments are evaluated, to determine whether
the design of the product and the production processes can be further optimized,
particularly in relation to cost of the product and the production processes.

Taguchi separates variables into two types. Control factors are those
variables which can be practically and economically controlled, such as a
controllable dimensional or electrical parameter. Noise factors are the variables
which are difficult or expensive to control in practice, though they can be
controlled in an experiment, e.g., ambient temperature, or parameter variation
with a tolerance range. The objective is then to determine the combination of
control factor settings (design and process variables) which will make the
product have the maximum robustness to the expected variation in the noise
factors.

13.11   Design Changes

Design changes occur throughout the design process. Often, assessing
the impact of changes of all aspects of the project can be very difficult. This is
particularly true for large projects involving multifunctional design teams. It is
important to have the design under revision control, so that the history of
changes may be tracked. To accomplish this, a design change methodology
should be employed. Each change to the design should be reviewed,
documented and approved before it is implemented. A simple change form, such
as that indicated in Figure 13-5 can be used. This type of form limits the number
of reviewers, but assures the appropriate personnel on the development team are
informed of the change.

The basic question for design change is when is a design put under
revision control. For example, the product specification changes frequently in
the beginning of the process, as will other documentation. To institute a

DESIGN REVISION CONTROL SHEET

Revision Control Number:_____

Subsystem:		Old Revision:	
Origination Date:		New Revision:	
Origination Site:			

Summary (additional information may be attached):

Change Description:
Reason for the Change:

Functional Review:

Function	Signature
Project Leader	
System Coordinator	
Validation Coordinator	

Non-Approval (additional information may be attached):

Reason for Non-Approval:

Document Information:

Effectivity Date:	
Originator Signature:	

Figure 13-5   Sample design change form.

change process too early will cause an excessive amount of documentation to become part of the project file. It is far better for all design activity that revision control be instituted after the initial flurry of changes has occurred. The activity, whether a specification, drawing, program, etc., should be fairly stable and have been reviewed at least once. This will allow for an orderly control of the design without excessive documentation.

13.12   Design Reviews

Despite disciple, training, and care, it is inevitable that occasional oversights or errors will occur in new designs. Design reviews are held to highlight critical aspects of the design and to focus attention on possible shortfalls. Design review are held to:

- review the progress of a design
- monitor reliability growth
- assure all specifications are being addressed
- peer review the design approach.

The primary purpose of the design review is to make a choice among alternative design approaches. The output of the review should include an understanding of the weak areas in the design and the areas of the design in need of special attention. Topics to be covered in a design review include:

- redundancy versus derating
- redesign of weak areas versus high reliability parts
- review of Failure Mode and Effects Analysis
- review of potential product misuse
- review overstressed areas.

The design review should follow a structured order and be well documented with topics discussed, decisions reached, and resulting action items.

There are three overall types of design reviews:

Informal Design Reviews: To address detailed technical design and performance issues, usually for an isolated part of the product.

Formal Design Review: To address technical performance issues for the entire product and correlate activities with the project objectives and the product specifications.

Program Review: To examine the project relative to budget nd schedule performance, technical discoveries or limitations. Program reviews, also known as progress (or project) reviews, are generally conducted by senior managers and do not concern themselves with technical reviews of design.

Formal design reviews are generally held according to the project plan and are convened to support major project milestones. Plenty of time should be allowed for the review meeting. People should be invited who will challenge the design, including experts. The purpose is to review theory, technical design specs, implementation, and performance to specification. The design review should be held to challenge the design, not familiarize people with it. If familiarization is needed, a separate session should be held prior to the actual review. People should be allowed to talk freely. Criticism should be expected and accepted.. A dedicated person not expected to participate in the review should be asked to take the minutes.

Informal design reviews are generally not scheduled per the project plan and are convened when the need arises to address specific concerns. Informal design reviews are generally not scheduled per the project plan and are convened when the need arises to address specific concerns. Generally, only local reviewers are invited. The informal reviews are used to brainstorm a particularly tough problem or to analyze alternate design approaches. These reviews are generally extremely detailed and focus on a particular sub-system, module or component. Informal review results are usually documented in lab notebooks or supporting memos.

For all design reviews, it is optimal to assure the design review personnel have not taken part in the actual design activity. This gives a fresh and unbiased look at the design. Some of the guidelines for design reviewers include:

- design reviewers have a serious responsibility to comment on the potential outcome of the project

- when notice of review meetings are announced, reviewers should plan ahead and take time to prepare for the reviews
- the reviewers should assure they understand project objectives and the product specification
- reviewers should attend all formally planned learning sessions
- if possible, reviewers should submit concerns and questions to the review chair in advance of the design review meeting. The issues and concerns can be discussed in depth at the meeting.
- reviewers should help the design review leader during the meeting by questioning the design's performance relative to the product specification, design specification, project objectives, safety, effectiveness, and reliability of the product's functioning.

References

Fries, Richard C., *Reliable Design of Medical Devices.* New York: Marcel Dekker, Inc., 1997.

Government - Industry Data Exchange Program, *Program Summary.* June, 1979.

Jensen, F. and N. E. Peterson, *Burn-In.* New York: John Wiley and Sons, 1982.

Lloyd, D. K., and M. Lipow, *Reliability Management, Methods and Management.* 2nd Edition. Milwaukee, WI: American Society for Quality Control, 1984.

Logothetis, N. and H. P. Wynn, *Quality Through Design.* London, England: Oxford University Press, 1990.

Mason, R. L., W. G. Hunter, and J. S. Hunter, *Statistical Design and Analysis of Experiments.* New York: John Wiley & Sons, 1989.

MIL-STD-202, *Test Methods for Electronic and Electrical Component Parts.* Washington, DC: Department of Defense, 1980.

MIL-HDBK-217, *Reliability Prediction of Electronic Equipment.* Washington, DC: Department of Defense, 1986.

MIL-STD-750, *Test Methods for Semiconductor Devices.* Washington, DC: Department of Defense, 1983.

MIL-STD-781, *Reliability Design Qualification and Production Acceptance Tests: Exponential Distribution.* Washington, DC: Department of Defense, 1977.

MIL-STD-883, *Test Methods and Procedures for Microelectronics.* Washington, DC: Department of Defense, 1983.

Montgomery, D. C., *Design and Analysis of Experiments.* 2nd Edition. New York: John Wiley & Sons, 1984.

O'Connor, Patrick D. T., *Practical Reliability Engineering.* 3rd Edition. Chichester, England: John Wiley & Sons, 1991.

Reliability Analysis Center, *Nonelectronic Parts Reliability Data: 1995.* Rome, NY: Reliability Analysis Center, 1994.

Ross, P. J., *Taguchi Techniques for Quality Engineering.* New York: McGraw-Hill, 1988.

Taguchi, Genichi, *Introduction to Quality Engineering.* Unipub/Asian Productivity Association, 1986.

Taguchi, Genichi, *Systems of Experimental Design.* Unipub/Asian Productivity Association, 1978.

Chapter 14

Software Design

Sherman Eagles – Medtronic, Inc.
Minneapolis, Minnesota

Many medical devices are rapidly becoming software intensive. Software controls their operation, collects and analyzes information to help make treatment decisions and provides a way for users to interface with the medical device. In these devices, the software transforms a general-purpose computer into a special-purpose medical device component. As in hardware design, specifying the software requirements, creating a sound software design and correctly implementing it are difficult intellectual challenges. Software has additional challenges. It is nearly impossible to measure software to determine if it meets the first test of quality: that it exists as specified. And software provides a great deal of flexibility to work around hardware or other problems, particularly those discovered late in development. We can only address these challenges with a disciplined, methodical approach to the creation of software, i.e., software engineering.

Software engineering has both managerial and technical aspects. There are certain fundamental activities that are necessary for each of these aspects. Executing these fundamental activities well is the key to successful medical device software design.

It must be noted that the term software design has multiple meanings. Design used in the context of the medical device encompasses all the activities that occur before manufacturing of the device begins. Since software is entirely abstract, all of the software development activities occur before the manufacturing phase begins. So all of the activities done for software development are part of the device's software design. This is the meaning of the term as used in the title of this chapter. There are also specific technical activities that are performed during the software development that are called software design. These activities translate what the software must do into how these requirements will be accomplished by the software. They also organize the software to take into account the use of the details of the physical features of the medical device in accomplishing the device's purpose.

14.1   Fundamentals of Software Engineering Management

Good management of software development is critical to delivering a high quality, reliable product. There are many skills necessary to be a good manager. The intent here is not to try to describe what is required to be a good manager, but to identify some fundamental management activities that must be accomplished for software developers to be successful in their tasks. These fundamental management activities are:

- Planning
- Estimating
- Tracking progress.

14.2   Planning Software Development

After the Normandy invasion, Dwight Eisenhower reportedly said "Plans are worthless, but planning is everything." As soon as the action starts, a plan must start to change. None of us can ever foresee how all the variables in a project will turn out. Our plans can never be entirely correct. If we are to have any hope of keeping control of a project once it is underway, we must have done good planning. Good planning requires a clear understanding of the problem, a recognition of the assumptions being made, a definition of what success will be and an in-depth knowledge of the resources available and their strengths and weaknesses.

Planning encompasses more than just documenting resources needed for the project and creating a schedule. It includes looking at the project from a management view including schedule and resources, as well as looking at how the work will be done. What development model should be used? What methodology? What programming language and tools? Planning also includes identifying how the software will be controlled, and how it will be tested.

A key input to planning for medical device software is safety risk. The most important factor is the greatest severity of injury that can result from a software failure. The United States Food and Drug Administration calls this the "level of concern" of the software. Since the software can pose no greater risk of injury than the medical device it is a part of, the software level of concern cannot be greater than the risk of the device. It can possibly be lower if the software is not used to control critical device functions and if a software failure could only cause a lesser severity of injury than the device itself could. Understanding the software level of concern is important, because some choices in software methods and process are not appropriate for software with a high level of concern.

Often when a software development project is planned, some of the most important considerations aren't even discussed because everyone believes they are so obvious. These are the objectives for the project and the assumptions that the project team is making. Making these explicit and clear allows the project team to recognize when objectives change or assumptions are not being fulfilled. This allows the team to adjust, rather than continuing down a path that is unlikely to succeed.

Another area that good planning addresses is relationships between groups. A project may depend on the work of others. Without thinking through and getting agreement on how knowledge and information will be shared, or how deliverables are to be made available, much time and effort may be used in managing communication breakdowns that have a high level of emotion. Actions as simple as asking questions may become a problem if the person being asked is on the critical path of another project. Thinking through a process for resolving issues between groups before the project gets underway is a beneficial exercise that is too frequently overlooked or left to be thought about "when it gets to be a problem."

Sub-contractors are often used for developing parts of the software. This can be a very useful approach, reducing development time and adding expertise in an area where the development team may not have much experience. On the other hand, managing the contract may not be simple. The developer of the medical device is responsible for all the components used in it, and must make sure that the software being developed by the contractor is of sufficient quality for its intended purpose. Once again, careful planning before the work begins will allow for adjustments to be made when unexpected situations arise.

Project risks are another topic that planning should address. Establishing the four Cs for all significant foreseeable risks will provide a great deal of help should one or more of them become a problem: chronology (when will the risk be quantified), contingencies (what are the possible courses of action that could be followed), consequences (what are the likely results of each action), and criteria (how will the course of action be chosen). Having gone through the process of analyzing potential project risks during the planning phase of the project will also provide help for dealing with unexpected problems that may come up after the project is underway.

14.3   Choosing the Software Development Process Model

A software development process model is the portion of a software life cycle model that occurs before the first release of the software. For any software development, there are some fundamental activities that always are performed, and some optional activities that are included to improve the likelihood of meeting specific project objectives such as short development schedule, high reliability, or high conformance with customer desires. The sequence in which these activities are performed, and the formality with which they are performed and documented may vary. A software development process describes the activities to be performed and defines the chronological ordering of these activities. In order to define the development schedule, a software development process model must be selected.

There are a number of basically different software development process models, with many variations. Whether a particular model is appropriate depends on the goals of the project and the level of concern of the software.

14.4   Development Process Models for High Level of Concern

If the requirements of the software are established and reliability is a major objective, such as for software with a higher level of concern, these software development process models should be considered.

14.4.1   Waterfall Model

This was the first documented software life cycle model. It divides the development process into steps, each of which reduces the level of abstraction of the solution. Each step includes a verification task and an exit criteria that must be met before moving on to the next step. As much as possible, iterations of a step are performed during the subsequent step.

The waterfall model's advantages are that it helps find errors early and provides a well understood structure. Its difficulties are that the requirements must be fully specified at the beginning of the project, before any design work has started. Finding out that requirements are wrong or incomplete late in the project can lead to extensive rework.

The waterfall model works best for complex systems where the requirements and technical methodologies are well understood. Many variations have been defined, such as overlapping steps, breaking implementation steps into parallel subprojects, and adding an introductory risk analysis step.

14.4.2   Incremental Delivery Model

The incremental delivery model is a modification of the waterfall model. It starts like the waterfall by analyzing requirements and creating an architectural design. Instead of delivering all of the software functionality at the end of the project, the functionality is divided up into increments that are delivered successively through out the project. Each increment refines the requirements and architectural design, then does detailed design, implementation, verification and release of its functionality.

This model works well when there is a need to deliver partial functionality before all of the functionality is needed. For example, a new medical device might need some software functionality for early hardware testing, additional functionality for validating expected clinical results in animals, more functionality when a human clinical study is performed, and the complete functionality for the market release of the device.

14.4.3   Spiral Model

The spiral model was developed by Boehm to address some of the difficulties with the waterfall model. The spiral model iterates a set of steps, creating in effect a series of mini projects. Each of these mini projects completes a loop around the spiral. The first step in each of these mini projects is to determine the objectives, alternatives and constraints for the portion of the product being developed. The next step is to determine risks and resolve them. Then the alternatives are evaluated, the deliverables for the iteration are developed and verified and a plan for the next iteration is created.

The main advantages of the spiral model are its flexibility and that it is risk driven, and as the project progresses and costs increase, the risks decrease. The disadvantage is that the spiral model requires expertise in risk management.

14.4.4   Cleanroom Model

The cleanroom model was created to develop software that has a predictable reliability. It combines a set of techniques that depend on verifying the correctness of each step in the development process model. This results in more formality in specifying requirements, performing design and implementing the design in code. Since each step is verified as correct, cleanroom eliminates structural testing. It uses a statistical approach to functional testing to demonstrate that the requirements were implemented and to measure the software reliability in terms of mean time to failure.

Since the design is verified against the requirements, the requirements specification must be complete before design can begin. The requirements specification must also be written with sufficient formality that functional correctness verification of the design can be supported. This can best be achieved by using a formal specification language. The design must proceed in small steps, each being verified to be equivalent with its predecessor. Verification based inspections, which inspect for correctness rather than defects, are used to provide independent confirmation of the design's correctness.

Software coding proceeds in a similar manner of stepwise implementation and verification using inspections. Since the code is verified for correctness to the design, no developer debugging or unit testing is needed for demonstrating that the code implements the design. Cleanroom eliminates this activity, and the developers do not execute their code.

Cleanroom relies on independent testing to ensure that the requirements were implemented correctly. It also uses statistical testing techniques, sampling inputs based on probability of usage, to determine the software's reliability. It adds a feedback loop driven by continuously measuring reliability to the incremental delivery development process model in order to improve the reliability of each incremental delivery. The result is a final product with very high quality and a predictable reliability.

14.5   Development Process Models for Low Level of Concern

For low level of concern software, where there is no safety risk, other
objectives may lead to different development process models. If the
requirements are understood, but the primary objective is time to market,
the design to schedule development process model may be appropriate.
If the requirements are not well understood and the primary objective is to
demonstrate functionality, the evolutionary delivery model may be the best
choice. These models are probably not acceptable for higher level of
concern software.

14.5.1   Design to Schedule Model

This model prioritizes functionality and then develops it incrementally,
with the early increments having the highest priority features. The difference
between this model and the incremental delivery model is that with the design to
schedule model you quit when the deadline is reached no matter how much has
been delivered. At the beginning of the project, it is unclear how many of the
planned increments will be completed.

14.5.2   Evolutionary Delivery Model

This model is used when requirements are changing rapidly or are not
understood very well at the beginning of the project. The portions of the system
that are best understood are developed and delivered. Feedback is gathered from
users or potential users and the additional understanding is used to evolve the
product to another version, which is developed and delivered. This iterative
process is repeated until the users are satisfied that the necessary functionality is
present in the software.

14.5.3   Code and Fix Model

If no planning is done, the default that gets used is called the code and
fix model. It is not really a software development process model, but more the
lack of one. With the code and fix model, you start with an idea of what you
want to build, maybe write some specifications, then start coding, debugging
and testing. As problems are found, they are fixed and sent back for more
testing. When the number of problems being found in test falls to an acceptable
level, or you run out of time to do more testing and fixing, you release the
product. This model is not recommended for any type of software development,
and is clearly not acceptable for any development in which software could
result in loss of safety.

14.6   Choosing a Design Method

As with development process models, there are a number of basically
different software design methods with many variations. They each provide
criteria for expressing and refining the principles of good software design. As
with life cycle models, each work best for certain types of problems. Whether a
particular method is appropriate depends on the characteristics and level of
concern of the software.

Most software design methods take one of three approaches:

- Top-down structured analysis and design
- Data-driven analysis and design
- Object-oriented analysis and design.

All these methods use decomposition to divide a complex problem into
parts that are small enough to be understood and implemented correctly. They
differ in what is being decomposed. Top-down structured analysis and design
uses algorithmic decomposition, data-driven analysis and design uses data
structure decomposition and object-oriented analysis and design uses object
decomposition.

14.6.1   Structured Analysis and Structured Design

Structured analysis and structured design grew from the ideas of structured programming and was popularized in the 1970s. It is a top down refinement approach that presents details in a layered fashion, hiding the detailed information regarding the design until the appropriate level. Structured analysis shows how data logically moves through a system being transformed by processes. Each process is decomposed into another set of processes and data flows providing more detail. The logical building blocks are algorithms, and the system is decomposed until the function of each process is a simple algorithm performing a single function.

Structured design partitions the system physically into modules that are organized into hierarchies with defined interfaces. Each module should solve one piece of the problem. Each module should be easy to understand. Connections between the modules should be as simple as possible. Each module has four attributes: input and output, function, internal logic and internal data.

14.6.2   Data-driven Analysis and Design

Data-driven analysis and design derives the structure of the software from the structure of the data that is input to the software and the structure of the data that is output by the software. These input and output structures are first modeled using a graphical notation. They then are converted into a program structure that maps inputs to outputs. The processing necessary to make the transformation from the input to output can be identified and associated with the program structure. The processing can then be decomposed as necessary. Data-driven design has been applied primarily to systems where input and output structures can be well defined and which have little concern for time-critical events, such as information management systems.

14.6.3   Object-oriented Analysis and Design

Object-oriented analysis and design groups data and the functions performed on that data into a single entity called an object. Rather than identifying data structures and process structures separately and then decomposing each, the object-oriented approach models systems in the real world as collections of objects which collaborate to perform some behavior. Objects can be identified, they can take action, and the current values of their properties can be determined. These characteristics are called identity, behavior and state. Objects communicate by messages which cause the receiving object to take an action.

14.7   Choosing a Programming Language

Programming languages are the tools used to transform the software design into executable instructions for the computer. The manner in which the programming language chooses to implement fundamental design concepts impacts the usability of the language. The trade-offs between programming languages are on characteristics such as ease of use, flexibility, performance, size of code generated, ease of maintenance and availability of development tools. The choice of programming language depends on the type of problem, the availability of tools for the target hardware, the design method chosen and the objectives of the project.

There is no such thing as a "safe" programming language. The responsibility for producing safe software rests with the software engineering team. A major consideration in the selection of a programming language is the availability of programmers with experience using the language. Programmers who are experienced with a language are more likely to know the potential problems and avoid them. There are however, some attributes of programming languages that make it easier for experienced programmers to produce dependable code. These include:

- Strong data typing - Will the data typing prevent misuse of variables?
- Exception handling - Do mechanisms exist to recover from runtime malfunctions?

- Separate compilation - Can modules be compiled separately? Is there type checking across module boundaries?
- Exhaustion of memory - Are there ways to guard against running out of memory at runtime?

When available, programming languages that provide these facilities would be a better choice for software which has safety as a primary objective.

14.8   Estimating and Scheduling

Once the choices of development process, design method and programming language have been made, it is possible to estimate the size of the software and the effort required for developing it. Of course, the more that is understood about the requirements, the more precise the estimates can be. Often, estimates must be made very early in the project, long before the details are known. There are several techniques and heuristics that can be used to help produce early estimates for planning the project.

One technique that is valuable is to use more than one method to estimate. This may include estimating the effort for each module based on past experience with similar modules, design and programming language. These estimates can be summed to provide an overall estimate for the project. A second method would be to estimate the size of the modules using lines of code or function points and then using one of the parametric tools available, such as COCOMO or SLIM. These tools will provide estimated effort for the project based on size and other parameters. If the estimates from different methods differ widely, more work must be done to understand why and which estimate needs modification.

Another technique that is valuable is to have more than one person provide estimates. Achieving a consensus from several estimators can greatly improve the estimate. The Delphi method can be used to achieve this consensus even when the estimators can't meet to discuss their estimates. In this method, anonymous estimates are provided by multiple software engineers. If there is no consensus, the results are anonymously reported back to the estimators and they are asked to refine their estimates and provide rationale for them. These steps are repeated until a consensus emerges. While the Delphi method may be excessive for all but very large projects, at minimum, having a peer review of all estimates before they are used can help ensure that major items are not overlooked.

Being able to compare what has been estimated to actual results from similar development is extremely valuable. Having data from historical projects organized and available is a great advantage, but even if the data hasn't been formally collected, a little detective work can uncover a great deal of useful information. It is well worth the time to do it.

It is important to be careful about expecting too much in productivity improvements from new technology or methods. Most organizations follow a similar development process model on every similar project. New tools or even changing the design method or programming language will not have a large immediate impact on the overall productivity for a project.

One of the most important factors to consider in the estimate is the impact of any system resource constraints placed upon the software. Limits on memory, mass storage, processing time or other resources can greatly increase the time and effort needed to develop the software. In some cases, getting the software to work can be done quickly, but getting it to work within the constraints may take a great deal of effort.

A similar concern is the case where the hardware that the software will execute on is being developed concurrently with the software. In this case, integrating the system will be a challenge, and seems to almost always take more time and effort than planned.

14.9   Tracking Progress

Once the estimate is complete and a schedule in place, tracking progress to the schedule is necessary to control the project. The most common way of tracking and communicating progress is called earned value accounting. It integrates scope, cost, and schedule measures to assess performance. Earned value involves calculating three key values for each activity:

- The planned cost of the activity. This is called the budgeted cost of work scheduled (BCWS)
- The actual cost of the activity. This is called the actual cost of work performed (ACWP)
- The earned value, also called the budgeted cost of work performed (BCWP). This is a percentage of the total budget equal to the percentage of the work actually completed.

These values can be used to calculate the cost variance (CV = BCWP - ACWP) and the schedule variance (SV = BCWP - ACWP) at the time of the progress report. They can also be used to forecast the project cost at completion and the project completion date.

14.10 Necessary Technical Software Development Activities

Software development is done in the context of systems engineering. What the system is to do must be determined first. These system requirements are then used to develop a system architecture, identifying which functions will be performed by which component of the system. The decisions about how to allocate functions to various components are made based on the objectives for the system, such as performance, cost, reliability, weight, power consumption, etc. The functions that are allocated to the software become the starting point for the software requirements analysis.

Technical software development activities produce work products that must be verified. Static analysis techniques such as reviews, walkthroughs and inspections, and dynamic techniques such as unit testing and system testing are used to verify the work products. These techniques will be discussed in the chapter on software verification and validation.

14.11 Software Requirements Analysis

This is the first technical step in the software engineering development process. Software requirements analysis refines the system requirements allocated to software to provide a model of the software behavior. The first task in software requirements analysis is to fully understand the basic elements of the problem that the software must solve. This includes identifying the exact purpose of the system, who will use it, and what the constraints are on the possible solutions. Once the problem is completely recognized, the functionality and data necessary for a solution are identified. Various alternative solutions can be analyzed and evaluated based on the criteria most important for the particular application. The results of this analysis is a set of function, data, performance and external interface requirements that define precisely what to build. These requirements make up the software requirements specification. The SRS plays many roles in a large development project.

1. It is the contract between management and the development team on exactly what is to be built.
2. It records the results of the analysis. It shows where the requirements are complete and where additional work is needed.
3. It defines what properties the software must have, and where there are constraints that limit the design choices.
4. It is used for estimating size and determining cost and schedule.
5. It is used by testers to determine acceptable behavior of the software.
6. It provides the standard definition of the expected behavior of the software for the system's maintainers.

If any commercially available off-the-shelf software is being included in the medical device software, it must be fully identified in the software requirements specification.

14.12 Software Hazard Analysis

For medical device software, software requirements analysis must also specify safety requirements. Identified system hazards that have been traced down to software must be mitigated by requirements or constraints on the software's behavior. These requirements and constraints are also documented in the software requirements specification and must be consistent with the rest of the software requirements.

The most direct way to trace system hazards to software is with a top-down fault tree analysis. How the software can contribute to the hazard condition is determined, and then requirements or constraints are identified that will prevent this software condition from occurring. When the software condition can be prevented by adding functionality, a requirement is written. If the software condition can only be prevented by constraining something from happening, a design constraint is written. Requirements are much easier to implement and verify than constraints and should be used to mitigate the software condition if possible. After these safety requirements and constraints are documented, it must be shown that the software requirements specification satisfies them. To do this, the software requirements specification must completely describe the behavior of the software under all conditions. Checking the software requirements specification for completeness requires analysis of states, transitions between states, inputs and outputs, values and timing. Some examples of criteria for checking specification completeness are:

- Every software state must be reachable from the initial software state
- Every software state must have a behavior specified for every possible input
- All information from sensors should be used somewhere in the specification
- Interlock failures should result in the halting of hazardous functions
- All incoming values should be checked and a response specified in the event of an out-of-range or unexpected value
- The response to excessive inputs must be specified
- Safety-critical outputs should be checked for reasonableness and for hazardous values.

14.13 Requirements Traceability

To assure that all requirements are implemented in the product, each requirement should be traced to the component of the design where it is implemented. In order to accomplish this, each requirement and each design component must be uniquely identified.

Traceability information can be maintained in traceability tables or in traceability lists. A traceability table is a matrix with requirements on one axis and design components on the other. The cell that is at the intersection of the requirement and the associated design component contains an entry showing the relationship. In a traceability list, each requirement is identified, along with a list of the design components that implement it.

To assure that all hazard mitigations result in requirements that are included in the software requirements specification, the hazard mitigations should be traced to the software requirements specification in the same manner that the requirements are traced to design components.This level of traceability makes it easy to see that each mitigation in the hazard analysis is identified in the software requirements and included in the software design. By extending this traceability to verification, it can be shown that all hazards mitigated by software have been specified, implemented and verified.

14.14 Software Architectural Design

Software architectural design defines the major structural elements of the software, their externally visible properties and the relationship among them. It partitions the real world problem (the software requirements) into elements of a software solution and organizes the relationships between these elements. The primary objective is to achieve an abstract representation of the structure, both of control and data. If the behavior of an element can impact other elements, that behavior should be described in the architecture. A modular program structure defining the control relationships between components and an organization of the logical relationship among the data elements is the starting point for software design. Some rules of thumb for good architectures:

- Well defined modules with functionality based on the principles of information hiding and separation of concerns
- Hardware specifics should be encapsulated
- Dependencies on commercial tools or products should be encapsulated
- Separate modules that are producers of data from those that are consumers of data

- Modules should be defined so they can be implemented independently.

Safety must be designed into a system. Trying to add safety on at the end of development can increase risk due to added complexity. Architectural decisions are extremely important for implementing safety requirements. The concept of modularity, allocating design decisions into separate components, is a characteristic of a good design that is almost essential to be able to verify that safe operation has been achieved. Without understanding (and documenting) the behavior of a component that may impact other components, it will be nearly impossible to show that the system is safe.

14.15 Detailed Design

Detailed design refines the abstract architectural design, filling in the details necessary to construct the final product. Detailed design must specify algorithms, data representations, connections between different processing elements and between processing elements and data structures. Detailed design must also be concerned with the packaging of the software product. Detailed design is performed using the chosen methodology. No matter what design methods and techniques are used, there are a number of fundamental design concepts that are important.

Modularity - The design should identify components or modules, and each module should solve one well-defined piece of the problem. The purpose of each module should be well defined. Each module should include the functional processing, data structures and control mechanisms necessary to achieve its purpose. Modules should communicate with each other using well-defined interfaces.

Information hiding - The internal processing details and data used by a module should not be observable from outside the module. The design decisions and their implementation should be hidden from other modules. This allows the detailed design and implementation decisions to be changed without impacting other modules.
Structure - This determines how the processing in a module is organized and controlled. If the software is thought of as a network,

made up of processing nodes connected by control or data links, the logical path through the network is the structure. Examples of structure include hierarchical ordering and concurrent ordering. In hierarchically ordered modules, the processing elements are related by "uses" and "is used by" relationships. In a hierarchy, process nodes execute sequentially , the relationships are directed, and a node is not allowed to use a node that precedes it in the sequence. In a concurrent structure, process nodes execute in parallel and control is maintained by use of shared variables and message passing, using mechanisms such as semaphores and queues.

Encapsulation - If a data structure can only be accessed by routines packaged with it in a single module it is said to be encapsulated. Other routines that use the data structure do so by using the access routines. They do not need to know how the data structure is implemented.

Cohesion - This measures the strength of the relatedness of elements within a module. Maximizing cohesion will reduce the number of interconnections between modules. Cohesion is described as (from weakest or least desirable to strongest or most desirable):

1. Coincidental cohesion - elements within the module have no apparent relationship to one another
2. Logical cohesion - elements within the module perform similar functions
3. Temporal cohesion - all elements are executed at the same time
4. Communication cohesion - all elements refer to the same set of input/output data
5. Sequential cohesion - the output of one element is used as the input for the next element
6. Functional cohesion - all elements are related to the performance of a single function
7. Informational cohesion - each element performs a single function and all elements refer to a single data structure.

Coupling - This is the measure of the strength of connections between modules. It measures how well information hiding has been achieved.

The stronger the coupling between two modules, the more likely that a change in one of the modules will require a change in the other. Coupling is ranked from strongest (least desirable) to weakest (most desirable).

1. Content coupling - the module modifies internal data or instructions in the other module
2. Common coupling - all modules share global data items
3. Control coupling - a module passes control flags that determine the sequence of processing in another module
4. Stamp coupling - only modules that require the data share global data
5. Data coupling - data items are passed between modules via parameters.

14.16 Implementation (Coding)

After a module has been designed, the design must be translated into source code. This is a detailed, labor intensive task. The primary goals are to write the code so that its purpose is clear, so that it correctly implements the design, and so that it will integrate easily into the system. Simplicity and clarity are desirable characteristics, complexity and cleverness are to be avoided. This is especially true in any software that is critical to safety. In this case, standard techniques should be used that are easy to understand and are easily documented.

To consistently achieve the desirable code characteristics, coding standards are used to specify a preferred coding style. Coding standards usually include items such as:

1. Naming conventions for variables and functions
2. Guidelines for scope of data
3. Guidelines for using specific types of data
4. Guidelines for control structures
5. Use of assertions and other error detection practices

6. Specific items to be aware of in the particular programming language

7. Documentation conventions.

Documentation that is included with the source code should provide the information necessary to maintain the module. This documentation should address how the module accomplishes its function and illuminate any portion of the code that may not be sufficiently self-documenting. The documentation generally consists of a prologue or header which has a standard format and comments embedded in the code that explain major data manipulations or end cases and exception handling.

14.17 Integration

Integration is the combining of code that has been implemented independently into a single system where it must work together. One approach to integration is to have a specific integration phase in the development process model. The individual software modules are built in the previous phases and then combined into a system in the integration phase. This is often referred to as "big bang" integration. While it is possible to wait until all the code has been developed to put it together as a system, the effort required to get everything working may be very great. In practice it is much more efficient to integrate the code a small piece at a time. This approach is called incremental integration, or sometimes continuous integration. Incremental integration requires establishing an initial system and then adding just a little additional code at a time, while making sure that the system continues to operate. This requires careful planning and tight control over the order in which code is added to the system since modules must be integrated after other modules which they depend upon. The integration control process must include criteria for including new code in each version of the system.

Incremental integration has several additional advantages. Each software element can be tested as part of the system, eliminating the need to develop a special testing bed to test the new software element. Incremental integration also provides a focus on the source of problems. If a problem appears, it is probably related to the new module being added to the system, either in the new module itself or in the interfaces between it and the rest of the system. Incremental integration also provides flexibility, since it is possible to easily revert to the previous system if adding a new module results in a problem.

14.18 Software Configuration Management

The goal of software configuration management is to control and track changes in the software to assure that nothing is lost or destroyed. Change will occur during all phases of the software development process. The reason change occurs is that the more is known about the customers needs, the device requirements, the software design, etc. These changes are necessary and valuable, but can lead to a great deal of confusion and rework if they are not coordinated and controlled.

All of the work products that make up a software product need to have changes controlled. This includes the software requirements and design as well as the code and tests. The controlled work products are called configuration items. In order to control change to these configuration items, each version of a configuration item must be identifiable. Part of software configuration management is to establish an identification scheme that provides both a unique name and a unique version identifier for each configuration item. Individual configuration items are often combined into groups to produce a software product. Another part of configuration management is to identify this collection of specific versions of configuration items.

Configuration control means that any version of a single configuration item or a named collection of configuration items can be retrieved or recreated at any time. Configuration control is often achieved by use of a version control library, which contains all revisions to each configuration item and a record of which versions are combined for each named collection version.

Another important element of configuration management is change control itself. Once a configuration item is placed under configuration management, a process must be identified as to how it can be modified. The key elements of the process are why a change is needed, who is making the change, who reviews and approves the change and when the change was made.

Once testing has begun, it is crucial to know what changes have been made so that appropriate re-testing can be done. An important part of configuration management is the ability to provide reports on the status of the configuration items and the changes. Each new version of the software work products should be able to show that all necessary changes were implemented and tested and that no unapproved changes were made.

In a safety critical system, it is also important to know that the changes did not negatively affect mitigation of hazards. Each change should be analyzed to determine if it affected a requirement that specifies a hazard mitigation, or a design component that implements a safety requirement.

14.19 Conclusion

Software is becoming a key technology in medical devices. To produce safe, reliable software requires a methodical engineering approach. The management activities of software engineering; planning, estimating, scheduling and tracking progress, are required before the technical software engineering activities can be successful.

Planning for software development includes documenting the software's role in the medical device system and understanding the level of concern of the software. Objectives and assumptions must be identified and dependencies on other groups specified. Key decisions to be made during the planning include what software development process model to use, what design method will be followed and what programming language will be used to implement the software.

After deciding how the software will be developed, estimates must be made for effort and schedule. At least two different methods of estimating should be used and the results compared. After establishing the overall estimates, a detailed plan is necessary which breaks the project down into small pieces of work that can be assigned and measured. Overall project progress should be tracked to control the project. The most common method of tracking project progress is the earned value accounting method.

The technical activities in developing software that are always necessary, regardless of the development process model are:

- Software requirements analysis
- Software hazard analysis
- Software architectural design
- Software detailed design
- Software implementation
- Software integration
- Software configuration management.

Executing the basic tasks of these activities using defined methods and established criteria is the best way to create reliable, safe medical device software that meets its requirements and intended use.

References

Bass, Len, Paul Clements and Rick Kazman, *Software Architecture in Practice*. Reading, Massachusetts: Addison Wesley Longman, Inc., 1998.

Boehm, Barry W., "A Spiral Model of Software Development and Enhancement," *Computer*. May, 1988.

Boehm, Barry W., *Software Engineering Economics*. Englewood Cliffs, New Jersey: Prentice-Hall, Inc. 1981.

Booch, Grady, *Object-Oriented Analysis and Design with Applications - Second Edition*. Redwood City, California: The Benjamin Cummings Publishing Company, Inc. 1994.

Booch, Grady, Ivar Jacobson and James Rumbaugh, *The Unified Modeling Language User Guide*. Reading, Massachusetts: Addison Wesley Longman, Inc., 1998.

Deutsch, Michael S. and Ronald R. Willis, *Software Quality Engineering - A Total Technical and Management Approach.* Englewood Cliffs, New Jersey. Prentice-Hall, 1988.

Dyer, Michael, *The Cleanroom Approach to Quality Software Development.* New York: John Wiley & Sons, Inc., 1992.

Fairley, Richard E., *Software Engineering Concepts.* New York: McGraw-Hill Book Company, 1985.

Hatley, Derek J. and Imtiaz A. Pirbhai, *Strategies for Real-Time System Specification.* New York: Dorset House Publishing, 1987.

Humphrey, Watts S., *Managing the Software Process.* Reading, Massachusetts: Addison-Wesley Publishing Company, 1989.

Kan, Stephen H., *Metrics and Models in Software Quality Engineering.* Reading, Massachusetts: Addison Wesley Longman, Inc., 1995.

Leveson, Nancy G., *Safeware.* Reading, Massachusetts: Addison-Wesley Publishing Company, 1995.

McConnell, Steve., *Code Complete.* Redmond, Washington: Microsoft Press, 1993.

McConnell, Steve., *Rapid Development.* Redmond, Washington: Microsoft Press, 1996.

Page-Jones, Meilir, *The Practical Guide to Structured Systems Design - Second Edition.* Englewood Cliffs, New Jersey. Prentice-Hall, Inc., 1988.

Pressman, R., *Software Engineering.* New York: McGraw-Hill Book Company, 1987.

Putnam, Lawrence H. and Ware Myers, *Measures for Excellence.* Englewood Cliffs, New Jersey: P T R Prentice-Hall, Inc., 1992.

Rakos, John J., *Software Project Management for Small to Medium Sized Projects.* Englewood Cliffs, New Jersey: Prentice-Hall, 1990.

Rumbaugh, James, et al., *Object-Oriented Modeling and Design.* Englewood Cliffs, New Jersey: Prentice-Hall, 1991.

Rumbaugh, James, Ivar Jacobson and Grady Booch, *The Unified Modeling Language Reference Manual.* Reading, Massachusetts: Addison Wesley Longman, Inc., 1998.

Sommerville, Ian and Pete Sawyer, *Requirements Engineering.* Chichester, England: John Wiley & Sons, Inc., 1997.

Storey, Neil, *Safety-Critical Computer Systems.* Harlow, England: Addison Wesley Longman, 1996.

Thayer, Richard H. and Merlin Dorfman, editors, *Software Requirements Engineering - Second Edition.* Los Alamitos, California: IEEE Computer Society Press, 1997.

Yourdon, Edward., *Modern Structured Analysis.* Englewood Cliffs, New Jersey: Yourdon Press, 1989.

Chapter 15

Human Factors Engineering

Richard C. Fries, PE, CRE – Datex-Ohmeda, Inc.
Madison, Wisconsin

In 1989, a study conducted at Brigham and Womens Hospital, in Boston, attempted to determine the causes of medical device failures within the hospital environment over an eleven month period. The results of the study indicated 41% of device problems or failures were caused by user problems or errors. The use and/or misuse of a medical device is thus seen to have an important impact on the overall reliability of the device. The methodology that addresses such user issues is Ergonomics or Human Factors.

15.1   What Is Human Factors?

Human Factors is defined as the application of the scientific knowledge of human capabilities and limitations to the design of systems and equipment to produce products with the most efficient, safe, effective, and reliable operation. This definition includes several interesting concepts.

Although humans are capable of many highly technical, complex or intricate activities, they also have limitations to these activities. Of particular interest to the medical designer are limitations due to physical size, range of motion, visual perception, auditory perception, and mental capabilities under stress. Although the user may be characterized by these limitations, the designer cannot allow them to adversely affect the safety, effectiveness, or reliability of the device. The designer should therefore identify and address all possible points of interface between the user and the equipment, characterize the operating environment, and analyze the skill level of the intended users.

Interface points are defined as those areas that the user must control or maintain in order to derive the desired output from the system. Interface points include control panels, displays, operating procedures, operating instructions, and user training requirements.

The environment in which the device will be used must be characterized to determine those areas that may cause problems for the user, such as lighting, noise level, temperature, criticality of the operation, and the amount of stress the user is experiencing while operating the system. The design must then be adjusted to eliminate any potential problems.

The skill level of the user is an important parameter to be analyzed during the design process and includes such characteristics as educational background, technical expertise, and computer knowledge. To assure the user's skill levels have been successfully addressed, the product should be designed to meet the capabilities of the least skilled potential user. Designing to meet this worst case situation will assure the needs of the majority of the potential users will be satisfied.

The final and most important activity in Human Factors Engineering is determining how these areas interact within the particular device. The points of interface are designed based on the anticipated operating environment and on the skill level of the user. The skill level may depend not only on the education and experience of the user, but on the operating environment, as well. To design for such interaction, the designer must consider the three elements that comprise human factors: the human element, the hardware element, and the software element.

15.1.1   The Human Element in Human Factors Engineering

The human element addresses several user characteristics, including memory and knowledge presentation, thinking and reasoning, visual perception, dialogue construction, individual skill level, and individual sophistication. Each is an important factor in the design consideration.

A human being has two types of memory. Short-term memory deals with sensory input, such as visual stimuli, sounds, and sensations of touch. Long term memory is composed of our knowledge database. If the human-machine interface makes undue demands on either short- or long-term memory, the performance of the individual in the system will be degraded. The speed of this degradation depends on the amount of data presented, the number of commands the user must remember, and/or the stress involved in the activity.

When a human performs a problem-solving activity, they usually apply a set of guidelines or strategies based on their understanding of the situation and their experiences with similar types of problems, rather than applying formal inductive or deductive reasoning techniques. The human-machine interface must be specific in a manner enabling the user to relate to their previous experiences and develop guidelines for a particular situation.

The physical and cognitive constraints associated with visual perception must be understood when designing the human-machine interface. For example, studies have shown that since the normal line of sight is within 15 degrees of the horizontal line of sight, the optimum position for the instrument face is within a minimum of 45 degrees of the normal line of sight (Figure 15-1). Other physical and cognitive constraints have been categorized and are available in references located at the end of this chapter.

When people communicate with one another, they communicate best when the dialogue is simple, easy to understand, direct, and to the point. The designer must assure device commands are easy to remember, error messages are simple, direct, and not cluttered with computer jargon and help messages are easy to understand and pointed. The design of dialogue should be addressed to the least skilled potential user of the equipment.

The typical user of a medical device is not familiar with hardware design or computer programming. They are more concerned with the results

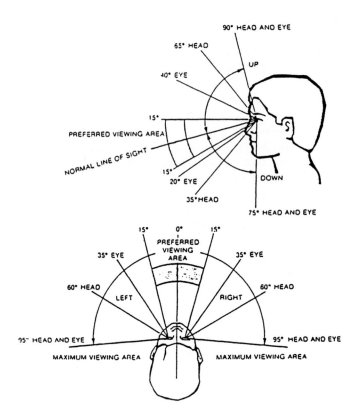

		MAXIMUM*		
	PREFERRED	EYE ROTATION	HEAD ROTATION	HEAD AND EYE ROTATION
UP	15°	40°	65°	90°
DOWN	15°	20°	35°	75°
RIGHT	15°	35°	60°	95°
LEFT	15°	35°	60°	95°

* Display area on the console defined by the angles measured from the normal line of sight.

Figure 15.1   Normal line of sight.   (From Fries, 1997.)

obtained from using the device, than about how the results were obtained. They want a system that is convenient, natural, flexible and easy to use. They don't want a system that looks imposing, is riddled with computer jargon, requires them to memorize many commands, or has unnecessary information cluttering the display areas.

In summary, the human element requires a device that has inputs, outputs, controls, displays and documentation that reflect an understanding of the user's education, skill, needs, experience, and the stress level when operating the equipment.

15.1.2   The Hardware Element in Human Factors

The hardware element considers size limitations, the location of controls, compatibility with other equipment, the potential need for portability, and possible user training. It also addresses the height of the

preferred control area and the preferred display area when the operator is standing (Figure 15-2), when the operator is sitting (Figure 15-3) and the size of the human hand in relation to the size of control knobs or switches (Figure 15-4).

Hardware issues are best addressed by first surveying potential customers of the device to help determine the intended use of the device, the environment in which the device will be used, and the optimum location of controls and displays. Once the survey is completed and the results analyzed, a cardboard, foam, or wooden model of the device is built and reviewed with the potential customers. The customer can then get personal, hands-on experience with the controls, displays, the device framework, and offer constructive criticism on the design. Once all changes have been made, the model can be transposed into a prototype, using actual hardware.

15.1.3   Software Element in Human Factors

The software element of the device must be easy to use and understand. It must have simple, reliable data entry, it should be menu driven if there are many commands to be learned, displays must not be

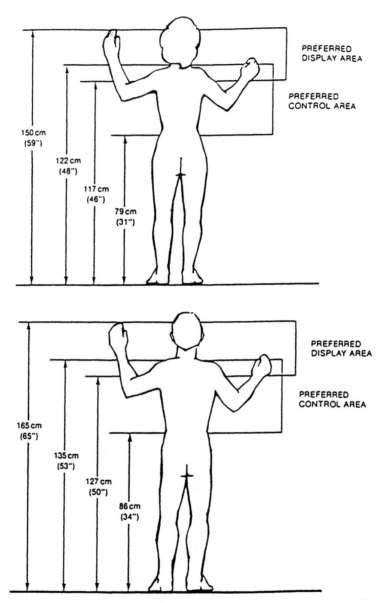

Figure 15-2   Display area when standing. (From Fries, 1997.)

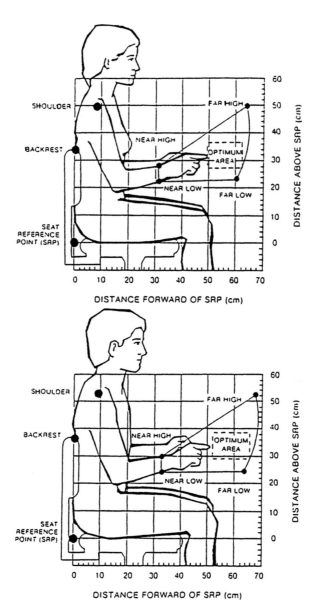

Figure 15-3   Display area when sitting. (From Fries, 1997.)

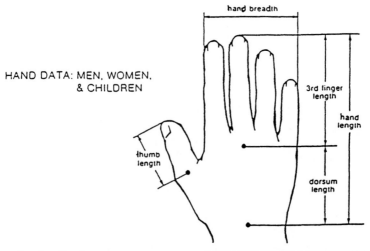

HAND DATA: MEN, WOMEN,
        & CHILDREN

HAND DATA	MEN			WOMEN			CHILDREN			
	2.5% tile	50.% tile	97.5% tile	2.5% tile	50.% tile	97.5% tile	6 yr.	8 yr.	11 yr.	14 yr.
hand length	173mm (6.8")	191mm (7.5")	208mm (8.2")	157mm (6.2")	175mm (6.9")	191mm (7.5")	130mm (5.1")	142mm (5.6")	160mm (6.3")	178mm (7.0")
hand breadth	81mm (3.2")	89mm (3.5")	97mm (3.8")	66mm (2.6")	74mm (2.9")	79mm (3.1")	58mm (2.3")	64mm (2.5")	71mm (2.8")	—
3rd finger lg.	102mm (4.0")	114mm (4.5")	127mm (5.0")	91mm (3.6")	100mm (4.0")	112mm (4.4")	74mm (2.9")	81mm (3.2")	89mm (3.5")	102mm (4.0")
dorsum lg.	71mm (2.8")	75mm (3.0")	81mm (3.2")	66mm (2.6")	74mm (2.9")	79mm (3.1")	56mm (2.2")	61mm (2.4")	71mm (2.8")	75mm (3.0")
thumb length	61mm (2.4")	69mm (2.7")	75mm (3.0")	56mm (2.2")	61mm (2.4")	66mm (2.6")	46mm (1.8")	51mm (2.0")	56mm (2.2")	61mm (2.4")

ADDITIONAL DATA: AVERAGE MAN

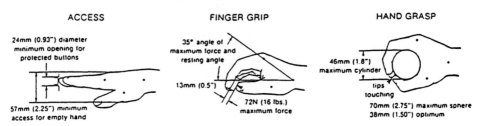

Figure 15.4   Hand sizes. (From Fries,, 1997.)

overcrowded, and dialogue must not be burdened with computer jargon. The software must provide feedback to the user through error messages and help messages. An indication that the process is involved in some activity is also important, as a blank screen leads to the assumption that nothing is active, and the user starts pushing keys or buttons.

Software must consider the environment in which it is to be used, especially with regard to colors of displays, type of data to be displayed, format of the data, alarm levels to be used, etc. Stress and fatigue can be reduced by consideration of color and the intensity of the displayed data. Operator effectiveness can be improved by optimizing the location of function keys, displaying more important data in the primary viewing area, and placing secondary data in the secondary display area. The inclusion of device checkout procedures and menus also improves operator effectiveness and confidence.

15.2   Human Factors Process

Human Factors is the sum of several processes including the analytic process that focuses on the objectives of the proposed device and the functions that should be performed to meet those objectives; the design and development process that converts the results of the analyses into detailed equipment design features; and the test and evaluation process which verifies that the design and development process has resolved issues identified in the analytic process.

Human Factors Engineering integrations begins with early planning and may continue throughout the lifecycle of the device. As a minimum, Human Factors should continue until the device is introduced commercially. Human Factors efforts following commercial introduction are important to the enhancement of the device and the development of future devices.

15.2.1   Planning

A Human Factors plan should be developed as an integral part of the overall plan for device development. The plan should guide Human Factors efforts in the interrelated processes of analysis, design and development, and test and evaluation. The plan should describe Human Factors tasks necessary to complete each process, the expected results of those tasks, the means of coordinating those tasks with the overall process for device development, and the schedule for that coordination. The plan should address the resources necessary for its accomplishment including levels of effort, necessary for its management and coordination as well as for accomplishment of its individual tasks.

The plan should assure that results of Human Factors tasks are available in time to influence the design of the proposed device as well as the conduct of the overall project. Analysis tasks should begin very early. Iterations of analysis tasks that refine earlier products may continue throughout the project. Design and development build on the products of early analysis, and iterations may also continue throughout the project. Test and evaluation should begin with the earliest products of design and development. The results of test and evaluation should influence subsequent iterations of analysis, design and development, and test and evaluation tasks.

15.2.2 Analysis

Successful Human Factors is predicated on careful analyses. Early analyses should focus on the objectives of the proposed device and the functions that should be performed to meet those objectives. Later analysis should focus on the critical human performance required of specific personnel as a means of establishing the Human Factors parameters for design of the device and associated job aids, procedures, and training and for establishing Human Factors test and evaluation criteria for the device. Analyses should be updated as required to remain current with the design effort.

15.2.3 Conduct User Studies

The goal of user studies is to learn as much as possible within a reasonable time frame about the customer's needs and preferences as they relate to the product under development. Several methods are available for getting to know the customer.

15.2.3.1 Observations

Observations are a productive first step toward getting to know the user. By observing people at work, a rapid sense for the nature of their jobs is developed, including the pace and nature of their interactions with the environment, co-workers, patients, equipment and documents. Such observations may be conducted in an informal manner, possibly taking notes and photographs. Alternatively, a more formal approach may be taken that includes rigorous data collection. For example, it may be important to document a clinician's physical movements and the time they spend performing certain tasks to determine performance benchmarks. This latter approach is referred to as a time-motion analysis and may be warranted if one of the design goals is to make the customer more productive.

Enough time should be spent observing users to get a complete sense for how they perform tasks related to the product under development. A rule of thumb in usability testing is that 5-8 participants provide 80-90 percent of the information you seek. The same rule of thumb may be applied to observations, presuming that you are addressing a relatively homogenous user population. Significant differences in the user population (i.e., a heterogenous user population) may warrant more extensive observations. For example, it may become necessary to observe people who have different occupational backgrounds and work in different countries.

Designers and engineers should conduct their own observations. For starters, such observations increase empathy for the customer. Also, first-hand experience is always more powerful than reading a marketing report.

15.2.3.2 Interviews

Similar to observations, interviews provide a wealth of information with a limited investment of time. Structured interviews based on scripted questions are generally better than unstructured interviews (i.e., a free flowing conversation). This is because a structured interview assures that the interviewer will ask everyone the same question, enabling a comparison of answers. Structured interviews may include a few open-ended questions to produce evoke comments and suggestions that could not be anticipated. The interview script should be developed from a list of information needs.

Generally, questions should progress from general to more specific design issues. Care should be taken to avoid mixing marketing and engineering related concerns with usability concerns.

Interviews can be conducted just after observations are completed. Conducting the interviews prior to the observations can be problematic as it tends to alter the way people react.

15.2.3.3 Focus Groups

Conducting interviews with people in their working environment (sometimes referred to as contextual interviewing) is generally best. Interviewees are likely to be more relaxed and opinionated. Interviews conducted at trade shows and medical conferences, for example, are more susceptible to bias and may be less reliable.

Conducting interviews with a group of 5-10 people at a time enables easy determination of a consensus on various design issues. In preparation for such a focus group, a script should be developed from a set of information requirements. Use the script as a guide for the group interview, but feel free to let the discussion take a few tangents if they are productive ones. Also, feel at liberty to include group exercises, such as watching a video or ranking and rating existing products, as appropriate.

Conduct enough focus groups to gain confidence that an accurate consensus has been developed. Two focus groups held locally may be enough if regional differences of opinion are unlikely and the user group is relatively homogenous. Otherwise, it may be appropriate to conduct up to 4 groups each at domestic and international site that provides a reasonable cross section of the marketplace.

Document the results in a focus groups report. The report can be an expanded version of the script. Begin the report with a summary section to pull together the results. Findings (i.e., answers to questions) may be presented after each question. The findings from various sites may be integrated or presented separately, depending on the design issue and opportunity to tailor the product under development to individual markets. Results of group exercises may be presented as attachments and discussed in the summary.

15.2.3.4 Task Analysis

The purpose of task analysis is to develop a detailed view of customer interactions with a product by dividing the interactions into discrete actions and decisions. Typically, a flow chart is drawn that shows the sequence and logic of customer actions and decisions. The task analysis is extended to include tables that define information and control requirements associated with each action and decision. In the course of the task analysis, characterize the frequency, urgency and criticality of integrated tasks, such as "checking the breathing circuit."

15.2.3.5 Benchmark Usability Test

The start of a new product development effort is a good time to take stock of the company's existing products. An effective way to do this is to conduct a benchmark usability test that yields, in a quantitative fashion, both objective and subjective measures of usability. Such testing will identify the strengths and weaknesses of the existing products, as well as help establish usability goals for the new product.

15.2.3.6 User Profile

To culminate the user study effort, write a so-called user profile. A user specification (2-5 pages) summarizes the important things learned about the customers. The profile should define the user population's demographics (age, gender, education level, occupational background, language), product-related experience, work environment and motivation level. The user profile is a major input to the user specification that describes the product under development from the customer's point of view.

15.2.3.7 Setup an Advisory Panel

To assure early and continued customer involvement, set up an advisory panel that equitably represents the user population. The panel may include 3-5 clinicians for limited product development efforts, or be twice as large for larger efforts. The panel participants are usually compensated for their time. Correspond with members of the panel on an as needed basis and meet with them periodically to review the design in progress. Note that advisory panel reviews are not an effective replacement for usability testing.

15.2.4   Set Usability Goals

Usability goals are comparable to other types of engineering goals in the sense that they are quantitative and provide a basis for acceptance testing. Goals may be objective or subjective. A sample objective goal might be: on average, users shall require 3 seconds to silence an alarm. This goal is an objective goal because the user's performance level can be determined simply by observation. For example, you can use a stop watch to determine task times. Other kinds of objective goals concentrate on the number of user errors and the rate of successful task completion.

A sample subjective goal is: on average, 75% of users shall rate the intuitiveness of the alarm system as 5 or better, where 1 = poor and 7 = excellent. This goal is subjective because it requires asking the user's opinion about their interaction with the given product. A rating sheet can be used to record their answers. Other kinds of subjective goals concentrate on mental processing and emotional response attributes, such as learning, frustration level, fear of making mistakes, etc.

Every usability goal is based on a usability attribute, e.g., task, speed or intuitiveness, includes a metric such as time or scale and sets a target performance level, such as 3 seconds or a rating of 5 or better.

Typically, up to 50 usability goals may be written, two-thirds of which are objective and one-third which are subjective. The target performance level on each goal is based on findings from preceding user studies, particularly the benchmark usability testing. If there is no basis for comparison, i.e., there are no comparable products, then engineering judgement must be used to set the initial goals and adjust them as necessary to assure they are realistic.

15.2.5   Design User Interface Concepts

Concurrent design is a productive method of developing a final user interface design. It enables the thorough exploration of several design concepts before converging on a final solution. In the course of exploring alternative designs, limited prototypes should be built of the most promising concepts and user feedback obtained on them. This gets users involved in the design process at its early stages and assures that the final design will be closely matched to user's expectations.

Note that the design process steps described below assume that the product includes both hardware and software elements. Some steps would be moot if the product has no software user interface.

15.2.5.1 Develop Conceptual Model

When users interact with a product, they develop a mental model of how it works. This mental model may be complete and accurate or just the opposite. Enabling the user to develop a complete and accurate mental model of how a product works is a challenge. The first step is developing so-called conceptual models of how to represent the product's functions. This exercise provides a terrific opportunity for design innovation. The conceptual model may be expressed as a bubble diagram, for example, that illustrates the major functions of the product and functional interrelationships as you would like the users to think of them. You can augment the bubble diagram with a narrative description of the conceptual model.

15.2.5.2 Develop User Interface Structure

Develop alternative user interface structures that compliment the most promising 2-3 conceptual models. These structures can be expressed in the form of screen hierarchy maps that illustrate where product functions reside and how many steps it will take users to get to them. Such maps may take the form of a single element, a linear sequence, a tree structure (cyclic or acyclic) or a network. In addition to software screens, such maps should show which functions are allocated to dedicated hardware controls.

15.2.5.3 Define Interaction Style

In conjunction with the development of the user interface structures, alternative interaction styles should be defined. Possible styles include question and answer dialogs, command lines, menus and direct manipulation.

15.2.5.4 Develop Screen Templates

Determine an appropriate size display based on the user interface structure and interaction style, as well as other engineering considerations. Using computer-based drawing tools, draw the outline of a blank screen. Next, develop a limited number (perhaps 3-5) of basic layouts for the information that will appear on the various screens. Normally, it is best to align all elements, such as titles, windows, prompts, numerics according to a grid system.

15.2.5.5 Develop Hardware Layout

Apply established design principles in the development of hardware layouts that are compatible with the evolving software user interface solutions. Assure that the layouts reinforce the overall conceptual model.

15.2.5.6 Develop a Screenplay

Apply established design principles in the development of a detailed screenplay. Do not bother to develop every possible screen at this time. Rather, develop only those screens that would enable users to perform frequently used, critical and particularly complex functions. Base the screen designs on the templates. Create new templates or eliminate existing templates as required while continuing to limit the total number of templates. Assure that the individual screens reinforce the overall conceptual model. You may choose to get user feedback on the screenplay (what some people call a paper prototype).

15.2.5.7 Develop a Refined Design

Steps 5 and 6 describe prototyping and testing the user interface. These efforts will help determine the most promising design concept or suggest a hybrid of two or more concepts. The next step is to refine the preferred design. Several reiterations of the preceding steps may be necessary, including developing a refined conceptual model, developing a refined user interface structure and developing an updated set of screen templates. Then, a refined screenplay and hardware layout may be developed.

15.2.5.8 Develop a Final Design

Once again, steps 5 and 6 describe prototyping and testing the user interface. These efforts will help you determine any remaining usability problems with the refined design and opportunities for further improvement. It is likely that design changes at this point will be limited in nature. Most can be made directly to the prototype.

15.2.6   Model the User Interface

Build a prototype to evaluate the dynamics of the user interface. Early prototypes of competing concepts may be somewhat limited in terms of their visual realism and how many functions they perform. Normally, it is best to develop a prototype that 1) presents a fully functional top-level that allows users to browse their basic options, and 2) enables users to perform a few sample tasks, i.e., walkthrough a few scenarios. As much as possible, include tasks that relate to the established usability goals.

User interface prototypes may be developed using conventional programming languages or rapid prototyping languages such as SuperCard, Altia Design, Visual Basic, Toolbook, and the like. The rapid prototyping languages are generally preferable because they allow for faster prototyping and they are easier to modify based on core project team and user feedback.

Early in the screenplay development process, it may make sense to prototype a small part of the user interface to assess design alternatives or to conduct limited studies, such as how frequently to flash a warning. Once detailed screenplays of competing concepts are available, build higher fidelity prototypes that facilitate usability testing. Once a refined design is developed, build a fully functional prototype that permits a verification usability test. Such prototypes can be refined based on final test results and serve as a specification.

15.2.7   Test the User Interface

There are several appropriate times to conduct a usability test, including:

- at the start of a development effort to develop benchmarks

- when you have paper-based or computer-based prototypes of competing design concepts

- when you have a prototype of your refined design

- when you want to develop marketing claims regarding the performance of the actual product.

While the rigor of the usability test may change, based on the timing of the test, the basic approach remains the same. You recruit prospective users to spend a concentrated period of time interacting with the prototype product. The users may undertake a self-exploration or perform directed tasks. During the course of such interactions, you note the test participants comments and document their performance. At intermittent stages, you may choose to have the test participant complete a questionnaire or rating/ranking exercise. Videotaping test proceedings is one way to give those unable to attend the test a first-hand sense of user-product interactions. Sometimes it is useful to create a 10-15 minute highlight tape that shows the most interesting moments of all test sessions.

During testing, collect the data necessary to determine if you are meeting the established usability goals. This effort will add continuity and objectivity to the usability engineering process.

15.3   Specifying the User Interface

15.3.1   Style Guide

The purpose of a style guide is to document the rules of the user interface design. By establishing such rules, you can check the evolving design to determine any inconsistencies. Also, it assures the consistency of future design changes. Style guides, usually 10-15 pages in length, normally include a description of the conceptual model, the design elements and elements of style.

15.3.2   Screen Hierarchy Map

The purpose of a screen hierarchy map is to provide an overview of the user interface structure. It places all screens that appear in the screenplay in context. It enables the flow of activity to be studied in order to determine if it reinforces the conceptual model. It also helps to determine how many steps users will need to take to accomplish a given task. Graphical elements of the screen hierarchy map should be cross-indexed to the screenplay.

15.3.3   Screenplay

The purpose of a screenplay is to document the appearance of all major screens on paper. Typically, screen images are taken directly from the computer-based prototype. Ideally, the screenplay should present screen images in their actual scale and resolution. Each screen should be cross-indexed to the screen hierarchy map.

15.3.4   Specification Prototype

The purpose of the specification prototype is to model accurately the majority of user interface interactions. This provides the core project team with a common basis for understanding how the final product should work. It provides a basis for writing the user documentation. It may also be used to orient those involved in marketing, sales and training.

15.3.5   Hardware Layouts

The hardware layout may be illustrated by the specification prototype. However, the hardware may not be located proximal to the software user interface. If this is the case, develop layout drawings to document the final hardware layout.

15.4   Additional Human Factors Design Considerations

The design of medical devices should reflect human factors engineering design features that increase the potential for successful performance of tasks and for satisfaction of design objectives.

15.4.1   Consistency and Simplicity

Where common functions are involved, consistency is encouraged in controls, displays, markings, codings, and arrangement schemes for consoles and instrument panels.

Simplicity in all designs is encouraged. Equipment should be designed to be operated, maintained, and repaired in its operational environment by personnel with appropriate but minimal training. Unnecessary or cumbersome operations should be avoided when simpler, more efficient alternatives are available.

15.4.2   Safety

Medical device design should reflect system and personnel safety factors, including the elimination or minimization of the potential for human error during operation and maintenance under both routine and non-routine or emergency conditions. Machines should be designed to minimize consequence of human error. For example, where appropriate, a design should incorporate redundant, diverse elements arranged in a manner that increases overall reliability when failure can result in the inability to perform a critical function.

Any medical device failure should immediately be indicated to the operator and should not adversely affect safe operation of the device. Where failures can affect safe operation, simple means and procedures for averting adverse effects should be provided.

When the device failure is life-threatening or could mask a life-threatening condition, an audible alarm and a visual display should be provided to indicate the device failure. Wherever possible, explicit notification of the source of failure should be provided to the user. Concise instructions on how to return to operation or how to invoke alternate backup methods should be provided.

15.4.3 Environmental/Organizational Considerations

The design of medical devices should consider the following:

- the levels of noise, vibration, humidity, and heat that will be generated by the device and the levels of noise, vibration, humidity, and heat to which the device and its operators and maintainers will be exposed in the anticipated operational environment
- the need for protecting operators and patients from electric shock, thermal, infectious, toxicologic, radiologic, electromagnetic, visual, and explosion risks, as well as from potential design hazards, such as sharp edges and corners, and the danger of the device falling on the patient or operator
- the adequacy of the physical, visual, auditory, and other communication links among personnel and between personnel and equipment
- the importance of minimizing psychophysiological stress and fatigue in the clinical environment in which the medical device will be used
- the impact on operator effectiveness of the arrangement of controls, displays and markings on consoles and panels (Figure 15-5)

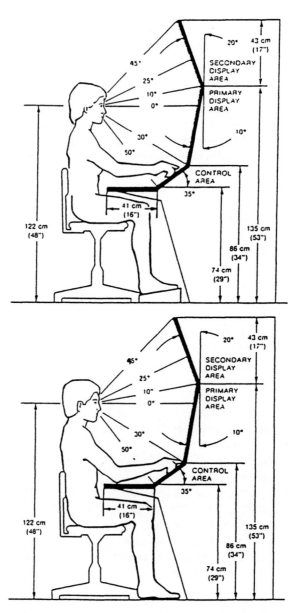

Figure 15-5   Arrangement of controls and displays. (From Fries, 1997.)

- the potential effects of natural or artificial illumination used in the operation, control, and maintenance of the device
- the need for rapid, safe, simple, and economical maintenance and repair
- the possible positions of the device in relation to the users as a function of the user's location and mobility
- the electromagnetic environment(s) in which the device is intended to be used.

15.5   Documentation

Documentation is a general term that includes operator manuals, instruction sheets, online help systems, and maintenance manuals. These materials may be accessed by many types of users. Therefore, the documentation should be written to meet the needs of all target populations.

Preparation of instructional documentation should begin as soon as possible during the specification phase. This assists device designers in identifying critical human factors engineering needs and in producing a consistent human interface. The device and its documentation should be developed together.

During the planning phase, a study should be made of the capabilities and information needs of the documentation users, including:

- the user's mental abilities
- the user's physical abilities
- the user's previous experience with similar devices
- the user's general understanding of the general principles of operation and potential hazards associated with the technology
- the special needs or restrictions of the environment.

As a minimum, the operator's manual should include detailed procedures for setup, normal operation, emergency operation, cleaning and operator troubleshooting.

The operator manual should be tested on models of the device. It is important that these test populations be truly representative of end-users and that they not have advance knowledge of the device.

Maintenance documentation should be tested on devices that resemble production units.

Documentation content should be presented in language free of vague and ambiguous terms. The simplest words and phrases that will convey the intended meaning should be used. Terminology within the publication should be consistent. Use of abbreviations should be kept to a minimum, but defined where they are used.

Information included in warnings and cautions should be chosen carefully and with consideration of the skills and training of intended users. It is especially important to inform users about unusual hazards and hazards specific to the device.

Human Factors Engineering design features should assure that the device functions consistently, simply, and safely, that the environment, system organization and documentation are analyzed and considered in the design, thus increasing the potential for successful performance of tasks and for satisfaction of design objectives.

15.6   Anthropometry

Anthropometry is the science of measuring the human body and its parts and functional capacities. Generally, design limits are based on a range of values from the 5th percentile female to the 95th percentile male for critical body dimensions. The 5th percentile value indicates that five percent of the population will be equal to or smaller than that value and 95 percent will be larger. The 95th percentile value indicates that 95 percent of the population will be equal to or smaller than that value and five percent will be larger. The use of a design range from the 5th to the 95th percentile values will theoretically provide coverage from 90 percent of the user population for that dimension.

15.6.1 Functional Dimensions

The reach capabilities of the user population play an important role in the design of the controls and displays of the medical device. The designer should take into consideration both one- and two-handed reaches in the seated and standing positions (Figures 15-6 and 15-7).

Body mobility ranges should be factored into the design process. Limits of body movement should be considered relative to the age diversity and gender of the target user population.

The strength capacities of the device operators may have an impact on the design of the system controls. The lifting and carrying abilities of the personnel responsible for moving and/or adjusting the device need to be considered to assure the device can be transported and adjusted efficiently and safely.

15.6.2 Psychological Elements

It is crucial to consider human proficiency in perception, cognition, learning, memory, and judgement when designing medical devices to assure that operation of the system is as intuitive, effective, and safe as possible. This is discussed in Chapter 1.

15.6.3 Workstation Design Considerations

Successful workstation design is dependent on considering the nature of the tasks to be completed, the preferred posture of the operator, and the dynamics of the surrounding environment. The design of the workstation needs to take into account the adjustability of the furniture, clearances under work surfaces, keyboard and display support surfaces, seating, footrests, and accessories.

The effectiveness with which operators perform their tasks at consoles or instrument panels depends in part on how well the equipment is designed to minimize parallax in viewing displays, allow ready manipulation of controls, and provide adequate space and support for the operator.

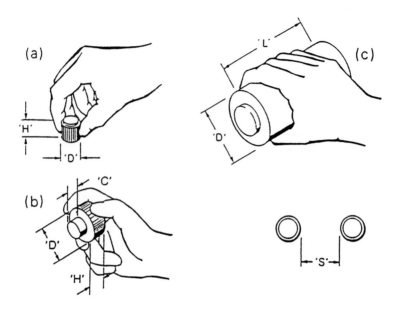

	DIMENSIONS						
	(a) Finger Grasp		(b) Thumb and Fingers Encircled			(c) Palm/Hand Grasp	
	'H' Height	'D' Diameter	'H' Height	'D' Diameter	'C' Clearance	'D' Diameter	'L' Length
Minimum	13 mm (0.5")	10 mm (0.375")	13 mm (0.50")	25 mm (1.0")	16 mm (.625")	38 mm (1.5")	75 mm (3.0")
Maximum	25 mm (1.0")	100 mm (4")	25 mm (1.0")	75 mm (3.0")	—	75 mm (3")	—

	TORQUE		'S' SEPARATION
	*	**	One Hand Individually
Minimum	—	—	25 mm (1.0")
Preferred	—	—	50 mm (2.0")
Maximum	32 mN-m (4.5 in.-oz.)	42 mN-m (6.0 in.-oz.)	—

* To and including 25 mm (1.0") diameter knobs.
** Greater than 25 mm (1.0") diameter knobs.

Figure 15-6   Example of functional dimensions. (From Fries, 1997.)

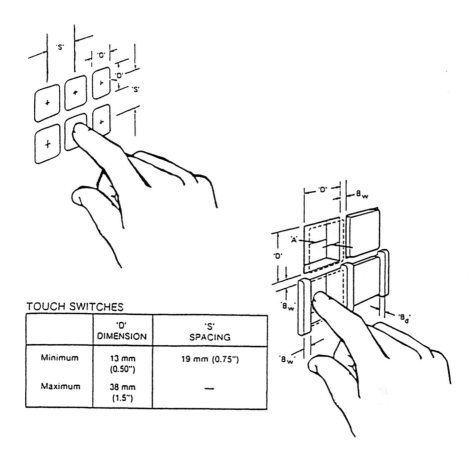

TOUCH SWITCHES

	'D' DIMENSION	'S' SPACING
Minimum	13 mm (0.50")	19 mm (0.75")
Maximum	38 mm (1.5")	—

PUSHBUTTON SWITCHES

	'D' DIMENSION	'A' Displacement	SEPARATION/BARRIERS *		RESISTANCE
			'Bw'	'Bd'	
Minimum	19 mm (0.75")	3 mm** (0.125")	3 mm (0.125")	5 mm (0.187")	280 mN (10 oz.)
Maximum	38 mm (1.5")	6 mm (0.250")	6 mm (0.250")	6 mm (0.250")	16.6 N (60 oz.)

* Barriers shall have rounded edges.
** 5 mm (.188") for positive position switches.

Figure 15-7   Example of functional dimensions. (From Fries, 1997.)

A horizontal or nearly horizontal work surface serves primarily as a work or writing surface or as a support for the operator's convenience items. Certain types of controls, such as joysticks or tracking controls, can also be part of the surface design.

Controls should have characteristics appropriate for their intended functions, environments, and user orientations, and their movements should be consistent with the movements of any related displays or equipment components. The shape of the control should be dictated by its specific functional requirements. In a bank of controls, those controls affecting critical or life-supporting functions should have a special shape and, if possible, a standard location.

Controls should be designed and located to avoid accidental activation. Particular attention should be given to critical controls whose accidental activation might injure patients or personnel or might compromise device performance. Feedback on control response adequacy should be provided as rapidly as possible.

15.7   Alarms and Signals

The purpose of an alarm is to draw attention to the device when the operator's attention may be focused elsewhere. Alarms should not be startling but should elicit the desired action from the user. When appropriate, the alarm message should provide instructions for the corrective action that is required. In general, alarm design will be different for a device that is continuously attended by a trained operator, such as an anesthesia machine, than for a device that is unattended and operated by an untrained operator, such as a patient-controlled analgesia device. False alarms, loud and startling alarms, or alarms that recur unnecessarily can be a source of distraction for both an attendant and the patient and thus be a hindrance to good patient care.

Alarm characteristics are grouped in the following three categories:

- high priority: a combination of audible and visual signals indicating that immediate operator response is required
- medium priority: a combination of audible and visual signals indicating that prompt operator response is required

- low priority: a visual signal, or a combination of audible and visual signals indicating that operator awareness is required.

A red flashing light should be used for a high priority alarm condition unless an alternative visible signal that indicates the alarm condition and its priority is employed. A red flashing light should not be used for any other purpose.

A yellow flashing light should be used for a medium priority alarm condition unless an alternative visible signal that indicates the alarm condition and it priority is employed. A yellow flashing light should not be used for any other purpose.

A steady yellow light should be used for a low priority alarm condition unless an alternative visible signal that indicates the alarm condition and its priority is employed.

Audible signals should be used to alert the operator to the status of the patient or the device when the device is out of the operator's line of sight. Audible signals used in conjunction with visual displays should be supplementary to the visual signals and should be used to alert and direct the user's attention to the appropriate visual display.

Design of equipment should take into account the background noise and other audible signals and alarms that will likely be present during the intended use of the device. The lowest volume control settings of the critical life support audible alarms should provide sufficient signal strength to preclude masking by anticipated ambient noise levels. Volume control settings for other signals should similarly preclude such masking. Ambient noise levels in hospital areas can range from 50 dB in a private room to 60 dB in intensive care units and emergency rooms, with peaks as high as 65 to 70 dB in operating rooms due to conversations, alarms, or the activation of other devices. The volume of monitoring signals normally should be lower than that of high priority or medium priority audible alarms provided on the same device. Audible signals should be located so as to assist the operator in identifying the device that is causing the alarm.

The use of voice alarms in medical applications should normally *not* be considered for the following reasons:

- voice alarms are easily masked by ambient noise and other voice messages
- voice messages may interfere with communications among personnel who are attempting to address the alarm condition
- the information conveyed by the voice alarm may reach individuals who should not be given specific information concerning the nature of the alarm
- the types of messages transmitted by voice tend to be very specific, possibly causing complication and confusion to the user
- in the situation where there are multiple alarms, multiple voice alarms would cause confusion
- different languages may be required to accommodate various markets.

The device's default alarm limits should be provided for critical alarms. These limits should be sufficiently wide to prevent nuisance alarms, and sufficiently narrow to alert the operator to a situation that would be dangerous in the average patient.

The device may retain and store one or more sets of alarm limits chosen by the user. When more than one set of user default alarm limits exists, the activation of user default alarm limits should require deliberate action by the user. When there is only one set of user default alarm limits, the device may be configured to activate this set of user default alarm limits automatically in place of the factory default alarm limits.

The setting of adjustable alarms should be indicated continuously or on user demand. It should be possible to review alarm limits quickly. During user setting of alarm limits, monitoring should continue and alarm conditions should elicit the appropriate alarms. Alarm limits may be set automatically or upon user action to reasonable ranges and/or percentages above and/or below existing values for monitored variables. Care should be used in the design of such automatic setting systems to help prevent nuisance alarms or variables that are changing within an acceptable range.

An audible high- or medium-priority signal may have a manually operated, temporary override mechanism that will silence it for a period of time, e.g., 120 seconds. After the silencing period, the alarm should begin sounding again if the alarm condition persists or if the condition was temporarily corrected but has now returned. New alarm conditions that develop during the silencing period should initiate audible and visual signals. If momentary silencing is provided, the silencing should be visually indicated.

An audible high or medium priority signal may be equipped with a means of permanent silencing, that may be appropriate when a continuous alarm is likely to degrade user performance of associated tasks to an unacceptable extent and in cases when users would otherwise be likely to disable the device altogether. If provided, such silencing should require that the user either confirm the intent to silence a critical life support alarm or take more than one step to turn the alarm off. Permanent silencing should be visually indicated and may be signalled by a periodic audible reminder. Permanent silencing of an alarm should not affect the visual representation of the alarm and should not disable the alarm.

Life support devices and devices that monitor a life-critical variable should have an audible alarm to indicate a loss of power or failure of the device. The characteristics of this alarm should be the same as those of the highest priority alarm that becomes inoperative. It may be necessary to use battery power for such an alarm.

15.8   Labeling

Controls, displays, and other equipment items that need to be located, identified, or manipulated should be appropriately and clearly marked to permit rapid and accurate human performance. The characteristics of markings should be determined by such factors as the criticality of the function labeled, the distance from which the labels have to be read, the illumination level, the colors, the time available for reading, the reading accuracy required, and consistency with other markings.

Receptacles and connectors should be marked with their intended function or their intended connection to a particular cable. Convenience receptacles should be labeled with maximum allowable load in amperes or watts. The current rating of fuses should be permanently marked adjacent to the fuse holder. Fuse ratings should be indicated either in whole number, common fractions, or whole number plus common fractions. Labeling of fuses and circuit breakers should be legible in the ambient illumination range anticipated for the maintainer's location.

Operators and maintenance personnel should be warned of possible fire, radiation, explosion, shock, infection or other hazards that may be encountered during the use, handling, storage, or repair of the device. Electromedical instruments should be labeled to show whether they may be used in the presence of flammable gases or oxygen-rich atmospheres. Hazard warnings should be prominent and understandable.

Normally, labels should be placed above panel elements that users grasp, press, or otherwise handle so the label is not obscured by the hand. However, certain panel element positions, user postures, and handling methods may dictate other label placements. Labels should be positioned to ensure visibility and readability from the position in which they should be read.

Labels should be oriented horizontally so that they may be read quickly and easily from left to right. Although not normally recommended, vertical orientation may be used, but only where its use is justified in providing a better understanding of intended function. Vertical labels should be read from top to bottom. Curved labels should be avoided except when they provide setting delimiters for rotary controls.

Labels should not cover any other information source. They should not detract from or obscure figures or scales that should be read by the operator. Labels should not be covered or obscured by other units in the equipment assembly. Labels should be visible to the operator during control activation. All markings should be permanent and should remain legible throughout the life of the equipment under anticipated use and maintenance conditions.

The words employed in the label should express exactly what action is intended. Instructions should be clear and direct. Words that have a commonly accepted meaning for all intended users should be utilized. Unusual technical terms should be avoided. Labels should be consistent within and across pieces of equipment in their use of words, acronyms, abbreviations, and part/system numbers. No mismatch should exist between the nomenclature used in documentation and that printed on the labels.

Symbols should be used only if they have a commonly accepted meaning for all intended users. Symbols should be unique and distinguishable from one another. A commonly accepted standard configuration should be used.

Human Factors Engineering hardware design considerations should include functional dimensions, workstation architecture considerations, alarms and signals, and labeling, and should always take the operator's psychological characteristics into account. Chapter 6 discusses Human Factors Engineering software design considerations.

15.9   Software

Computerized systems should provide a functional interface between the system and users of that system. This interface should be optimally compatible with the intended user and should minimize conditions that can degrade human performance or contribute to human error. Thus, procedures for similar or logically related transactions should be consistent. Every input by a user should consistently produce some perceptible response or output from the computer. Sufficient online help should be provided to allow the intended but uninitiated user to operate the device effectively in its basic functional mode without reference to a user's manual or experienced operator. Users should be provided appropriate information at all times on system status either automatically or upon request. Provision of information about system dysfunction is essential.

In applications where users need to log-on to the system, log-on should be a separate procedure that should be completed before a user is required to select among any operational options. Appropriate prompts for log-on should be displayed automatically on the user's terminal with no special action required other than turning on the terminal. Users should be provided feedback relevant to the log-on procedure that indicates the status of the inputs. Log-on processes should require minimum input from the user, consistent with system access security.

In the event of a partial hardware/software failure, the program should allow for orderly shutdown and establishment of a checkpoint so restoration can be accomplished without loss of data.

Where two or more users need to have simultaneous access to a computer system, under normal circumstances, operation by one person should not interfere with the operations of another person. For circumstances in which certain operators require immediate access to the system, an organized system for insuring or avoiding preemption should be provided. Provisions should be made so that preempted users are notified and can resume operations at the point of interference without data loss.

15.9.1   Data Entry

Manual data entry functions should be designed to establish consistency of data entry transactions, minimize user's input actions and memory load, ensure compatibility of data entry with data display, and provide flexibility of user control of data entry. The system should provide feedback to the user about acceptance or rejection of an entry.

When a processing delay occurs, the system should acknowledge the data entry and provide the user with an indication of the delay. If possible, the system should advise the user of the time remaining for process completion.

Data entry should require an explicit completion action, such as the depression of an ENTER key to post an entry into memory. Data entries should be checked by the system for correct format, acceptable value, or range of values. Where repetitive entry of data sets is required, data validation for each set should be completed before another transaction can begin.

Data should be entered in units that are familiar to the user. If several different systems of units are commonly used, the user should have the option of selecting the units either before or after data entry. Transposition of data from one system of units to another should be accomplished automatically by the device. When mnemonics or codes are used to shorten data entry, they should be distinctive and have a relationship or association to normal language or specific job-related terminology.

Data deletion or cancellation should require an explicit action, such as the depression of a DELETE key. When a data delete function has been selected by a user, a means of confirming the delete action should be provided, such as a dialogue box with a delete acknowledgement button or a response to a question such as, Are you sure? (Y/N). In general, requiring a second press of the DELETE key is not preferred because of the possibility of an accidental double press. Similarly, after data have been entered, if the user fails to enter the data formally, for instance by pressing an ENTER key, the data should not be deleted or discarded without confirmation from the user.

Deleted data should be maintained in a memory buffer from which they can be salvaged, such as the UNDELETE option. The size and accessibility of this buffer should depend on the value of the data that the user can delete from the system.

The user should always be given the opportunity to change a data entry after the data have been posted. When a user requests change or deletion of a data item that is not currently being displayed, the option of displaying the old value before confirming the change should be presented. Where a data archive is being created, the system should record both the original entry and all subsequent amendments.

15.9.2   Displays

Visual displays should provide the operator with a clear indication of equipment or system status under all conditions consistent with the intended use and maintenance of the system. The information displayed to a user should be sufficient to allow the user to perform the intended task, but should be limited to what is necessary to perform the task or to make decisions. Information necessary for performing different activities, such as equipment operation versus troubleshooting, should not appear in a single display unless the activities are related and require the same information to be used simultaneously. Information should be displayed only within the limits of precision required for the intended user activity or decision making and within the limits of accuracy of the measure.

Graphic displays should be used for the display of information when perception of the pattern of variation is important to proper interpretation. The choice of a particular graphic display type can have significant impact on user performance. The designer should consider carefully the tasks to be supported by the display and the conditions under which the user will view the device before selecting a display type.

Numeric digital displays should be used where quantitative accuracy of individual data items is important. They should not be used as the only display of information when perception of the variation pattern is important to proper interpretation or when rapid or slow digital display rates inhibit proper perception.

Displays may be coded by various features, such as color, size, location, shape, or flashing lights. Coding techniques should be used to help discriminate among individual displays and to identify functionally related displays, the relationship among displays, and critical information within a display.

Display formats should be consistent within a system. When appropriate for users, the same format should be used for input and output. Data entry formats should match the source document formats. Essential data, text, and formats should be under computer, not user, control. When data fields have a naturally occurring order, such as chronological or sequential, such order should be reflected in the format organization of the fields. Where some displayed data items are of great significance, or require immediate user response, those items should be grouped and displayed prominently. Separation of groups of information should be accomplished through the use of blanks, spacing, lines, color coding, or other similar means consistent with the application.

The content of displays within a system should be presented in a consistent, standardized manner. Information density should be held to a minimum in displays used for critical tasks. When a display contains too much data for presentation in a single frame, the data should be partitioned into separately displayable pages. The user should not have to rely on memory to interpret new data. Each data display should provide the needed context, including the recapitulation of prior data from prior displays, as necessary.

An appropriate pointing device, such as a mouse, trackball, or touch screen, should be used in conjunction with applications that are suited to direct manipulation, such as identifying landmarks on a scanned image or selecting graphical elements from a palette of options. The suitability of a given pointing device to user tasks should be assessed.

15.9.3   Interactive Control

General design objectives include consistency of control action, minimized need for control actions, and minimized memory load on the user, with flexibility of interactive control to adapt to different user needs. As a general principle, the user should decide what needs doing and when to do it. The selection of dialogue formats should be based on anticipated task requirements and user skills.

System response times should be consistent with operational requirements. Required user response times should be compatible with required system response time. Required user response times should be within the limits imposed by the total user task load expected in the operational environment.

Control-display relationships should be straightforward and explicit, as well as compatible with the lowest anticipated skill levels of users. Control actions should be simple and direct, whereas potentially destructive control actions should require focused user attention and command validation/confirmation before they are performed. Steps should be taken to prevent accidental use of destructive controls, including possible erasures or memory dump.

Feedback responses to correct user input should consist of changes in the state or value of those elements of the displays that are being controlled. These responses should be provided in an expected and logical manner. An acknowledgement message should be employed in those cases where the more conventional mechanism is not appropriate. Where control input errors are detected by the system, error messages and error recovery procedures should be available.

Menu selection can be used for interactive controls. Menu selection of commands is useful for tasks that involve the selection of a limited number of options or that can be listed in a menu, or in cases when users may have relatively little training. A menu command system that involves several layers can be useful when a command set is so large that users are unable to commit all the commands to memory and a reasonable hierarchy of commands exists for the user.

Form-filling interactive control may be used when some flexibility in data to be entered is needed and when the users will have moderate training. A form-filling dialogue should not be used when the computer has to handle multiple types of forms and computer response is slow.

Fixed-function key interactive control may be used for tasks requiring a limited number of control inputs or in conjunction with other dialogue types.

Command language interactive control may be used for tasks involving a wide range of user inputs and when user familiarity with the system can take advantage of the flexibility and speed of the control technique.

Question and answer dialogues should be considered for routine data entry tasks when data items are known and their ordering can be constrained, when users have little or no training, and when the computer is expected to have moderate response speed.

Query language dialogue should be used for tasks emphasizing unpredictable information retrieval with trained user. Query languages should reflect a data structure or organization perceived by the users to be natural.

Graphic interaction as a dialogue may be used to provide graphic aids as a supplement to other types of interactive control. Graphic menus may be used that display icons to represent the control options. This may be particularly valuable when system users have different linguistic backgrounds.

15.9.4   Feedback

Feedback should be provided that presents status, information, confirmation, and verification throughout the interaction. When system functioning requires the user to standby, WAIT or similar type messages should be displayed until interaction is again possible. When the standby or delay may last a significant period of time, the user should be informed. When a control process or sequence is completed or aborted by the system, a positive indication should be presented to the user about the outcome of the process and the requirements for subsequent user action. If the system rejects a user input, feedback should be provided to indicate why the input was rejected and the required corrective action.

Feedback should be self-explanatory. Users should not be made to translate feedback messages by using a reference system or code sheets. Abbreviations should not be used unless necessary.

15.9.5   Prompts

Prompts and help instructions should be used to explain commands, error messages, system capabilities, display formats, procedures, and sequences, as well as to provide data. When operating in special modes, the system should display the mode designation and the file(s) being processed. Before processing any user requests that would result in extensive or final changes to existing data, the system should require user confirmation. When missing data are detected, the system should prompt the user. When data entries or changes will be nullified by an abort action, the user should be requested to confirm the abort.

Neither humor or admonishment should be used in structuring prompt messages. The dialogue should be strictly factual and informative. Error messages should appear as close as possible in time and space to the user entry that caused the message. If a user repeats an entry error, the second error message should be revised to include a noticeable change so that the user may be certain that the computer has processed the attempted correction.

Prompting messages should be displayed in a standardized area of the display. Prompts and help instructions for system-controlled dialogue should be clear and explicit. The user should not be required to memorize lengthy sequences or refer to secondary written procedural references.

15.9.6   Defaults

Manufacturer's default settings and configurations should be provided in order to reduce user workload. Currently defined default values should be displayed automatically in their appropriate data fields with the initiation of a data entry transaction. The user should indicate acceptance of the default values. Upon user request, manufacturers should provide a convenient means by which the user may restore factory default settings.

Users should have the option of setting their own default values for alarms and configurations on the basis of personal experience. A device may retain and store one or more sets of user default settings. Activation of these settings should require deliberate action by the user.

15.9.7   Error Management/Data Protection

When users are required to make entries into a system, an easy means of correcting erroneous entries should be provided. The system should permit correction of individual errors without requiring reentry of correctly entered commands or data elements.

References

Association for the Advancement of Medical Instrumentation (AAMI), *Human Factors Engineering Guidelines and Preferred Practices for the Design of Medical Devices.* Arlington, VA: Association for the Advancement of Medical Instrumentation, 1993.

Backinger, C. and P. Kingsley, *Write It Right: Recommendations for Developing User Instruction Manuals for Medical Devices Used in Home Health Care.* Rockville, MD: U. S. Department of Health and Human Services, 1993.

Bogner, M. S., *Human Error in Medicine.* Hillsdale, NJ: Lawrence Erlbaum Associates, 1994.

Brown, C.M., *Human-Computer Interface Design Guidelines.* Norwood, NJ: Ablex Publishing Company, 1989.

Fries, Richard C., "Human Factors and System Reliability", in *Medical Device Technology.* Volume 3, Number 2, March, 1992.

Fries, Richard C., *Reliable Design of Medical Devices*. New York: Marcel Dekker, Inc., 1997.

Hartson, H. Rex, *Advances in Human-Computer Interaction*. Norwood, N J: Ablex Publishing Corporation, 1985.

Le Cocq, Andrew D., "Application of Human Factors Engineering in Medical Product Design", *Journal of Clinical Engineering*. Volume 12, Number 4, July-August, 1987.

Mathiowetz, V. et al, "Grip and Pinch Strength: Normative Data for Adults", in *Archives of Physical Medicine and Rehabilitation*. Volume 66, 1985.

MIL-HDBK-759, *Human factors Engineering Design for Army Material*. Washington, DC: Department of Defense, 1981.

MIL-STD-1472, *Human Engineering Design Criteria for Military Systems, Equipment and Facilities*. Washington, DC: Department of Defense, 1981.

Morgan, C.T., *Human Engineering Guide to Equipment Design*. New York: Academic Press, 1984.

Philip, J. H., "Human Factors Design of Medical Devices: The Current Challenge", *First Symposium on Human Factors in Medical Devices*, December 13-15, 1989. Plymouth Meeting, PA: ECRI, 1990.

Pressman, R. S., *Software Engineering*. New York: McGraw Hill, 1987.

Weinger, Matthew B. and Carl E. Englund, "Ergonomic and Human Factors Affecting Anesthetic Vigilance and Monitoring Performance in the Operating Room Environment", *Anesthesiology*. Volume 73, Number 5, November, 1990.

Wiklund, Michael E., "How to Implement Usability Engineering," in *Medical Device and Diagnostic Industry*. Volume 15, Number 9, 1993.

Wiklund, Michael E., *Medical Device and Equipment Design - Usability Engineering and Ergonomics*. Buffalo Grove: Interpharm Press, Inc., 1995.

Woodson, W. E., *Human Factors Design Handbook*. New York: McGraw Hill, 1981.

Yourdon, E., *Modern Structured Analysis*. Englewood Cliffs, NJ: Yourdon Press, 1989.

Chapter 16

Biocompatibility

Richard C. Fries, PE, CRE – Datex-Ohmeda, Inc.
Madison, Wisconsin

Biological evaluation of medical devices is performed to determine the potential toxicity resulting from contact of the component materials of the device with the body. The device materials should not, either directly or through the release of their material constituents:

- produce adverse local or systemic effects
- be carcinogenic
- produce adverse reproductive and developmental effects.

Therefore, evaluation of any new device intended for human use requires data from systematic testing to ensure that the benefits provided by the final product will exceed any potential risks produced by device materials.

When selecting the appropriate tests for biological evaluation of a medical device, one must consider the chemical characteristics of device materials and the nature, degree, frequency and duration of its exposure to the body. In general, the tests include:

- acute
- sub-chronic and chronic toxicity
- irritation to skin, eyes and mucosal surfaces
- sensitization
- hemocompatibility
- genotoxicity
- carcinogenicity
- effects on reproduction including developmental effects.

However, depending on varying characteristics and intended uses of devices as well as the nature of contact, these general tests may not be sufficient to demonstrate the safety of some specialized devices. Additional tests for specific target organ toxicity, such as neurotoxicity and immunotoxicity may be necessary for some devices. For example, a neurological device with direct contact with brain parenchyma and cerebrospinal fluid (CSF) may require an animal implant test to evaluate its effects on the brain parenchyma, susceptibility to seizure, and effects on the functional mechanism of choroid plexus and arachnoid villi to secrete and absorb CSF. The specific clinical application and the materials used in the manufacture of the new device determines which tests are appropriate.

Some devices are made of materials that have been well characterized chemically and physically in the published literature and have a long history of safe use. For the purposes of demonstrating the substantial equivalence of such devices to other marketed products, it may not be necessary to conduct all the tests suggested in the FDA matrix of this guidance. FDA reviewers are advised to use their scientific judgement in determining which tests are required for the demonstration of substantial equivalence under section 510(k). In such situations, the manufacturer must document the use of a particular material in a legally marketed predicate device or a legally marketed device with comparable patient exposure.

16.1   The FDA and Biocompatibility

In 1986, FDA, Health and Welfare Canada, and Health and Social Services UK issued the Tripartite Biocompatibility Guidance for Medical Devices. This Guidance has been used by FDA reviewers, as well as by manufacturers of medical devices, in selecting appropriate tests to evaluate the adverse biological responses to medical devices. Since that time, the International Standards Organization (ISO), in an effort to harmonize biocompatibility testing, developed a standard for biological evaluation of medical devices (ISO 10993). The scope of this 12-part standard is to evaluate the effects of medical device materials on the body. The first part of this standard "Biological Evaluation of Medical Devices: Part 1: Evaluation and Testing", provides guidance for selecting the tests to evaluate the biological response to medical devices. Most of the other parts of the ISO standard deal with appropriate methods to conduct the biological tests suggested in Part 1 of the standard.

The ISO Standard, Part 1, uses an approach to test selection that is very similar to the currently-used Tripartite Guidance, including the same seven principles. It also uses a tabular format (matrix) for laying out the test requirements based on the various factors discussed above. The matrix consist of two tables: Initial Evaluation Tests for Consideration (Table 16-1) and Supplementary Evaluation Tests for Consideration (Table 16-2). In addition, FDA is in the process of preparing toxicology profiles for specific devices. These profiles will assist in determining appropriate toxicology tests for these devices.

To harmonize biological response testing with the requirements of other countries, FDA will apply the ISO standard, Part 1, in the review process in lieu of the Tripartite Biocompatibility Guidance.

FDA notes that the ISO standard acknowledges certain kinds of discrepancies. It states "due to diversity of medical devices, it is recognized that not all tests identified in a category will be necessary and practical for any given device. It is indispensable for testing that each device shall be considered on its own mertis: additional tests not indicated in the table may be necessary." In keeping with this inherent flexibility of the ISO standard, FDA has made several modifications to the testing required by ISO 10993-Part 1. These modifications are required for the category of surface devices permanently

Device Categories			Biological Effect							
Body Contact		Contact Duration	C	S1	I1	S2	S3	G	I2	H
X = ISO evaluation tests for consideration O = Additional tests which may be applicable		A: 24 hrs B: 24 hrs to 30 days C: >30 days								
Surface devices	Skin	A	X	X	X	.	.	.	.	.
		B	X	X	X	.	.	.	.	.
		C	X	X	X	.	.	.	.	.
	Mucosal membrane	A	X	X	X	.	.	.	.	.
		B	X	X	X	O	O	.	O	.
		C	X	X	X	O	X	X	O	.
	Breached or compromised surfaces	A	X	X	X	O	.	.	.	.
		B	X	X	X	O	O	.	O	.
		C	X	X	X	O	X	X	O	.
External communicating devices	Blood path, indirect	A	X	X	X	X	.	.	.	X
		B	X	X	X	X	O	.	.	X
		C	X	X	O	X	X	X	O	X

Legend:

C	Cytotoxicity	I2	Implantation
G	Genotoxocity	S1	Sensitization
H	Hemocompatibility	S2	System Toxicity
I1	Irritation	S3	Sub-chronic Toxicity

Table 16-1   Initial Evaluation Tests for Consideration

Device Categories			Biological Effects							
Body Contact	Contact Duration	Cytoto xicity	S 1	I 1	S 2	S 3	G	I 2	H	
X = ISO evaluation tests for consideration O = Additional tests which may be applicable	A: 24 hrs B: 24 h rs to 30 days C: >30 days									
	Tissue/bone/dentin communicating	A	X	X	X	O	.	.	.	.
		B	X	X	O	O	O	X	X	.
		C	X	X	O	O	O	X	X	.
	Circulating blood	A	X	X	X	X	.	O	.	X
		B	X	X	X	X	O	X	O	X
		C	X	X	X	X	X	X	O	X
Implant devices	Tissue/bone	A	X	X	X	0	.	.	.	.
		B	X	X	O	O	O	X	X	.
		C	X	X	O	O	O	X	X	.
	Blood	A	X	X	X	X	.	.	X	X
		B	X	X	X	X	O	X	X	X
		C	X	X	X	X	X	X	X	X

Table 16-1   (continued)

Device Categories			C 1	C 2	R	B
Body Contact		Contact Duration				
X = ISO evaluation tests for consideration		A: 24 hrs				
O = Additional tests which may be applicable		B: 24 h rs to 30 days				
		C: >30 days				
Surface devices	Skin	A	.	.	.	.
		B	.	.	.	.
		C	.	.	.	.
	Mucosal membrane	A	.	.	.	.
		B	.	.	.	.
		C	O	.	.	.
	Breached or compromised surfaces	A	.	.	.	.
		B	.	.	.	.
		C	O	.	.	.
External communicating devices	Blood path, indirect	A	.	.	.	.
		B	.	.	.	.
		C	X	X	.	.

Legend:

B	Biodegradable
C1	Chronic Toxicity
C2	Carcinogenicity
R	Reproductive Development

Table 16-2   Supplementary Evaluation Tests for Consideration

Device Categories		Chronic Toxicity	C2	R	B	
Body Contact	Contact Duration					
X = ISO evaluation tests for consideration	A: 24 hrs	y				
O = Additional tests which may be applicable	B: 24 h rs to 30 days					
	C: >30 days					
	Tissue/bone/dentin communicating	A	.	.	.	.
		B	.	.	.	.
		C	O	X	.	.
	Circulating blood	A	.	.	.	.
		B	.	.	.	.
		C	X	X	.	.
Implant devices	Tissue/bone	A	.	.	.	.
		B	.	.	.	.
		C	X	X	.	.
	Blood	A	.	.	.	.
		B	.	.	.	.
		C	X	X	.	.

Table 16-2   (continued)

contacting mucosal membranes (e.g., IUDs). The ISO standard would not require acute, sub-chronic, chronic toxicity and implantation tests. Also, for externally communicating devices, tissue/bone/dentin with prolonged and permanent contact (e.g., dental cements, filling materials etc.), the ISO standard does not require irritation, systemic toxicity, acute, sub-chronic and chronic toxicity tests. Therefore, FDA has included these types of tests in the matrix. Although several tests were added to the matrix, reviewers should note that some tests are commonly requested while other tests are to be considered and only asked for on a case-by-case basis. Thus, the modified matrix is only a framework for the selection of tests and not a checklist of every required test. Reviewers should avoid proscriptive interpretation of the matrix. If a reviewer is uncertain about the applicability of a specific type of test for a specific device, the reviewer should consult toxicologists in ODE.

FDA expects that manufacturers will consider performing the additional tests for certain categories of devices suggested in the FDA-modified matrix. This does not mean that all the tests suggested in the modified matrix are essential and relevant for all devices. In addition, device manufacturers are advised to consider tests to detect chemical components of device materials which may be pyrogenic. The FDA believes that ISO 10993, Part 1, and appropriate consideration of the additional tests suggested by knowledgeable individuals will generate adequate biological data to meet it's requirements.

Manufacturers are advised to initiate discussions with the appropriate review division in the Office of Device Evaluation, CDRH, prior to the initiation of expensive, long-term testing of any new device materials to ensure that the proper testing will be conducted. We also recognize that an ISO standard is a document that undergoes periodic review and is subject to revision. ODE will notify manufacturers of any future revisions to the ISO standard referenced here that affect this document's requirements and expectations.

16.2   International Regulatory Efforts

ISO is in the process of publishing a series of standards on the biological evaluation of medical devices—ISO 10993. Many parts of this series have been accepted as international standards, while the rest are under development (see Table 16-3). The subject of the first part, ISO 10993-1, is the categorizing and performance of safety testing. Part 2 of the standard, ISO 10993-2, is concerned with animal welfare requirements; another section, ISO 10993-12, deals with sample preparation and reference materials. Most of the remaining parts of the standard treat the individual tests.

The EU has issued a council directive—93/42/EEC, 1993—
concerning medical devices. All medical devices to be sold on the EU market
must comply with this directive after June 14, 1998. The European Committee
for Standardization (CEN) is currently in the process of adopting the ISO
10993 standard as the European standard. In 1986 the responsible authorities
in the United Kingdom, United States, and Canada issued the Tripartite
document, which was a guidance on the selection of toxicological tests for
medical device safety testing. This document has now been replaced by ISO
10993-1 as a first step in the process of international harmonization. In 1995
FDA chose to accept the ISO 10993-1 standard, with a modification of the
matrix listing (see below). Japanese authorities have also issued a guideline for
toxicological   testing of medical devices. This document is available in an
unofficial translation as Guidelines for Basic Biological Tests of Medical
Materials and Devices. It resembles ISO 10993 in structure and content, but
recommends modified tests and sample preparations.

The procedure for using the ISO 10993-1 standard is illustrated by the
flowchart in Figure 16-1. The standard is applicable only for devices that are
directly or indirectly in contact with the body or body fluids. If a device is to be
subjected to the standard, the first step is to characterize the material. Such
characterization need not always be followed by biological evaluation, because
there may be sufficient historical data to verify that the device meets the
requirements of the standard. If the material and/or the intended use of the
device is different from any historical safe device, biological evaluation has to
be performed. By following the standard, a suitable test program can be chosen
depending on the type and duration of body contact. Within the EU, all new
medical devices must carry the CE mark from June 14, 1998. This should
ensure the availability of relevant documentation regarding biocompatibility
and the lack of health problems associated with the use of a device. It is
noteworthy that the approval of such documentation is not, as it was previously,
accorded by the national health authorities, but rather by the so-called notified
bodies, whose experts review the products and production facilities of medical
device manufacturers.

16.3   Device Category and Choice of Test Programs

The need to evaluate a medical device biologically depends on the
material used in the device, the intended body contact, and the duration of that

Part	Title
1	Evaluation and Testing
2	Animal Welfare Requirements
3	Tests for Genotoxicity, Carcinogenicity, and Reproductive Toxicity
4	Selection of Tests for Interactions with Blood
5	Tests for Cytotoxicity – In Vitro Methods
6	Tests for Local Effects after Implantation
7	Ethylene Oxide Sterilization Residuals
8	Clinical Investigation of Medical Devices
9	Degradation of Materials Related to Biological Testing
10	Test for Irritation and Sensitization
11	Test for Systemic Toxicity
12	Sample Preparation and Reference Material
13	Identification and Quantification of Degradation Products from Polymers
14	Identification and Quantification of Degradation Products from Ceramics
15	Identification and Quantification of Degradation Products from Coated and Uncoated metals and Alloys
16	Toxicokinetic Study Design for Degradation Products and Leachables
17	Glutaraldehyde and Formaldehyde Residues in Industrially Sterilized Medical Devices

Table 16-3   Listing of Individual Parts of ISO 10993

contact. A device designed for surface contact for a limited time is not as likely to be bioincompatible as a permanent-exposure implant device made of the same material. The ISO 10993-1 standard divides medical devices into three main categories: surface devices, externally communicating devices, and implant devices. Each category is further divided into subcategories according to the type of contact to which the patient is exposed (see Table 16-4).

The choice of test program for a device in a given category depends on the duration of the contact. Three different time spans are given: limited contact (<24 hours), prolonged contact (24 hours - 30 days), and permanent contact (>30 days). ISO 10993-1 lists the tests that must be considered for each category.

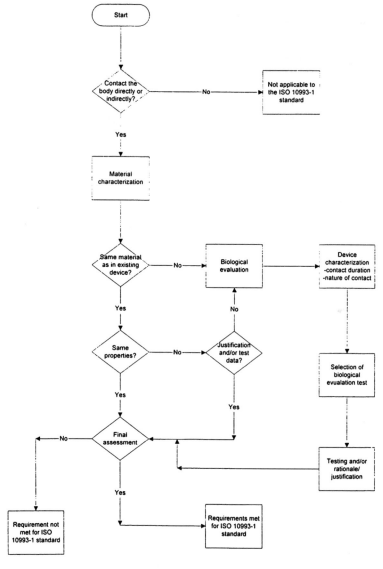

Figure 16-1   Steps in the biological evaluation of medical devices.

The ISO test matrix should not be considered as a checklist for the different tests that have to be performed, but rather as a guide for qualified toxicologists who also take into consideration material information and historical data from similar devices. The certifying authorities in most countries (e.g., notified bodies, FDA, Japanese authorities) are generally cooperative when a company must decide on a test program for a device. It is therefore advisable to maintain close contact with the relevant authorities during the entire process. However, testing should not be performed simply to meet regulatory requirements. This is important not only to lessen the risk of overtesting and excessive use of experimental animals, but also because a strict regulatory approach may mask potential negative health effects that might be identified via optional or nonroutine testing procedures.

As regards CE marking of existing products on the market or safety evaluation of medical devices already in clinical use, appropriate historical or clinical data should be employed whenever possible to avoid unnecessary testing.

16.4   Preparation of Extracts

ISO 10993-12 describes how samples for biological evaluation should be selected, prepared, and extracted. Other guidelines provide similar descriptions, which differ slightly in the specifics of the extraction procedures.

The device to be tested (the test article) should be a representative specimen of the mass-produced device. It should also be finished or treated (e.g., coated or sterilized) in the same way as the mass-produced device.

Because the toxic potential of materials and devices depends to a substantial degree on the leachability and toxicity of soluble components, extracts of the device are normally used in the tests. In some tests, however, an evaluation under normal-use conditions is mimicked by using the device or a piece of the device directly. Ideally, extraction media should constitute a series of media with decreasing polarity to ensure the extraction of components of widely different solubility properties. The most commonly used extraction media are physiological saline, vegetable oil, dimethylsulfoxide, and ethanol. Other extraction media such as polyethylene glycol or aqueous dilutions of

Device Categories		Examples
Surface Devices	Skin	Electrodes, external prostheses, fixation tapes, compression bandages, monitors various types
	Mucous membrane	Contact lenses, urinary catheters, intravaginal and intraintestinal devices, endotracheal tubes, bronchoscopes, dental protheses, orthodontic devices
	Breached or compromised surfaces	Ulcer, burn, and granulation tissue dressings or healing devices, occlusive patches
Externally Communicating Devices	Blood path indirect	Solution administration sets, extension sets, transfer sets, blood administration sets
	Tissue/bone/dentin communicating	Laparoscopes, arthroscopes, draining systems, dental cements, dental filling materials, skin staples
	Circulating blood	Intravascular catheters, temporary pacemaker electrodes, oxygenators, extracorporeal oxygenator tubing and accessories, dialyzers, dialysis tubing and accessories, hemoadsorbents and immunoadsorbents
	Tissue/bone implant devices	Orthopedic pins, plates, replacement joints, bone protheses, cements and intraosseous devices, pacemakers, drug-supply devices, neuromuscular sensors and simulators, replacement tendons, breast implants, artificial larynxes, subperiosteal implants, ligation clips
	Blood	Pacemaker electrodes, artificail arteriovenous fistulae, heart fvalves, vascular graafts, internal drug-delivery catheters, ventricular-assist devices

Table 16-4   Device Categories and Examples According to ISO 10993-1

ethanol may be selected in certain cases. For in vitro cytotoxicity testing, complete cell-culture medium is most often employed. The various guidelines also differ somewhat with respect to the temperature at which the extraction is conducted. Some leachable compounds may be chemically altered at high temperatures, and it is now generally recommended that extraction be conducted at 37°C—simulating body temperature—for 72 hours. This procedure will probably become increasingly accepted as the most appropriate

extraction method. For in vitro cytotoxicity tests, extraction at 37°C for 24
hours is usually recommended, since certain constituents of the media are
relatively labile.

The amount of leachable substances released to the extraction media is
related to the surface area and thickness of the product to be extracted.
Recommendations vary from 1.25 to 6 cm2 of product per milliliter of
extraction medium, depending on the size and shape of the product, or from 0.1
to 0.2g of product per milliliter of extraction medium when a surface area
cannot readily be estimated (e.g., for powders or granulates). In any case, the
specific properties of the product must be taken into account in order to make
usable extracts.

For cases in which a medical device comprises several components
made from different materials, the ideal procedure from a toxicological point of
view would be to test extracts of the components separately. However, in some
situations this is not practical, and extracts of the whole device may be used
instead.

16.5   Biological Control Tests

Biological control tests are not described in the ISO 10993 standard
for biological evaluation of medical devices, since these particular tests are
designed primarily for batch-control purposes. Such tests are also used during
the product development phase to identify sources of contamination and to
establish procedures that ensure the intended quality of the end product.

16.5.1   Microbiological Control Tests

Microbiological control tests are necessary to establish the
microbiological status of an end product—factors such as sterility, absence of
pathological bacteria, or limits for microbial counts. Furthermore, it is often
necessary to monitor the microbiological load of raw materials and
intermediary products, or to check the efficiency of production and sterilization
processes. The tests are performed by rinsing the materials or products in

physiological saline and assessing the rinsing medium for microbes, or by directly incubating the products in growth media.

16.5.2   Tests for Endotoxins

Even sterile medical devices may contain cell-wall lipopolysaccharides originating from gram-negative bacteria. Such so-called endotoxins or pyrogens can cause an abrupt fever reaction after entering directly into the body from sources such as venous catheters, syringes, or implant components. Two different biological assays can be used to measure the presence of endotoxins: the rabbit pyrogen test and the Limulus test. In both cases, an eluate is prepared—normally by rinsing the surfaces of the product with water—and then tested for endotoxins. In the rabbit pyrogen test, the eluate is injected intravenously and the rectal temperature of the animal is measured after the injection. In the Limulus test, the eluate is incubated together with lysate from the blood of the horseshoe crab (Limulus polyphemus), which contains a substance that forms a gel in the presence of endotoxins.

16.5.3   Test for Nonspecific Toxicity

This test is designed to assess any nonspecific adverse effect that occurs following intravenous injection of a device eluate in mice. The test is often performed with the same eluate used for the pyrogen test. The mice are inspected regularly for any signs of ill health, which can indicate the presence of toxic substances leaching from the product.

16.6   Tests for Biological Evaluation

This section provides a brief description of the individual tests included in the ISO 10993/EN 30993 standard.

16.6.1   Cytotoxicity

The aim of in vitro cytotoxicity tests is to detect the potential ability of a device to induce sublethal or lethal effects as observed at the cellular level.

According to ISO 10993-1, the in vitro cytotoxicity assay is one of two tests--
the other is the sensitization test described below--that must be considered in
the evaluation of all device categories.

Three main types of cell-culture assays have been developed:

- the elution test
- the direct-contact test
- the agar diffusion test.

In the elution test, an extract (eluate) of the material is prepared and added in
varied concentrations to the cell cultures. Growth inhibition is a widely used
parameter, but others may also be used. In the direct-contact test, pieces of test
material are placed directly on top of the cell layer, which is covered only by a
layer of liquid cell-culture medium. Toxic substances leaching from the test
material may depress the growth rate of the cells or damage them in various
ways. In the agar diffusion test, a piece of test material is placed on an agar
layer covering a confluent monolayer of cells. Toxic substances leaching from
the material diffuse through the thin agar layer and kill or disrupt adjacent cells
in the monolayer. As always, the physical and chemical properties of the test
material should be considered before the choice of the test system is made.

There is usually a good qualitative correlation between results from
cell-culture tests and studies performed in vivo with respect to cytotoxicity
versus primary tissue effects. It is important to recognize, however, that
although cell-culture toxicity is in general a good and sensitive indicator of
primary tissue compatibility, exceptions may arise in cases where leaching
substances cause tissue damage in vivo through more complex mechanisms. At
present, the in vitro cytotoxicity assays should be used as screening tests and
considered primarily as supplements to the various in vivo tests.

16.6.2 Sensitization

The sensitization test recognizes a potential sensitization reaction
induced by a device, and is required by the ISO 10993-1 standard for all device

categories. The sensitization reaction is also known as allergic contact dermatitis, which is an immunologically mediated cutaneous reaction. This is in contrast to irritant contact dermatitis (skin irritation)--a skin reaction caused by the primary and direct effect of a substance on the skin. In animals, the sensitization reactions manifest themselves as redness (erythema) and swelling (edema).

The preferred animal species for sensitization testing is the albino guinea pig. There is no reliable alternative in vitro test that can predict the sensitizing potential of a substance. The various available guinea pig methods have certain features in common: an induction (sensitization) phase, when the potential allergen is presented to the organism, followed by a rest period and a subsequent challenge phase to determine whether or not sensitization has occurred.

One of the most recognized and validated assays is the guinea pig maximization test (GPMT). A test design very similar to the GPMT is widely used for assessing the sensitizing potential of medical devices. After a challenge period, the skin reactions are graded on a ranking scale according to the degree of erythema and edema.

Predictive tests in guinea pigs are important tools in identifying the possible hazard to a population repeatedly exposed to a substance. Nevertheless, results from sensitization tests in guinea pigs have to be evaluated carefully. A positive test result in this assay may rate a substance as a stronger sensitizer than it appears to be during actual use. On the other hand, a negative result in such a sensitive assay ensures a considerable safety margin regarding the potential risk to humans.

16.6.3 Skin Irritation

The ISO 10993-10 standard describes skin-irritation tests for both single and cumulative exposure to a device. The preferred animal species is the albino rabbit, whose highly sensitive, light skin makes it possible to detect even very slight skin irritation caused by a substance. Skin-irritation tests of medical devices are performed either with two extracts obtained with polar and nonpolar solvents or with the device itself.

In the single-exposure test, rabbits are treated for several hours only, whereas for the cumulative test the same procedure is repeated for several days. All extracts and extractants are applied to intact skin sites. Skin reaction is seen as redness or swelling and is graded according to a specified classification system.

Dermal irritation is the production of reversible changes in the skin following the application of a substance, whereas dermal corrosion is the production of irreversible tissue damage (scar formation) in the skin. Materials that leak corrosive substances are not likely candidates for medical device production.

16.6.4   Intracutaneous Reactivity

The intracutaneous reactivity test is designed to assess the localized reaction of tissue to leachable substances. The test is required for consideration in nearly all the device categories in ISO 10993-1 (see Table III). Polar and nonpolar solvent extracts are administered as intracutaneous injections to rabbits. Undesirable intracutaneous reactivity includes redness or swelling.

16.6.5   Acute Systemic Toxicity

Acute systemic toxicity is the adverse effect occurring within a short time after administration of a single dose of a substance. ISO 10993-1 requires that the test for acute systemic toxicity be considered for all device categories that indicate blood contact. For this test, extracts of medical devices are usually administered intravenously or intraperitoneally in rabbits or mice.

Determining acute systemic toxicity is usually an initial step in the assessment and evaluation of the toxic characteristics of a substance. By providing information on health hazards likely to arise from short-term exposure, the acute systemic toxicity test can serve as a first step in the establishment of a dosage regimen in subchronic and other studies, and can also supply initial data on the mode of toxic action of a substance. The test is similar to the nonspecific toxicity test. Normally, only one of these two procedures is included in a test battery.

16.6.6   Genotoxicity

Genetic toxicology tests are used to investigate materials for possible mutagenic effects--that is, damage to the body's genes or chromosomes. The tests are performed both in vitro and in vivo. ISO 10993- 1 requires the genotoxicity (mutagenicity) test to be considered for all device categories indicating permanent (>30 days) body contact (except for surface devices with skin contact only).

A mutation is a change in the formation content of the genetic material (DNA code) that is propagated through subsequent generations of cells. Mutations can be classified into two general types:

- gene mutations
- chromosomal mutations.

Gene mutations are changes in nucleotide sequences at one or several coding segments within a gene; chromosomal mutations are morphological alterations or aberrations in the gross structure of the chromosomes.

The simplest and most sensitive assays for detecting induced gene mutations are those using bacteria. Gene mutations can also be detected in cultured mammalian cells. Current in vivo assays for gene mutations are cumbersome and not widely used. The simplest and most sensitive assays for investigating chromosomal aberrations are those that use cultured mammalian cells. However, two well-established in vivo procedures are also available: chromosomal aberrations can be studied in bone marrow or peripheral blood cells of rodents dosed with a suspect chemical or extract either by counting micronuclei in maturing erythrocytes (micronucleus test) or by analyzing chromosomes in metaphase cells.

In addition to these mutagenicity tests, various assays can measure the induction of an overall genotoxic response--an indirect indicator of potential damage to the genetic material.

16.6.7   Implantation

Implantation tests are designed to assess any localized effects of a device designed to be used inside the human body. Implantation testing methods essentially attempt to imitate the intended use conditions of an implanted material. Although different tests use various animal species, the rabbit has become the species of choice, with implantation performed in the paravertebral muscle. Implantation can be either surgical or nonsurgical: the surgical method involves the creation of a pouch in the muscle into which the implant is placed, while the nonsurgical method uses a cannula and stylet to insert a cylinder-shaped implant. Through a macroscopic examination (which may be supplemented with microscopic analysis), the degree of tissue reaction in the paravertebral muscle is evaluated as a measure of biocompatibility.

16.6.8   Hemocompatibility

The purpose of hemocompatibility testing is to look for possible undesirable changes in the blood caused directly by a medical device or by chemicals leaching from a device. Undesirable effects of device materials on the blood may include hemolysis, thrombus formation, alterations in coagulation parameters, and immunological changes. According to the ISO 10993-4 (EN 30993-4) standard, devices that only come into very brief contact with circulating blood--for example, lancets, hypodermic needles, or capillary tubes--generally do not require blood/device interaction testing.

ISO 10993-4 describes hemocompatibility tests in five different categories:

- thrombosis
- coagulation
- platelets

- hematology
- immunology.

Most of the individual tests are not discussed in detail, but they may be performed either in vivo or, preferably, in vitro. There is still some uncertainty with respect to what is actually required by the regulatory authorities for the hemocompatibility test.

16.6.9 Subchronic and Chronic Toxicity

Subchronic toxicity is the potentially adverse effect that can occur as a result of the repeated daily dosing of a substance to experimental animals over a portion of their life span. In the assessment and evaluation of the toxic characteristics of a chemical, the determination of subchronic toxicity is carried out after initial information on toxicity has been obtained by acute testing, and provides data on possible health hazards likely to arise from repeated exposures over a limited time. Such testing can furnish information on target organs and the possibilities of toxin accumulation, and provide an estimate of a no-effect exposure level that can be used to select dose levels for chronic studies and establish safety criteria for human exposure.

In subchronic or chronic toxicity studies, one or two animal species are dosed daily, usually for a period of 3 to 6 months; the rat is the standard animal species of choice. The animals are given the test substance in increasing doses. The dose level of the low-dose group should be at the level of human exposure. When extracts of medical devices are employed, one dose level (the highest practically applicable volume) is often sufficient, since strong toxicity is generally not expected.

16.6.10 Carcinogenicity

The objective of long-term carcinogenicity studies is to observe test animals over a major portion of their life span to detect any development of neoplastic lesions (tumor induction) during or after exposure to various doses of a test substance. Carcinogenicity testing is normally conducted with oral dosing. For implants and medical devices, however, only extracts can be tested and they must be administered intravenously, necessitating certain modifications of the standard procedure. There are only a very few products for which this comprehensive test can be justified.

In carcinogenicity studies, mice or rats are dosed every day for 18 to 24 months. For medical device extracts, one dose level (again the highest practically applicable volume) is usually sufficient. At the completion of the dosing period, all surviving animals are sacrificed and their organs and tissues examined microscopically for the presence of tumors. An increased incidence of one or more category of tumors in the dosed group would indicate that the product tested has the potential to induce tumors and could be considered a possible carcinogen in humans.

16.7   Alternative Test Methods

As mentioned previously, a major goal in international toxicological testing is to reduce not only the use of in vivo studies but also the number of animals employed in these tests. A few of the in vivo procedures used today for testing medical devices may be of questionable worth for safety evaluation. However, the availability of accepted and validated in vitro assays is still limited. Substantial resources have been made available for validation of alternative in vitro assays in toxicology as replacements for animal tests, but it may take years before validated methods can be implemented, and any goal of replacing all in vivo studies with in vitro assays will probably never be met.

Recently, a working group under the auspices of the European Center for Validation of Alternative Methods (ECVAM) has recommended a few alternative methods that can be used for safer testing of medical devices. These include two in vitro tests as potential substitutes for the in vivo assays for skin and eye irritation. However, the implementation of validated protocols and internationally accepted guidelines for these tests is likely to be delayed into the next century.

References

Biological Evaluation of Medical Devices, ISO 10993 Standard Series, Geneva, International Organization for Standardization, ongoing.

Bollen, Lise S. and Ove Svendsen, "Regulatory Guidelines for Biocompatibility Safety Testing," in *Medical Plastics and Biomaterials.* May, 1997.

Council Directive 93/42/EEC of 14 June 1993 Concerning Medical Devices, Official Journal of the European Communities, vol. 36, July, 1993.

Toxicology Subgroup, Tripartite Subcommittee on Medical Devices, "Tripartite Biocompatibility Guidance for Medical Devices," Rockville, MD, FDA, Center for Devices and Radiological Health (CDRH), 1986.

Guidelines for Basic Biological Tests of Medical Materials and Devices. Unofficial translation of Japanese guideline ISBN 4-8408-0392-7.

Svendsen O, Garthoff B, Spielmann H, et al., "Alternatives to the Animal Testing of Medical Devices (the Report and Recommendations of ECVAM Workshop 17)", in *ATLA*, 1996.

Chapter 17

Reliability Assurance

Richard C. Fries, PE, CRE – Datex-Ohmeda, Inc.
Madison, Wisconsin

The term reliability is a term that has been used extensively, but is often misunderstood. Reliability has been described by some as a group of statisticians spewing endless streams of data. Others have described it as testing a device "ad nauseam." Reliability is neither of these.

Reliability is a characteristic that describes how good a device really is. It is a measure of the dependability of the device. It is a characteristic that must be planned for, designed and manufactured into a device. The inclusion of reliability in manufacturing is important, because no matter how reliably a device is designed, it will not be a success unless it is manufactured and serviced reliably. Thus, reliability is the state of mind in which all personnel associated with a product must be. It is a philosophy that dictates how good a device will be.

17.1   Reliability versus Unreliability

If reliability is a measure of how good a device is, unreliability is a measure of the potential for the failure of a device. It is the result of the lack of planning for design and manufacturing activities. It is a philosophy that states the manufacturer does not care how good their device will be. The consequences of such a philosophy include:

- high cost
- wasted time
- customer inconvenience
- poor customer reputation.

Because reliability is preferable to unreliability, processes should be instituted to avoid the causes of unreliability, including:

- improper design
- improper materials
- manufacturing errors
- assembly and inspection errors
- improper testing
- improper packaging and shipping
- user abuse
- misapplication.

17.2   Quality versus Reliability

The terms "quality" and "reliability" are sometimes used interchangeably, although they are quite different. The difference grew out of the need for a time-based concept of quality. This distinction of time marks the difference between the traditional quality control concept and the modern approach to reliability.

The traditional concept of quality does not include the notion of a timebase. The term *quality* is defined in ISO 8402 as:

the totality of features or characteristics
of a product or service that bear on its
ability to satisfy stated or implied needs.

The definition refers to this totality at a particular instant of time. Thus, we may speak of the quality of a component at incoming, the quality of a subassembly in a manufacturing test, or the quality of a device at set-up.

In terms of this definition, a medical device is assessed against a specification or set of attributes. Having passed the assessment, the device is delivered to a customer, accompanied by a warranty, so that the customer is relieved of the cost implications of early failures. The customer, upon accepting the device, realizes that it might fail at some future time, hopefully far into the future. This approach provides no measure of the quality of the device outside the warranty period. It assumes this is the customer's responsibility and not the company's.

Reliability, on the other hand is quality over a specific time period, such as the five year expected life of a device or an eight hour operation. It has been described as the science of estimating, controlling and managing the probability of failure over time.

If the medical device is assessed against a specification or set of attributes, but was additionally designed for a Mean Time Between Failures of five years prior to being sent to the customer, reliability is being designed into the product (A Mean Time Between Failure of five years means 63% of the units in the field would have failed once within the five year period). A company must realize that, if they want to be successful and build a satisfied customer base, the responsibility for the quality of the device outside the warranty period belongs to them.

17.3   The Definition of Reliability

This idea of quality over a period of time is reflected in the more formal definition of reliability:

the probability, at a desired confidence level,
that a device will perform a required function,

without failure, under stated conditions, for
a specified period of time.

This definition contains four key requirements:

- to perform a required function, the function must have
  been established through such activities as customer
  and/or market surveys. Thus, reliability requires the
  device to be fully specified prior to design.
- to perform without failure, the normal operation of the
  device must be defined, in order to establish what a
  failure is. This activity also includes anticipating the
  misuse to which the device could be subjected and
  designing around it.
- to perform under stated conditions, the environment in
  which the device will operate must be specified. This
  includes typical temperature and humidity ranges,
  methods of shipping, shock and vibration experienced in
  normal usage and interference from associated equipment
  or to other equipment
- to operate for a specified period of time, the life
  expectancy of the device must be defined as well as the
  typical daily usage.

In summary, reliability assumes that preliminary thought processes
have been completed and that the device and its environment have been
thoroughly defined. These conditions make the task of the designer easier and
less costly in time and effort. It assumes that failure-free or failure-tolerant
design principles are used. It assumes manufacturing processes are designed so
that they will not reduce the reliability of the device.

Reliability, like any science, depends upon other technical areas as a
base for its functionality. These include:

- Basic mathematics and statistics
- Current regulatory standards
- Design principles
- Software Quality Assurance
- System interface principles

- Human factors
- Cost/benefit analysis
- Common sense.

17.4   History of Reliability

Reliability originated during World War II, when the Germans first introduced the concept to improve the operation of their V-1 and V-2 rockets. Prior to this time, most equipment was mechanical in nature and failures could usually be isolated to a simple part. Products were expected to be reliable and safety margins in stress-strength, wear or fatigue conditions were employed to assure it. Then, as electronics began to grow, so did reliability.

From 1945 to 1950, various military studies were conducted in the United States on equipment repair, maintenance costs and failure of electronic equipment. As a result of these studies, the Department of Defense established an ad hoc committee on reliability in 1950. This committee became a permanent group in 1952, known as the Advisory Group on the Reliability of Electronic Equipment (AGREE). In 1957, this group published a report that led directly to a specification on the reliability of military electronic equipment.

In the early sixties, the field of reliability experienced growth and widespread application in the aerospace industry, especially following the failure of Vanguard TV3 and several satellites. During this time engineers also began to realize that to really improve reliability, one must eliminate the source of failures. This led to the first Physics of Failure Symposium in 1962. This was followed by a period of growth in other highly technical areas, such as computers.

Today many industries and government agencies employ specialists in the area of reliability. Reliability is moving in the direction of more realistic recognition of causes and effects of failures, from the system to the component level. These companies have come to realize that poor reliability is costly, leads to poor customer reputation and the subsequent loss of market share. Industries that are regulated must also comply with reliability requirements established by the regulating agencies.

17.5   Types of Reliability

Reliability is composed of three primary subdivisions, each with their own particular attributes:

- Electronic reliability
- Mechanical reliability
- Software reliability.

17.5.1   Electronic Reliability

Electronic reliability (Figure 17-1) is a function of the age of a component or assembly. The failure rate is defined in terms of the number of malfunctions occurring during a period of time. As is evident from the figure, the graph is divided into three distinct time periods:

- Infant mortality
- Useful life
- Wearout.

17.5.1.1 Infant Mortality

Infant mortality is the beginning of the life of an electronic component or assembly. This period is characterized by an initial high failure rate, which decreases rapidly and then stabilizes. These failures are caused by gross, built-in flaws due to faulty workmanship, bad processes, manufacturing deviations from the design intent or transportation damage.
Examples of early failures include:

- Poor welds or seals
- Poor solder joints
- Contamination on surfaces or in materials
- Voids, cracks, or thin spots on insulation or protective coatings.

Many of these failures can be prevented by improving the control over the manufacturing process, by screening components or by burn-in procedures.

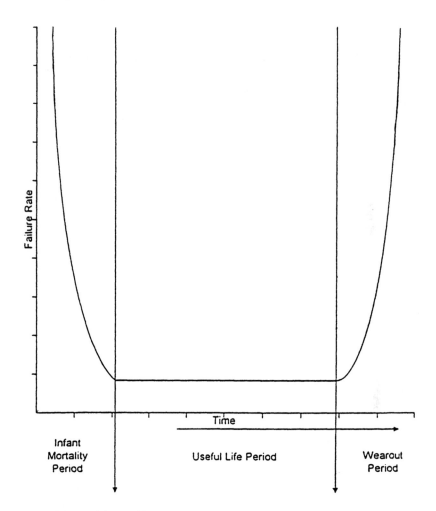

Figure 17-1   Electronic reliability curve. (From Fries, 1997.)

improvements in design or materials are necessary for these manufacturing
deviations.

17.5.1.2 Useful Life

The useful life period of a component or assembly is the largest
segment of the life cycle and is characterized by a constant failure rate. During
this period, the failure rate reaches its lowest level and remains relatively
constant. Failures occurring during this period are either stress related or occur
by chance. These are the most difficult to repeat or analyze.

17.5.1.3 Wearout

The final period in the life cycle occurs when the failure rate begins to
increase rapidly. Wearout failures are due primarily to deterioration of the
design strength of the components or assemblies, as a consequence of operation
and/or exposure to environmental fluctuations. Such deterioration may result
from:

- Corrosion or oxidation
- Insulation breakdown or leakage
- Ionic migration of metals on surfaces or in vacuum
- Frictional wear or fatigue
- Shrinkage and cracking in plastics.

Replacing components prior to reaching the wearout period through a
preventive maintenance program can prevent wearout failures.

17.5.2   Mechanical Reliability

Mechanical reliability (Figure 17-2) differs considerably from
electronic reliability in its reaction to the aging of a component or assembly.
Mechanical components or assemblies begin their life cycle at a failure rate of
zero and experience a rapidly increasing failure rate. This curve approximates
the wearout portion of the electronics life curve.

Mechanical failures are due primarily to deterioration of the design
strength of the component or assembly. Such deterioration may result from:

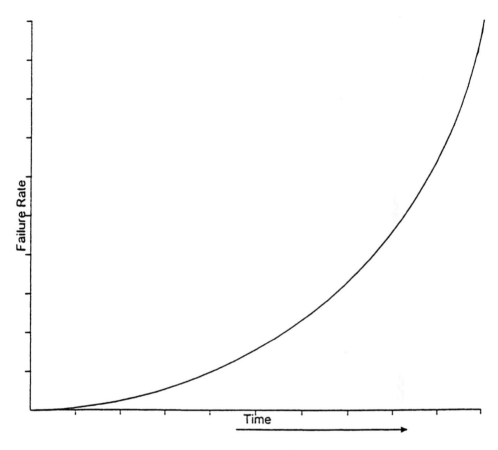

Figure 17-2   Mechanical reliability curve. (From Fries, 1997.)

- Frictional wear
- Shrinkage and/or cracking in plastics
- Fatigue
- Surface erosion
- Corrosion

- Creep
- Material strength deterioration.

Optimization of mechanical reliability occurs with timely elimination of components or assemblies through preventive maintenance, before the failure rate reaches unacceptably high levels.

17.5.3   Software Reliability

The following definition of reliability is given by the *IEEE Standard Glossary of Software Engineering Terminology*:

> The ability of a system or component to perform its required functions under stated conditions for a specified period of time.

In the case of medical device software, that definition should be expanded to include the concepts of safety and efficacy as follows:

> The ability of a system or component to perform its required functions in a safe and effective manner, under stated conditions, for a specified period of time.

The main point of this definition is that reliability, safety, and efficacy are inseparable requirements for medical device software.

In order to apply this definition, the software developer must know exactly what the "required functions" of the particular medical device are. Sometimes such functional definitions are obvious, but in general they are not. Such knowledge requires the existence of a formal software specification.

In addition, the software developer must know the "stated conditions." This means the environment in which the software is to operate must be fully defined. This may include whether the software will be operated during a stressful situation, the lighting and noise levels in the area of operation, and the technical knowledge of the user.

"For a specified period of time" indicates the reliability is being measured for a specific period of time, known as a mission time. This may be the length of a surgical case, the warranty period for the device, or the total operational life of the device.

Software reliability differs considerably from both electronic and mechanical reliability in that software is not subject to the physical constraints of electronic and mechanical components. Software reliability consists of the process of preventing failures through structured design and detecting and removing errors in the coding. Once all "bugs" are removed, the program will operate without failure forever (Figure 17-3). However, practically, the software reliability curve may be as shown in Figure 17-4, with early failures as the software is first used and a long period of constant failures, as bugs are fixed.

Software failures are due primarily to:

- Specification errors
- Design errors
- Typographical errors
- Omission of symbols.

17.6   Device Reliability

The life cycle of any medical device may be represented by a graph known as the Reliability Bathtub Curve (Figure 17-5). It is a graph of failure rate versus the age of the device.

The graph is identical to that for electronics described above. As with the electronics life curve, there are three distinct time periods:

Infant mortality
Useful life
Wearout

The discussion of the three life periods contained in the section on electronic reliability applies to device reliability as well.

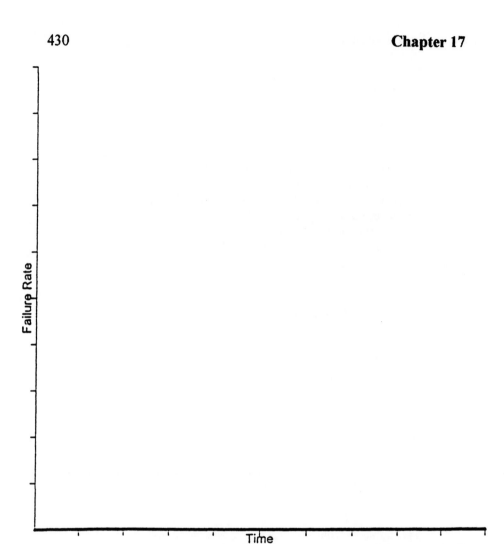

Figure 17-3   Ideal software reliability curve. (From Fries, 1997.)

17.7   Optimizing Reliability

Reliability optimization involves consideration of each of the life cycle periods. Major factors that influence and degrade a system's operational reliability must be addressed during design in order to control and maximize

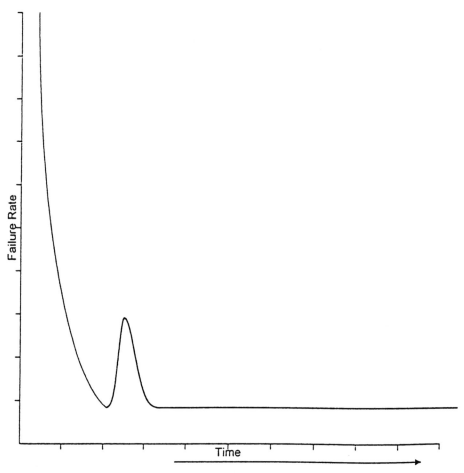

Figure 17-4   Practical software reliability curve. (From Fries, 1997.)

system reliability. Thus, early failures may be eliminated by a systematic
process of controlled screening and burn-in of components, assemblies and the
device. Stress related failures are minimized by providing adequate design
margins for each component and the device. Wearout failures may be
eliminated by conducting timely preventive maintenance on the device, with
appropriate replacement of effected components.

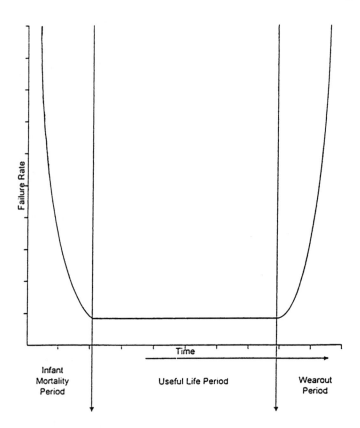

Figure 17-5　　Reliability bathtub curve.　(From Fries, 1997.)

17.8　Reliability's Effect on Medical Devices

Subjecting a medical device to a reliability program provides a structured approach to the product development process. It provides techniques that improve the quality of the device over a period of time as well as reduce development and redevelopment time and cost. It yields statistical data that quantifies the success, or lack of success, of the development process and predicts future performance. It also assures regulatory requirements are satisfied and gives confidence that regulatory inspections will produce no major discrepancies.

The use of the various reliability techniques results in decreased warranty costs and the resultant increase in customer acceptance. This naturally leads to an enhanced customer perception of the manufacturer and the resultant increase in market share. Reliability techniques also reduce the risk of liability by assuring safety has been the primary concern during the design and development process. By reducing up-front costs, limiting liability risks and increasing future profits, reliability is essential to the success of any company.

Most importantly, the inclusion of reliability gives development personnel a feeling of confidence that they have optimized the design to produce a device that is safe and effective for its intended use and will remain that way for a long period of time. This confidence will foster success in future products.

17.9   Initial Reliability Prediction

Once the design has proceeded to the point where parts have been defined and a parts list developed, an initial prediction based on the parts used may be performed to produce an initial MTBF value. This value may then be compared to the original reliability goal to determine if the design will meet the intended reliability. The initial prediction is also used to highlight certain areas of the design that have a high failure rate, such as a particular component or an assembly, such as a PC board or a pneumatic circuit. The prediction is also used to form the basis for future analysis, reliability growth and change.

Certain limitations exist with the prediction method. The first deals with the ability to accumulate data of known validity for the new application. The design may contain many new components, some of which are new to the marketplace and are not included in MIL-HDBK-217. Also, a component may be used in an application for which failure rate data has not been accumulated. In these cases, you may have to rely on vendor data or on the history of similar components in similar products.

A second limitation is the complexity of the predicting technique. It takes a long time to list each component, look up each failure rate and then calculate the MTBF for each assembly and then the device. As the complexity of the product increases, the length of time increases. Several companies have advertised computer programs that perform the prediction. The program takes the individual components and their quantity and determines the failure rates from tables residing in the computer, which are periodically updated. No matter the effort it takes to complete, the prediction must be done to get the basis for future activities.

MIL-HDBK-217 contains two methods of doing a prediction, a parts stress analysis and a part count analysis. The parts stress analysis requires a greater amount of detail to complete and thus is applicable at a later stage in development, when hardware testing has been completed. The parts count analysis requires a minimum of information, including the parts, quantities, quality levels and application environment. Because it does not require operational stress levels, it can be performed early in the design phase as soon as a parts list is developed. Only the parts count method will be discussed here. Details of the parts stress analysis may be found in MIL-HDBK-217.

17.9.1   Parts Count Prediction

There are four items necessary to begin a parts count prediction:

- a schematic
- a parts list
- MIL-HDBK-217
- marketing parameters.

The marketing parameters include 1) the use rate, i.e., the number of hours the device is in operation per day, the number of days per week and the number of weeks per year, 2) the desired MTBF goal, 3) the desired life of the device and 4) the desired warranty cost as a percentage of sales. These parameters are used for final calculations after the MTBF has been calculated.

The first step in completing a part count prediction is to choose the environment in which the product will be used from among the many listed in the handbook. The three most commonly experienced by medical devices, in order of increasing severity, are:

GF   Ground Fixed

Conditions less than ideal, such as installation in permanent
racks, with adequate cooling air and possible installations in
unheated buildings. An example would be a wall mounted
gas pressure alarm.

GB   Ground Benign

Nonmobile, laboratory environment, readily accessible to
maintenance. An example would be CAT scan residing in
one location or a monitor permanently set on a table or desk.

GM   Ground Mobile

Equipment installed on wheeled or tracked vehicles. An
example would be an evoked potential system that can be
rolled from the operating room into a patient's room or a
laboratory.

Where a question exists as to which of two environments should be chosen,
select the more severe of the two.

Once the environment is chosen, all parts, in one particular assembly,
such as a PC board or a pneumatic circuit, are listed on a form, such as
that shown in Figure 17-6. The form lists the type of component, the style
of part, where applicable, the quantity of that component in the assembly,
the failure rate for that component, and the total failure rate for the
quantity of that component.

When all parts are listed on the sheet, start the process of determining
the individual failure rates. The individual components are found in the
appropriate tables within the parts count analysis portion of
MIL-HDBK-217. The base failure rate is listed as well as the quality
factor and other parameters, where necessary. The component failure rate
is found by multiplying the base failure rate and the quality factor and

INITIAL RELIABILITY PREDICTION

Device_____

Subsystem_____   Date_____

Component	Style	Quantity	Individual Failure Rate	Total Failure Rate

Total Failure Rate_____

MTBF_____

Figure 17-6   Parts count prediction sheet.

other listed factors. This number is then listed in the individual
component failure rate. This number is multiplied by the quantity
included in the assembly and the total failure rate is determined. This
process continues for the remainder of the items in the assembly. When
all components are determined, the total failure rates are summed to
determine the failure rate for the assembly. This failure rate is listed
as failure per million hours. To calculate the MTBF for the assembly, the
total failure rate is divided by one million and the reciprocal taken.
This will be the MTBF in hours.

The above process is repeated for each assembly. When completed,
the total failure rates for each assembly are summed, yielding the total
failure rate for the device. The MTBF for the device is calculated as it
was above, for the assembly. An example will help illustrate the method.

17.9.2   Parts Count Prediction Example

A company is developing the model 3322 monitor. The device
consists of several PC boards and a display. Reliability Engineering has the
task of determining the MTBF of the device, based on the hardware
components used, for comparison to the reliability goal.

The device will be stationary during use. Thus the environment "GB"
is chosen from MIL-HDBK-217. The parts for each PC board are listed on
separate worksheets and the failure rates calculated. Figure 17-7 shows a
sample worksheet for the ADC board.

The PC board is listed in Figure 17-8 under the term "PCBs." Read
across the line until the column GB is found. The value there is 0.0027. The
Quality Factor for the interconnects is found in Figure 17-9. Since this board is
a MIL-SPEC board, the quality factor is 1. The total failure rate for the board
is then the product of the initial failure rate and the quality factor.

Total failure rate = component failure rate (quality factor)

Therefore, the failure rate for the PC board is 0.0027 failures per million hours.

INITIAL RELIABILITY PREDICTION

Device_____3322 Monitor_____

Subsystem____ADC Board_____ Date__5/3/95_____

Component	Style	Quantity	Individual Failure Rate	Total Failure Rate
PC Board		1	0.0027	0.0027
Resistors	RN	30	0.007	0.2100
Capacitors	CK	5	0.004	0.0200
Capacitors	CM	10	0.003	0.0300
Diodes	Zener	18	0.022	0.396
Transistors	Si NPN	8	0.003	0.024
54LS164		2	0.045	0.090
8259		1	0.055	0.055
54LS240		3	0.045	0.155
54LS00		5	0.030	0.150

Total Failure Rate 1.133 fr/million hours

MTBF   882,613 hours_____

Figure 17-7   Worksheet for the ADC board. (From Fries, 1997)

Part Type	ARW	AUT	CL	GB
SWITCHES				
Toggle & Pushbutton	0.046	0.01	1.2	0.001
Sensitive	6.9	1.5	180.0	0.15
Thumbwheel	26.0	5.6	670.0	0.56
Other Rotary	15.0	3.3	400.0	0.33
CIRCUIT BREAKERS				
Thermal	5.2	1.0	N/A	0.11
Magnetic	2,8	0.54	N/A	0.06
CONNECTORS				
Cir/Rack/Panel	0.56	0.34	5.1	0.0055
Coaxial	0.55	0.32	5.3	0.006
PCBs	0.096	0.014	2.6	0.0027
IC SOCKETS	0.048	0.019	1.3	0.0019
INTERCONNECT ASSY	0.78	0.62	21.0	0.041

Figure 17-8   Interconnects data. (From MIL-HDBK-217.)

The resistors are type "RN." The data for resistors are found Figure 17-10. Find style "RN" and the column GB. The value is 0.007. The quality value for resistors of two letter types found in Figure 17-11 is 1. Therefore the failure rate for the resistors is 0.007 failures per million hours.

To find integrated circuit data, for example 54LS164, the cross reference in Figure 17-12 is used. Locate 54LS164 in the table. It references the number 30605 in Figure 17-13. That table list the complexity for 30605 as 36 gates. Then turning to Figure 17-14, under MOS for 1-100 gates, look under the column marked GB and find the value 0.009. Since the integrated circuit is to be burned-in, Quality Level B-2 is used. Figure 17-15 lists the quality level as 5. The failure rate is then 0.045 failures per million hours.

Part Type	Quality MIL-SPEC	Level NON-MIL
Magnetrons	1	N/A
Inductive	1	3
Motors	1	6
Relays, Solid State	1	3
Relays, Time Delay	1	4
Relays, All Others	1	6
Switches, Toggle & Sensitive	1	20
Switches, Thumbwheel	1	1.5
Switches, Other Rotary Types	1	50
Circuit Breakers	1	8.4
Connectors	1	3
Interconnection Assemblies	1	10

Figure 17-9   Interconnects quality levels. (From MIL-HDBK-217.)

Other parts have their failure rates calculated in the same manner, using the appropriate MIL-HDBK-217 tables. Figure 17-7 lists the failure rates for the remaining components on the ADC board. They are then summed to give the total failure rate for the board. The failure rate is then divided by one million to yield the failure rate per hour. The reciprocal of this number yields the MTBF in hours.

The total failure rate for the device is calculated by summing the individual failure rates for the subassemblies and other components (Figure 17-16). The parts previously calculated are included along with other parts whose failure rate may be obtained from the vendor or component testing. The MTBF

RESISTORS, FIXED			USE ENVIRONMENT		
CONSTRUCTION	STYLE	MIL-SPEC	AUT	GMS	GB
Composition	RCR	39008	0.017	0.0006	0.0005
	RC	11	0.083	0.0030	0.0025
Film	RLR	39017	0.012	0.0015	0.0012
	RL	22684	0.060	0.0074	0.0062
	RNR	55182	0.014	0.0017	0.0014
	RN	10509	0.069	0.0083	0.0069
Film, power	RD	11804	0.210	0.0140	0.0120
Film, network	RZ	83401	0.630	0.0300	0.0250
Wirewound	RBR	39005	0.270	0.0100	0.0085
Accurate	RB	93	1.400	0.0510	0.0430
Wirewound	RWR	39007	0.150	0.0150	0.0140
Power	RW	26	0.760	0.0760	0.0690
Wirewound	RER	39009	0.094	0.0095	0.0080
Ch. Mount	RE	18546	0.470	0.0480	0.0400

Figure 17-10   Resistor data. (From MIL-HDBK-217.)

of the monitor is then calculated to be 39,626 hours. This indicates that 63% of the operational devices will have experience one failure within the first 39,626 hours of operation.

This value may then be compared to the reliability goal to determine if the values are comparable. It is also important to look at the individual subassemblies to determine which have the highest failure rates. The designer should then determine how the subassembly may be changed to reduce the failure rate. This may include using a component with a higher reliability or by using redundant components.

The prediction value may also be used to calculate the warranty cost for the device. To do this, several parameters for the device are necessary including:

Failure Rate Level	Quality Factor
L	1.5
M	1.0
P	0.3
R	0.1
S	0.03

For non-ER parts (styles with only 2 letters in Tables 5.2-27 and 5.2-28), the Quality Factor = 1 providing parts are procured in accordance with the part specification; if procured as commercial (NON-MIL) quality, the Quality Factor = 3. For ER parts (styles with 3 letters), use the Quality Factor value for the "letter" failure rate level procured.

Figure 17-11   Resistor quality levels.   (From MIL-HDBK-217.)

Operating time per year   2500 hours
Number of units sold per year   200 units
Selling price $58,000
Average charge for a service call $ 850

The following calculations can then be made:

Total sales per year = 200 units ($58,000 per unit)
= $11,600,000

The reliability of the device based on 2,500 hours operating time per year is:
Reliability = exp(-use time/MTBF)
= exp(-2500/39626)
= exp(-0.0631)
= 0.94

This means 94% of the 200 units will survive the first year of operation without a failure, while 5%, or 12 units, will fail. Therefore, the total Service charges are:
Service charge = 12 units ($850 per Service call)
= $10,200

COMMERCIAL	M38510/	COMMERCIAL	M38510/	COMMERCIAL	M38510/
5409	01602	54116	01503	54F151	33901
54S09	08004	5412	00106	54153	01403
54LS09	31005	54LS12	30006	54S153	07902
5410	00103	54121	01201	54LS153	30902
54L10	02003	54L121	04201	54F153	33902
54H10	02303	54122	01202	54154	15201
54S10	07005	54L122	04202	54155	15202
54LS10	30005	54LS122	31403	54LS155	32601
54F10	33003	54123	01203	54156	15203
54ALS10	37002	54LS123	31401	54LS156	32602
54HC10	65002	54LS124	31701	54157	01405
54ALS1000	38401	54125	15301	54S157	07903
54ALS1002	38402	54LS125	32301	54LS157	30903
54ALS1003	38403	54LS125A	32301	54F157	33903
54ALS1004	38409	54126	15302	54S158	07904
54ALS1005	38410	54LS126	32302	54LS158	30904
54ALS1008	38404	5413	15101	54F158	33904
54H101	02205	54LS13	31301	5416	00802
54ALS1010	38405	54132	15103	54160	01303
54ALS1011	38406	54LS132	31303	54LS160	31503
54ALS1020	38407	54HC132	65005	54LS160A	31503
54H103	02206	54S133	07009	54161	01306
54ALS1032	38408	54ALS133	37005	54LS161	31504
54ALS1034	38411	54S134	07010	54LS161A	31504
54ALS1035	38412	54S135	07502	54162	01305
54107	00203	54S138	07701	54LS162	31511
54LS107	30108	54LS138	30701	54LS162A	31511
54LS109	30109	54ALS138	37701	54163	01304
54F109	34102	54S139	07702	54LS163	31512
54ALS109	37102	54LS139	30702	54LS163A	31512
54S11	08001	5414	15102	54164	00903
54H11	15502	54LS14	31302	54L164	02802
54LS11	31001	54S140	08101	54LS164	30605
54F11	34002	54145	01005	54165	00904
54ALS11	37402	54147	15601	54LS165	30608
54S112	07102	54148	15602	54LS165A	30608
54LS112	30103	54LS148	36001	54LS166	30609
54F112	34103	54S15	08002	54LS168	31505
54ALS112A	37103	54LS15	31002	54LS169	31506
54S113	07103	54150	01401	54LS169A	31506
54LS113	30104	54151	01406	5417	00804
54S114	07104	54S151	07901	54170	01801
54LS114	30105	54LS151	30901	54LS170	31902

Figure 17-12   Integrated circuit data. (From MIL-HDBK-217.)

M38510/ XXXXX	COMPLEXITY (# of gates)	Np	M38510/ XXXXXX	COMPLEXITY (# of gates)	Np
30502	4	14	30903	15	16
30601	47	16	30904	15	16
30602	41	16	30905	17	16
30603	37	14	30906	15	16
30604	39	16	30907	15	16
30605	36	14	30908	16	16
30606	48	14	30909	15	16
30607	48	16	31001	3	14
30608	62	16	31002	3	14
30609	68	16	31003	2	14
30701	16	16	31004	4	14
30702	18	16	31005	4	14
30703	18	16	31101	31	16
30704	44	16	31201	42	16
30801	63	24	31202	42	16
30901	17	16	31301	2	14
30902	16	16			

Figure 17-13   Integrated circuit complexity. (From MIL-HDBK-217.)

DEVICE DESCRIPTION		APPLICATION ENVIRONMENT		
NUMBER OF GATES	TECHNOLOGY	GB	GF	GM
1 - 100	BIPOLAR	0.0061	0.0222	0.0349
	MOS	0.0094	0.0323	0.0517
>100 - 1,000	BIPOLAR	0.0115	0.0391	0.0608
	MOS	0.0179	0.0593	0.0945
>1,000 - 3,000	BIPOLAR	0.0225	0.0750	0.1164
	MOS	0.0354	0.1155	0.1837
>3,000 - 10,000	BIPOLAR	0.0604	0.2519	0.4039
	MOS	0.0863	0.3330	0.5386
>10,000 - 30,000	BIPOLAR	0.1066	0.4103	0.6507
	MOS	0.1584	0.5724	0.9200

Figure 17-14   Integrated circuit failure rates. (From MIL-HDBK-217.)

QUALITY LEVEL	DESCRIPTION	QUALITY FACTOR
S	Procured in full accordance with MIL-M-38510, Class S requirements. Class S listing on QPL-38510.	0.25
S-1	Procured in full compliance with the requirements of MIL-STD-975 or MIL-STD-1547 and have procuring activity specification approval.	0.75
B	Procured in full accordance with MIL-M-38510, Class B requirements. Class B listing on QPL-38510.	1.0
B-1	Fully compliant with all requirements of paragraph 1.2.1 of MIL-STD-883 and procured to a MIL drawing, DESC drawing or other government approved document.	2.0
B-2	Not fully compliant with requirements of paragraph 1.2.1 of MIL-STD-883 and procured to government approved documentation including vendor's equivalent Class B requirements.	5.0
D	Hermetically sealed parts with normal reliability screening and manufacturer's quality assurance practices. Non hermetic parts encapsulated with organic material must be subjected to 160 hours burn-in at 125 degrees C, 10 temperature cycles (-55 C to 125 C) with end point electricals and high temperature continuity test at 100 degrees C.	10.0
D-1	Commercial or non-mil standard part, encapsulated or sealed with organic materials (e.g., epoxy, silicone or phenolic)	20.0

Figure 17-15   Integrated circuit quality levels. (From MIL-HDBK-217.)

INITIAL RELIABILITY PREDICTION

SUMMARY SHEET

Device_____3322 Monitor_____

Date   5/15/95_____

Assembly	Quantity	Total Failure Rate (fr/million hours)
ADC Board	1	1.133
Mother Board	1	1.266
Display Board	1	1.587
Display	1	1.25
Power Supply	1	20.000

Total Device Failure Rate   25.2360 fr/million hours

Device MTBF   39,626 hours

Figure 17-16   Device total failure rate.

The warranty cost as a percentage of sales is thus:

Warranty Cost = (Service charges/Total Sales) 100
= ($10200/$11600000) 100
= 0.09% of sales

This value should be compared to the company standard for warranty cost.

17.9.3   Summary of Reliability Prediction

There are computer programs which will calculate a reliability prediction. The programs usually come with a database of components and failure rates. When such a program is purchased, it is essential to get periodic updates to the component database to assure the program is using the latest failure rate values.

Experience comparing initial predictions with actual field data has shown that the parts count value is approximately 10% to 20% below the actual value calculated from field data. However, the prediction values are good indicators of trends with regard to warranty costs, serve to highlight parts of the device with high failure rates, and provide valuable information for the Service department in planning the inventory of replacement parts.

Predictions can be updated after Reliability testing is completed to establish a greater confidence in the calculated value.

In addition to the Parts Count Prediction, MIL-HDBK-217 provides a second type of prediction, based on more detail of how the component operates. This second type of prediction requires information such as component current, component voltage, ambient temperature, etc. This prediction provides a more detailed calculation for the reliability, but would occur later in the development process because of the details required. The choice of the type of prediction will depend on the type of information desired and how early in the development process it is desired.

17.10   Design for Variation

During design, one may need to deal with the problem of assessing the combined effects of multiple variables on a measurable output or other characteristics of a product, by means of experiments. This is not a problem that is important in all designs, particularly when there are fairly large margins between capability and required performance, or for design involving negligible risk or uncertainty, or when only one or a few items are to be manufactured. However, when designs must be optimized in relation to variations in parameter values, processes, and environmental conditions, particularly if these variations can have combined effects, it is necessary to use methods that can evaluate the effects of the simultaneous variations.

Statistical methods of experimentation have been developed which enable the effects of variation to be evaluated in these types of situations. They are applicable whenever the effects cannot be theoretically evaluated, particularly when there is a large component of random variation or interactions between variables. For multivariable problems, the methods are much more economical than traditional experiments, in which the effect of one variable is evaluated at a time. The traditional approach also does not enable interactions to be analyzed, when these are not known empirically.

References

Dhillon, B. S., *Reliability Engineering in Systems Design and Operation*. New York: Van Nostrand Reinhold Company, 1983.

Fries, Richard C., *Reliability Assurance for Medical Devices, Equipment and Software*. Buffalo Grove, IL: Interpharm Press, Inc., 1991.

Fries, Richard C., *Reliable Design of Medical Devices*. New York: Marcel Dekker, Inc., 1997.

Goldberg, M. F. and J. Vaccaro, editors. *Physics of Failure in Electronics*. Spartan Books, Inc., 1963.

IEEE Std. 610.12, *Standard Glossary of Software Engineering Terminology*. New York: Institute of Electrical and Electronics Engineers, 1990.

ISO 8402, *Quality Vocabulary*. Switzerland: International Organization for Standardization, 1986.

Kececioglu, Dimitri, *Reliability Engineering Handbook*. Englewood Cliffs, NJ: PTR Prentice Hall Inc, 1991.

Langer, E. and J. Meltroft, editors. *Reliability in Electrical and Electronic Components and Systems*. North Holland Publishing Company, 1982.

Lloyd, D. K. and M. Lipow, *Reliability Management, Methods and Mathematics*. 2nd Edition, Milwaukee, Wisconsin: The American Society for Quality Control, 1984.

MIL-STD-721C, *Definition of Terms for Reliability and Maintainability*. Washington, DC: Department of Defense, 1981.

Niehoff, Ken, *Designing Reliable Software*. Medical Device & Diagnostic Industry, Volume 16, Number 9, September, 1994.

O'Connor, P. D. T. *Practical Reliability Engineering*. New York: John Wiley and Sons, 1984.

Reliability Analysis Center. *Reliability Design Handbook*. Chicago: ITT Research Institute, 1975.

Sandberg, J. B. "Reliability For Profit...Not Just Regulation", in *Quality Progress.*, August, 1987.

Chapter 18

Product User Guides

Margaret Rickard – Datex-Ohmeda, Inc.
Madison, Wisconsin

What if this chapter could answer all your questions about writing user documentation? What if this chapter could tell you the right way to write a user manual? If one definitive answer existed, the life of a technical writer would be greatly simplified. Unfortunately, there is no one right way to write user manuals. The guidelines in this chapter can only steer you toward the direction of ease-of-use and readability in a manual -- not perfection.

Writing user manuals is difficult, and along the way there are 101 places where something could go wrong. This chapter is not an exhaustive dissertation of any of specific topic. Providing some guidelines, this chapter shares some experiences and insights that may help you deal with the many challenges involved in completing a good, usable user manual.

The main thrust behind good user documentation is "knowing the user." The content and format of your guide depend on your product and your audience. Without this cornerstone, creating a quality manual is virtually impossible. Quality requires writing from the user's point of view.
As you read this chapter, you will see the different building blocks of the manual development process. The first few blocks involve building the team and including feedback from customers in the design process. The middle layer consists of gathering accurate information, good design and concise writing. The finishing layers consist of disseminating the information in its appropriate format to the audience.

From the following essential elements (the building blocks) of good user documentation, use what is appropriate to your company's products and processes.

- Why user documentation is important
- The teams
- User research
- How a manual evolves
- Style guides
- Writing tips
- References
- Bibliography.

18.1   Why User Documentation Is Important

Every company touts customer satisfaction in advertising and emphasizes it within the mission statement and company goals. Satisfaction is the customer's subjective response to a product. The user manual is part of the product and thereby affects how customer's view product usability, capability, performance, reliability, and maintainability.

A study by Smart and Sewright examined how customer's perceptions of manuals affect their perceptions of the quality of the product. Their test model had documentation as the dependent variable with product quality (measured by six variables) as the response variable. The results infer that documentation does indeed affect customer's perceptions of a product. For example, in respect to the usability variable, 72 percent of the respondents correlate usability of the manual to that of the system.

Today's health care finds more and more technical writers writing for the homecare market. One of the least acceptable results from the growing homecare market is an increase in user error. This increase is attributed, by some, to the difficulty lay users have in understanding the manuals that come with the devices they use. Are these home care device manuals being written for health care professionals rather than lay users because that is the audience for whom most have written? Designing and writing homecare device instructions for lay users is essential, and knowing your audience is the first step toward good, useful instructions. You need to provide the "least competent user" with the information necessary to use your device safely and effectively.

A good user manual enhances customer's satisfaction. A good user manual gives the customers the information they need, when they need it and in a format that is right for them. This is not an easy task; successful completion requires a team effort.

18.2   It's a Team Effort

Any successful team embraces the strengths and accepts the weaknesses of its members. A winning team draws from the experience and knowledge of each member. This holds true for a product and documentation team. In developing a good manual, two types of team interplay best assure a user manual that meets, or better yet, exceeds customer expectations. One team, the technical communication team, integrates the expertise of writing, design and illustration. The other team is the project team.

18.2.1 Technical Communication Team

The technical communication team integrates the expertise of writing, design and illustration. The people on the team need to act as a team; all working toward the same goals. Team work is not easy and requires certain personality traits and certain business and personal skills. You must:

- Participate as part of a team; be willing to pitch in and do your part
- Be an active listener; listen objectively and carefully
- communicate well
- Understand the products you are writing or illustrating about and the tools you are using
- Understand and handle the stress that comes with deadlines, criticism and unresponsive reviewers and contributors
- Adapt to the changes in today's business environment.

Core skills include writing, information flow, layout and design, delivery method (on-line versus print; reference versus user guide versus cookbook tutorial) and tool expertise. Writers take the complex theory of operation and reduce it to comprehensible, concise instructions. Illustrators work from the simplified text to create a visual cue or path for the customers to follow.

Common sense tells us that correct and well thought out illustrations enhance the reader's ability to learn, comprehend and retain information. Additionally, research supports the premise that a well-balanced combination of text and graphics out performs either alone.

Illustrations and text must complement each other. A poorly matched combination negatively affects learning and the readers willingness to pick up and read a manual. If the thickness and layout of a manual intimidate the readers, the completeness and accuracy of the information within do not matter. The writer and graphic artist must work as a well-oiled machine. Studies show that attractiveness and effectiveness of the product manual improve when this collaboration occurs early and often throughout the development of a manual.

This integrated collaboration takes time, requires face-to-face meetings and commitment from both visual and verbal experts. For this team to succeed, the members must know the collective talents and skills and use them; embracing the good and supporting the less developed areas. Members must take charge of their respective areas while working with the others toward the creation of an expertly designed and written user guide.

This user guide consists several essential elements that must flow seamlessly to achieve readability and retrievability. The elements include layout, page formats, sections, graphics, subjects. Readability is the degree of ease with which text is read and understood and retrievability is the degree of ease with which information can be found. Layout, the way text is presented on a page (chunking, sorting, ranking), should not be confused with page format. Formatting involves the physical attributes on the page, such as masthead, page number and section identifiers. These design elements must blend with the text and graphics to create a cohesive unit. This cohesive unit can only result through teamwork.

There must be a game plan that directs each facet of the technical communication team. This plan or process describes the steps and those responsible for the information and action along the way from the concept to launch and support phases of the product and the manual. Figure 18-1 illustrates potential building blocks.

A manual, even if developed through the best collaboration, is significantly enhanced and improved when other departments and customers are included in the process. Gathering contents requires writers and illustrators to leave their desks. Organizational support must exist for the writer's and designer's mission. If this support is missing, gathering information becomes a hit or miss operation. A fully integrated technical communication team provides useful synergy.

18.2.2   The Project Team

As documentation is a required part of a complete product, it needs to be an integrated part. In today's competitive world, the user guide affects the usefulness of the product and the product's acceptance by the customers. A successful product incorporates the skills, knowledge and sweat from departments such as marketing, research and development, service, training, manufacturing, regulatory and quality assurance and yes -- technical communications.

Writers and regulatory affairs personnel must work closely with the core team. This closeness is especially important for medical manufacturers because user error may result in more serious consequences than that of a user error in setting a VCR. Writers and graphic designers, working with hardware and software engineers, can be an advocate for the design of easy-to-use

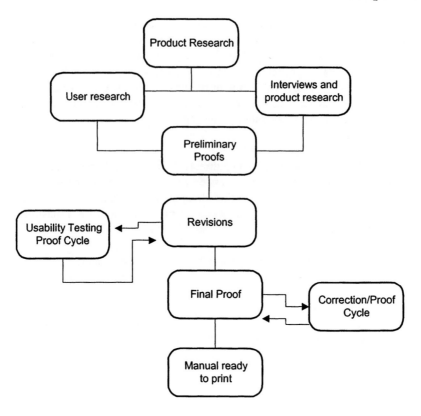

Figure 18-1   Initial building blocks in manual development process.

products. These types of products result in shorter and easier-to-use manuals, in fewer calls to the customer support department and in more satisfied customers.

18.3   How a Manual Evolves

"Nobody reads the manual"-- how many times have writers heard that statement in meetings, cubicles, hallways, offices and engineering labs. Studies show this is not true. They show that product manuals remain a much-needed (value-added) component of a product. One study of 34 test participants found that 74 percent skim the user guide and 15 percent thoroughly read at least the tutorials.

As products develop through a product development process, so does the supporting documentation. The manual process development cycle involves many steps. Entwined throughout the process are several concepts:

- User research
- User advocacy
- Instruction content outline and organization
- Writing, illustration and design procedures
- Writing warnings, cautions, notes
- Format and delivery design
- Testing, revision, approvals
- Distribution
- Revisiting the project.

18.3.1 User Research

This step is often overlooked for a variety of reasons -- tight schedule, lack of resources, lack of upper management support. The benefits of usable documentation support the integration of user research into the document development cycle. Well-developed manuals contribute significantly toward making a product easy to use.

- Clear and solidly indexed manuals help reduce technical support costs. If users can easily find the information they need to perform a task, they quickly complete a task, spend less time on problems and experience less frustration.
- Clearly written and well-organized manuals increase customer satisfaction by helping users perform their tasks more efficiently.
- Effective manuals and other product support tools can reduce training costs by helping the customer to learn and master tasks faster.

Reading preference	Percentage
Skim the user's guide	74%
Skim on-line documentation	50%
Run interactive tutorials	44%
Skim reference manual	41%
Skim reference or hint cards	26%
Thoroughly read reference cards	18%
Skim written tutorials	15%
Thoroughly read written tutorials	15%
Thoroughly read the user guide	9%
Read on-line documentation	9%
Thoroughly read reference manual	6%

Table 18-1   Reading Preferences

For medical products, a well-written manual that is useful to the user is not the only benefit of user research and testing of manuals. The FDA is redefining what they are looking for in product development in that they will be looking for human factors and testing throughout product and user interface design. The FDA defines the user interface broadly. "Description of the user interface includes all aspects of the device that a user operates, reads, uses, or comes in contact with, in the course of interacting with the device, including the controls, and displays, alarms, operating logic and all manuals, labeling and training materials necessary to operate and maintain the device."

The single most important rule in any kind of writing, but especially true for technical writing, is to know and write to your audience. To create manuals with the characteristics listed above, plan the tone, style, language, content and special format requirements from your knowledge of the audience. This means understanding the background, tasks and work environment of your audience.

Writing for the medical community helps define your audience. But even within the medical community, there are varying degrees of education, skill and learning behavior. More importantly, multiple users use the product for different tasks and in different ways. For example, users of an

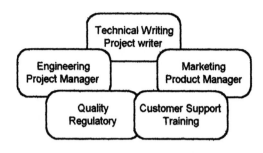

NO - Project team is not a
set of isolated experts

YES - Core team - disciplines
working together

Figure 18-2   Suggested team for integrated products and manuals.

anesthesiology machine may include anesthesiologists, nurse anesthetists and biomedical engineers. Each group typically expects different things from the machine, approaches the machine differently and performs different tasks. Adding to this equation and making the definition of an audience even more difficult, within these three groups, the users also vary by ability and knowledge.

Marketing, engineering and customer support often collect demographics of existing and potential users. Analyze this information by breaking it down: biological characteristics, literacy, technical sophistication, and learning preferences. Other characteristics and distinctions are important for your users, such as environment; e.g., do they typically work in dimly lit rooms.

This information should guide the choices you make in designing and writing the manual. You may need to manipulate current styles and elements to match your user's needs. For example, whether it is the anesthesiologist or biomedical engineer or a technician or clinician, you may manipulate elements like:

- Language and reading level
- Proportion of visual to verbal text
- Arrangements of segments/chapters

- Safety warnings

- Depth of instructions.

You can measure personal characteristics with questions like:

- Do you use this machine almost every day or only once in a while?
- Are you likely to have used other products like it?
- Do you do routine maintenance?
- Do you understand technical and medical terminology?
- Will you use the manual only to learn how to set up, use or operate the machine?
- Will you refer to the entire manual or only sections as necessary?
- Will you be able to look at the machine as you read the manual?
- What kinds of information do you want:
      basic instructions
      routine maintenance procedures
      troubleshooting
      explanation of concepts and theory.
- What kinds of manuals do you use:
      quick guides
      reference manuals
      technical manuals
      cheat sheets.

This section explained the need for user research, the benefits derived and listed several tools for gathering user information for the initial planning stages in manual development. The next section briefly explains a key role technical writers can play in gathering this information and in making sure the manuals and other product-support documentation meets the needs of the users.

18.3.2   User Advocate

In today's "lean" organizations, you often find hardware, software and mechanical engineers, technical writers, product managers, but usability specialists are rare. Often a member of the core team takes on the role of usability specialist, and more often than not, that member is the technical writer. That may mean learning new skills for the technical writer. The fit of knowledge and the motivation of a usability specialist and a writer are good for the "user friendliness and ease-of-use" of the product and the product's manual.

There are many tools to help with user research:

- Work practice observations -- you should always visit one or two potential users and observe them in their environment performing their everyday tasks.
- End user interviews -- this is when you can obtain personal characteristics and preferences.
- Focus groups -- provide valuable information on text organization and key tasks.
- Task analysis -- show the specifics of tasks performed.

18.3.3   Methods of User Research

There are many techniques for collecting information on the people who use our products. Type of product, development stage, schedule and management commitment to usability play a role in the technique used.

Usability and user research focus on how a product is used rather than on the functions and features. There are many ways to solicit this information:

- User and task observations -- watch user doing their tasks; analyze work processes
- Interviews, focus groups, questionnaires -- meet with users to solicit their preferences
- Benchmarking and competitive analysis – evaluate similar products
- Participatory design -- bring the user's perspective to design in early development stages
- Paper prototyping -- involve user's early in the development stage
- Usability testing -- watch actual users perform real tasks with the application.

There are many types of usability testing techniques. Select the one appropriate to your product and development process. You can find details of these techniques in many books. The next section briefly describes some details of a site visit, one of the most beneficial techniques.

18.3.4   Site Visit

Though one of other hardest techniques to implement, the visit to a customer site is one of the most beneficial. These visits often require coordination between marketing and maybe sales. Make sure the site your visit is approved by the product manager. Once the initial contact is made, follow up with a letter confirming the phone conversation. This letter should include:

- Purpose of study
- Expected outcomes
- Kinds of tasks you'll want to observe
- How long the visit will last
- What feedback they can expect
- What kind of equipment will be needed or that you will be bringing
- What assistance, if any, you will need from them
- A confirmation of the day and time
- A name and phone number if they have questions or need to reschedule.

If you are working on a confidential product where security is a requirement, you need to pick your sites carefully. You may also need the participants to sign a confidentiality or nondisclosure agreement.

Site plans and materials are key to a successful site visit. With the plan you determine the goals and develop the game plan or outline of what will happen during the visit. This chapter provides a brief account of test plans and site visits. You can find detailed information in many books and society literature, such as "Practical Approaches to Usability Testing for Technical Documentation," 1995, Society for Technical Communication.

Method	Use	Notes
Read and locate	Determine ease of navigation and organization	Need large sample of text and or illustrations. Be sure questions fit application and tasks.
Summary test	Comprehension and key concepts	Have users read specific sections of manual and then reflect back on what they think it means. Good for theory and concept sessions.
Usability edit	Users act as editors. They read through text and mark up things that are hard to understand, wordy or inconsistent.	This is good for procedures and step-by- step cookbooks.
Tasks	Test the clearness of instructions.	Select key procedures. Users complete tasks using text and illustrations. This is a good test for a preliminary manual
Telephone survey	General feedback.	Call before sending the information. Get the users to commit to a time frame they can commit to when assessing the data.
Training classes	Good for troubleshooting information, sequence of tasks and functions that may be used out of context.	Sit in on training classes. Listen to the types of questions asked and pay attention to the sequence in which the attendees do the tasks. Work with the instructor to train the class on the use of the manual(s).

Table 18-2   Examples of Documentation Usability Techniques

Method	Use	Notes
Paper and pencil testing	Initial feedback on structure, graphics, terminology, heading levels and task sequences.	Use this technique early on in manual development. Create samples of proposed manuals and walk users through tasks.
Field visits	Get a sense of the environment in which the manuals are used. Talk with many types of users with one visit -- nurses, doctor, and biomedical engineers.	Focus on important tasks and allow questions on the product as well as the manuals.
Customer support feedback	Hot issues from the field. Find out what customers are saying they need.	Customer support provides good input on user interface and documentation issues.

Table 18-2   (continued)

Site plan template

A plan may include:

- A brief introduction stating what the study is about.
- A list of questions you want to be able to answer after the study.
- What you want to accomplish with the study.
- Description of the participants.
- Description of the locations.
- Describe the visit -- what are the tasks, how much time is involved, milestones.
- A schedule of what will happen at each visit
- Description of the materials.
- Definition of what tools will be needed.

- A list the data analysis techniques you plan to use.
- Samples of materials, check lists, tasks.

Materials

The type of materials depends on the formality and nature of your visit. Contextual inquiry sessions differ in materials from visits focusing on task analysis or that of usability testing.

Some materials are common to most site visits, such as demographic questionnaires and observers' notebooks. The questionnaire confirms the characteristics you initially identified when you selected the participants and the notebook, which emphasizes what the observers should focus on, creates guidelines and task breakdowns to help the observer take notes.

Check list for visiting a site

Visit requirements:

- Audio and/or video tape recording. Although these are not mandatory for a successful visit, they can simplify the task of summarizing the event. Make sure you have extra batteries and blank tapes. You must ask permission before you tape a visit.
- Note taking. Two people visiting a site simplifies the information gathering and is less intrusive to the customers. Be sure to have plenty of paper and pencils. If you use a laptop, be sure the battery is charged should no outlet be easily accessible.
- Materials for the customers. Bring copies of the correspondence that went to that site, extra questionnaires, release and confidentiality forms (if required), supplies for the tasks, such as colored markers, sticky notes, diagrams, prototype, props.

The visit

The site visit provides you an opportunity for customer feedback and the customers a chance for creating a product that they can really use -- one that will make their tasks or jobs easier to do. If done right, the site visit provides a win-win situation. The guidelines for a visit are mostly common sense.

- Be on time
- Be courteous at all times (remember the customer is always right)
- Remind them you are there to find out information or to test a product; you are not there to test them -- they are not the ones being tested
- If you don't know the answer to a question, be sure to find it out and respond back to the participant
- Keep to the schedule and leave on time.

Although before you left the site you thanked them for their time and their efforts to help you, always send a follow-up thank you note.

Site visit report

The report is crucial and often follows the categories found in the site visit plan. The report is the basis for the structure of the product documentation. The report also provides feedback to the project team and concrete evidence to management that this type of activity is necessary and beneficial.

There are many ways to write a report. Write one that meets the needs of your development team. Essential elements of a report include:

- Issues or objectives and goals
- Statement of participants -- who they are and what are their characteristics
- Schedule and location
- List of who attended and what their roles were; for example, note taker, observer, test giver
- Executive summary

- Questionnaire and tabulated results
- Tasks and summary of results
- Post-questionnaire results and demographics
- Recommendations.

Once the report is distributed, call a meeting with the project to discuss the findings and arrive at the team's recommendations. If the recommendations are different from in the initial report, add the team's recommendations, redistribute and file for future reference.

18.3.5   What Goes into the Manual

Today, most people are overwhelmed by information and by tasks. There is always more to do than time in which to do it. Short and to-the-point quick guides are often the only manuals users pick up, leaving the user reference manuals to sit on the shelf.

Use the information from the team recommendations, the user site visits and the other user information collected in the user research stage to determine what goes into the manual and how it is organized. For example, a task analysis provides the sequence of tasks and helps the writer identify primary from secondary tasks.

Quick guides, cheat sheets, helpful hints assist the users in accomplishing their tasks. These can be on-line or hardcopy but usually there is a preference from the user. Some tasks, specially when operating medical equipment, need to be done quickly and with minimum interruption in the attention given to the patient. The best place for this type of information may be a cheat sheet that is attached to the machine -- not in on-line help or a manual.

A quick way to determine the most needed and most often accessed information is to look at what is printed on the "sticky notes" or other pieces of paper taped to the machine or walls. This is the type of information gathered through the various user research techniques.

Users need to know what to do, how to do it and when to do it. Your job is to meet these needs efficiently. Completing a task analysis early helps the writer design and organize the supporting tools to meet these needs.

Much research shows that step-by-step tutorials are the most read part of a manual. Based on this research and on your own, establish a format that incorporates an easy to use pattern. Place the procedures at the beginning of the chapters to save the readers from digging through the text. Make the procedures easy to find using visual cues and white space.

Cautions and warnings

Manufacturers have a duty and responsibility to warn users of potential dangers present in the system. On medical devices and in the manuals that support medical devices, there are always cautions and warnings. Each company has a Regulatory, Quality Control or a Legal department that provide input to what and where cautions and warnings must be in the manuals. Another statement often found at the beginning of the manual is the statement advising readers to read the entire instruction manual(s) before trying to operate the device.

General cautions and warnings provide information customers should know before they start operating the device. Place these statements in the beginning of the manual and at appropriate places throughout the manual, such as before a task or instruction.

There are several definitions of cautions and warnings according to the FDA:

Caution -- alerts the user to the possibility of a problem with the device associated with its use or misuse.

Warning -- alerts the user to the possibility of injury, death, or other serious adverse reactions associated with the use or misuse of the device.

Write your cautions and warnings to do four things:

- Identify the severity of the risk; will result in serious injury or death.
- Describe the nature of the risk: plugging in this cord while standing in water.
- Tell the user how to avoid the risk: make sure your hands are dry and you are standing on dry ground.
- Clearly communicate to the person exposed to the risk; be sure to write to the level of your audience.

Guidelines for writing cautions and warnings

- Include a signal word and color to convey the seriousness
- Include a symbol showing the nature of risk and consequences
- Clearly describe in words how to avoid the hazard
- Be consistent in terminology
- Keep cautions and warnings separate from general instructions
- Follow company and appropriate regulatory agency guidelines
- Place warnings and cautions throughout text wherever relevant.

18.3.6   Testing, Revisions, and Approvals

Once the manuals are completed, test them. Take them on site or simulate the environment and ask users or potential users to perform routine tasks using the manuals and other product tools. Set goals for the users; for example, can they perform a task using the instructions within so much time or with only a certain amount of rework or number of errors. The core team should decide what reasonable parameters for the response times.

- Calibrate the system for a pre-use check test.
- Set the system to mechanical ventilation.

- Turn off mechanical ventilation.
- Set the case parameters.

You can also test for the attributes of the manual, such as navigational cues, accuracy, applicability, attractiveness, completeness, consistency, retrievability and understandability. Table 18-3 shows the original outline of a quick reference guide and the resulting table of contents after testing six users.

Testing can also help catch errors of misinformation, steps that are missing (omissions can be just as dangerous as inaccurate text), and discrepancies. Quality has to be considered from the point of view of the user and these types of errors reflect poorly on the manual and the product.

While the writers can do all the right things--user research, succinct and accurate writing, document testing and rewriting--the quality of the manual cannot make up for a poorly developed product.

18.3.7 Distribution

You thoroughly researched the user needs, wrote a manual based on those needs and tested its usefulness. You created preliminary proofs, final proofs and received the input and approvals from the project team. Using the user research, you created a manual that meets the needs of the customers. This includes formatting and packaging. An example might be a pocket-size guide for pre-operation checkout information or setup information that clinicians might like to carry around in their pocket. To ensure meeting your customer's needs, you might want to send 5-10 copies of this manual with the system.

You design and package the documentation set to encourage the user to use and keep the manual. Make sure the appropriate instruction manual is the first thing a user sees when unpacking the product.

Remember the special someone who went the extra mile to make sure you got all the information you needed. Provide copies of the manuals to team members that may need copies.

Before testing	After testing
Control Basics	Control Basics
Setup, Mode and Pause	Pre-Op Checklist
Start/Stop	How to ....
Alarm Limits	How to ...
Disassembly/Assembly	How to ...
Adjust Arm Height	How to ...
	Top Ten Troubleshooting

Table 18-3   Before and After Table of Contents

18.3.8   Revisit the Project

There are two aspects to revisiting the project; team evaluation and customer follow-up. With the team evaluation, the writer and the illustrator think through their involvement; what went well and what didn't. A good idea would be for the writer and illustrator to meet with other team members to solicit their input on the process.

Another way to handle this part of revisiting the project would be to distribute an evaluation questionnaire. This questionnaire may question the process, communication, cooperation and commitment levels, and quality of the final results.

There are several ways to solicit customer feedback on the released manual.

- Site visits
- Questionnaires
- Phone surveys
- Customer support (evaluate customer calls)
- Feedback from marketing and field personnel.

Collecting this information is important, but what you do with the information is critical to the success of future projects.

- Distribute a summary of the feedback from both evaluations (team and customer) to co-workers and team members that were involved or may be involved on future projects.
- Make any necessary changes in the process.
- Note any necessary changes to the manuals -- to be implemented in next revision.
- Keep a record of the feedback for reference by other teams.
- Revise usability guidelines as needed or create them if they do not exist.

18.4   Style Guides

A style guide is a tool to set standards; it is not an instrument to stifle creativity. Everyone recognizes the need for standards, but creating them and following them are an entirely different matter. For a style guide to succeed, the guide must be created by everyone involved and commitment to the guide must start at the top and trickle down through the department.

Manuals, along with the product, represent your corporate image and level of commitment to the customers. A high quality message reflects positively on corporate image and employee morale. Often, the first contact a user may have with a product is the user documentation. And first impressions are lasting. Establishing consistent document design is one way to project an image of excellence and dependability for your company.

18.4.1   What and Why

A style guide is just that -- a guide. The essential element of any user guide is that it meets the requirements of the user in that it contains the information the users need in the form that they need it. Perception is reality, and if a manual looks difficult to use or looks like it does not contain the necessary information, then the manual fails. A style guide helps the writer write a consistent, clear manual.

A typical style guide provides standards for achieving consistent style and terminology. It contains specific information relating to the company-preferred page format, use of typeface and emphasizers, navigational tools, preferred spellings and acceptable abbreviations and terminology.

Writers and artists are creative people who constantly devise new ideas for improved learning tools. This creativity results in documentation tools meeting the specific needs of the product on which they are working. Since guidelines and standards grow and change as new developments and products arise, innovative ideas should be expected and welcome.

The guidelines provide a foundation for this creativity and advantages, both internal and external.

•	Consistency	Consistency conveys quality and dependability.
•	Consistency	Consistency in design provides a "company" look and feel. It also lessens the learning curve and is less intimidating for customers and support people.
•	Consistency	Consistency in organization increases readability, predictability and ease of use and reduces learning time.
•	Productivity	Manuals can be created or revised without guesswork.
•	Productivity	Projects can be taken over with little difficulty.
•	Productivity.	A ready reference for terms or issues reduces guesswork, increases consistency.

18.4.2   A Process

Indicative to a style guide is a manual development process. The manual production process may vary slightly depending on whether the manual is for a new or revised product. It is important that the writers, illustrators and in some cases, designers work together at the onset of product development. The flow chart in figure 18-4 depicts an example product development cycle.

Manual stages

Getting reviewed manuals returned is often one of the most frustrating parts of a writer's job. Specifying the differences between the proofs is important and can help with the quality of review comments. As with most things, there are black and white as well as gray areas in defining the differences between preliminary and final manuals.

Preliminary

During preliminary review, reviewers review for technical content, organization and completeness. Preliminary manuals:

- Are close (approximately 90% or more) to the final content and format.
- May or may not have associated art.
- May or may not have final art.
- May or may not have gone through regulatory approval process.

Final

During final review, reviewers only review for technical correctness. Final manuals:

- Are in final format
- Include final art
- Have gone through any regulatory approval process.

Publishing guidelines for preliminary and final review can support your efforts in timely and value-added proofs.

18.4.3   Templates and Organization

The official template evolves from input of end users, writers and artistic designers. This template must meet the needs of everyone involved. For the end users, the template must provide the information they need in the way they need to see it. For the writers and illustrators, it must accommodate the tools they use and allow for the most efficient manual development and revision process.

Manual Development Process

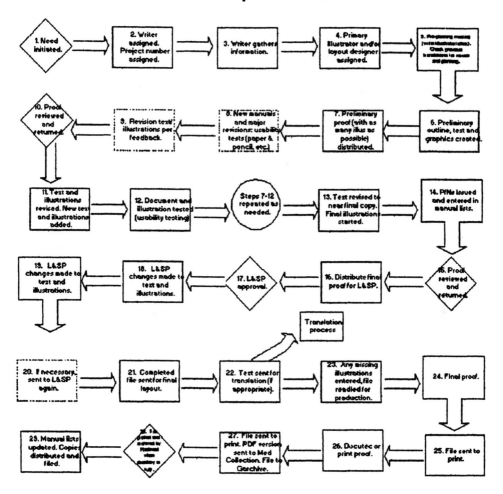

Figure 18-4 Manual development cycle.

The template includes styles for table of contents, section master page, headers, footers, figures, index and text pages. The original template could reside on the network and be downloaded for use by the individual writers and artists.

Covers and bindings

Walk into any bookstore. The variety of covers, size and binding of manuals and books is endless. What you choose must match the needs of your user, your process and your budget.

The trend today is toward smaller manuals, but the manual set may include a variety of sizes and types of information. For example, the main guides may be 81/2 by 11 with quick guide and cheat sheets being smaller. The main guides may be three-hole drilled for insertion into a binder that then sits on a shelf. The quick guide may be spiral bound or saddle stitched because it needs to fit into small spaces.

A trick often used to include color on the manual cover but to also stay within budget restrictions is the "pre-printed" cover. You can print volumes of covers with some artistic elements of color that help give the manual an inviting and friendly appearance. The covers may even match or contain some element of design used in the advertising and marketing of the product. This allows for consistency across the different types of information the user sees. To customize the cover to the manual or product, run the cover through color press and print the specifics in black.

Organizing the sections

While it may vary slightly based on the product, this list describes a general scheme of manual organization. Sectional table of contents include a brief "how to use" or "what's in this section" statement. There may be more than one manual, depending on the needs of the product. There may also be complementary guides, such as Quick reference, pocket guides, etc. The goal is to keep the text and illustrations consistent throughout the customer documentation.

The examples below reflect, in addition to the required legal
information, the results of a survey of anesthesiologists, nurse anesthetists and
biomedical engineers of how they would like to see the information organized.

User operations guide

> Cover
> Title page
> User responsibility
> Global table of contents
> Introduction
>> Table of contents
>> How to use the manual
>> Overview of system
>> Symbols/conventions used in manual and
>> on the product
> System controls (sections here depend on the system)
>> Table of contents
>> Overview
>> What are they
>> How to use
> Preoperative tests
>> Table of contents
>> Test intervals
>> Checklists
> Tutorial
>> Table of contents
>> Before a case
>> During a case
>> Other tasks
> Appendix
>> Additional sections (if required)
> Index (manuals more than 50 pages must include an
> index at least for English versions)

Setup, maintenance and troubleshooting guide

Cover
Title page
User responsibility
Global table of contents
Introduction
  Table of contents
  How to use the manual
System setup
  Table of contents
  How to set up the breathing circuit
  How to install gas cylinders
  How to use the shelves
Maintenance and troubleshooting (this may be
another whole manual)
  Table of contents
  Introduction
  Maintenance
  Troubleshooting
  Alarms
  User messages
  Other as appropriate
  Illustrated parts
  Specifications (this may be separate)
Appendix (if required)
Index (manuals more than 50 pages must include an
index at least for English versions)

Quick guide

Cover
"How to" sections on tasks most performed by the
users (keep the number of tasks to 10 or less to keep
the guide "quick")
Troubleshooting (abbreviated version from that in
the user guide; these reflect the "most likely"
troubleshooting situations).

18.4.4 The Drive Toward Consistency

The examples in this section are just that -- examples. Each writing department has rules and guidelines. These guidelines reflect years of writing experience and are gleaned from published style guide standards.

Illustrated steps

When an illustration is used before, after or within steps or procedures, any numbers on the illustration should reflect the steps.

If an illustration reflects only identifying text, the numbers on the illustration should reflect the associated legend; for example, "The following is an example of the ventilator display."

Bulleted lists

Use bullets, check marks, etc., to emphasize parts of a series.

- Introduce each list with a main clause followed by a colon.
- Capitalize the first word of each item.
- End with a period only if the item is a complete sentence.

Numbered lists

Use numbers for sequential steps or when you want to show a hierarchical relationship.

- Introduce each list with a main clause followed by a colon.
- Capitalize the first word of each item.
- End each item with a period.

An index

Each guide over 50 pages should have an index. In shorter guides, use your discretion.

- Use two 3-inch columns with a 0.25 gutter.
- Use a 0.5 point line to separate the columns.
- Use 10-point Helvetica for entries.
- Insert two spaces between index entry and page number.
- Indent two spaces for second level entries.

Intensifiers

Intensifiers are mechanical means of stressing ideas and concepts according to their importance. Use intensifiers with discretion. This section offers guidelines toward the effective use of common intensifiers such as boldface, underlining, italics, quotation marks, capital letters and centering.

Boldface
Use bold face for:
Section/chapter/subsection headings
The words: warning, caution and note
Display messages
Push knob to confirm change
Display functions when used as a user command
Select **2. Ventilation Setup** from main menu

Underlining
Use underlining sparingly. One instance of use may be for highlighting critical words in a message, such as <u>Do not</u> . . .

Italics
Use *italics* for:

- Figure titles and captions
- Highlighting special text
- Special effects
- Additional words (remember too many sentences in italics make for difficult reading).

Quotation marks

- Use "quotation marks" when:
- Identifying direct quotes
- Quotations appear in original
- Referring to a specific word, component or phrase ("absorber panel open" alarm)
- Identifying blank spaces (enter the tidal volume " ").

Remember,

- The period and comma always go inside the quotation marks (in Europe, they place them outside the marks)
- The dash, semicolon, question mark and exclamation point go within quotes only when apply to quoted matter.
- The dash, semicolon, question mark and exclamation point go outside the quotation marks when apply to the whole sentence.

Capital letters

Avoid unnecessary capitals.   Use a capital only if you can justify it. For example, do not say "The system switch turns ventilator and pneumatics On and Off." or "The indicator is On when the electrical power is on."

Use CAPITAL letters for:

- Acronyms
- Control panel & function names if they appear in with a capital letter or in all caps
- Product names
- Names of particular entities, such as Hewlett Packard
- Bullet lists, especially if the items are complete sentences
- The first word in headers, footers, figure titles, legends.

Center

Centering text or graphics has limited use -- with the best use being large figures.

18.4.5　General Rules of Grammar

- Spell out whole numbers below 10; use figures for 10 and above.
  (They have four four-room houses, 10 three-room houses, 12 10-
  room houses, 20 cars and two buses.)
  Spell out first through ninth when they indicate sequence in time or
  location (first base; First Amendment). Use 1st, 2nd, etc. when the
  sequence has been assigned in forming names (1st ward, 7th Fleet,
  etc.)
  Spell out a numeral at the beginning of a sentence. If necessary,
  rewrite the sentence. The one exception is a numeral that identifies
  a calendar year (1997 was a great year.).
  Spell out casual expressions (He walked a quarter of a mile. A
  thousand times no.).
  Use words or numerals according to an organization's practice
  (20th Century Fox, Big Ten football).
- Only use a comma in numbers with more than four digits (1000,
  10,000) unless you are representing a number on the display that
  includes a comma.
- Combine numerals and words for numbers greater than six digits
  (i.e., 1 million) unless you are referring to a specific number (for
  example, 165,700 bytes).
- Try to avoid using "will be." The message ~~will be~~ displayed. . .
  The message is displayed or The message appears.
- Avoid leaving orphans at ends of lines or paragraphs. For example,
  system.
- Use active voice.
- Speak directly to the reader, referring to her as "you" rather than as
  "the user."
- Include articles; write "Preparing the absorber" not "Preparing
  absorber."
- When in question, refer to The Associated Press Stylebook and
  Libel Manual.

18.4.6   Formatting Bibliographic Information

Journal article
Krikelas, J. "Information-Seeking Behavior: patterns and concepts." <u>Drexel Library Quarterly</u> 19, no, 2 (Spring 1983): 5-20.

Book
Eisenson, J. <u>The Improvement of Voice and Diction</u>. 2nd ed. New York: Macmillan. 1965.

Presentation
Allan, J., Punch, and Chi, C. "Signal Averaging in Measurements." Presented at ACM, New Orleans, November, 1987.

Internet
There is no set standard but until one is securely established, follow one of these examples:

> Krikelas, J. "Information-Seeking Behavior: patterns and Concepts."
> <u>Drexel Library</u>
> <u>Quarterly</u> 19, no, 2 (Spring 1983): 5-20.
> On-line. Internet. December 30, 1997 (date you accessed)
> Available http://www.article web address

or

> Hartman, Brian. (1996, July 9). Lamm to seek reform party nomination.
> *Now Politics* [On-line]. Available:
> http://www.politicsnow.com/news/July96/09/pn0709lamm/index.htm
> [1996, July 9]

18.4.7   Handling Grammatical Exceptions

The following alphabetical list covers preferred spellings and subject/verb agreement for unusual "gray area" words. Use what is appropriate and acceptable for use within your company.

accept the selection/change not confirm the selection/change

back up (v.)
backup (n.)
back-up (adj.)

criteria is, not criteria are

data is, not data are

double check (n.)
double-check (v.)

gray, not grey

on screen / on line (prep. phrases)
on-screen/ on-line (adj.)

owner's (guide/manual)

re-enter

save the selection/change, not confirm the selection/change

set up (v.)
setup (n.)
set-up (adj.)

user's (guide/manual)

18.4.8   Using Abbreviations and Acronyms

This section lists acceptable abbreviations and acronyms/initializations, but it is preferable to spell the word entirely. When using a shortened word form, always spell out or define it in the first reference. The following is just an example of basic acronyms, you'll need to customize to your company's products.

adjustable pressure limit	APL
American National Standards Institute	ANSI
analog/digital	A/D
common gas outlet	CGO
days	d
dual common gas outlet	DCGO
electronic gas delivery	EGD
electronic vaporization and mixing	EVM
field replaceable unit	FRU
floppy disk drive	FDD
fresh gas	FG
gas management system	GMS
hard drive	HD
Hewlett Packard	HP
hour	h
inspiratory to expiratory ratio	I:E ratio
intensive care unit	ICU
International Standards Organization	ISO
light emitting diode	LED
local area network	LAN
mean time between failure	MTBF
mean time to repair	MTTR
micro	μ
microsecond	μs
microvolt	μV
milli	m
milliampere	mA
millimeter	mm

millisecond	mS
minute	min
nano	n
ohm	☐
operating room	OR
original equipment manufacturer	OEM
parts per million	ppm
pound	lb
second	s
volt	V
watt	W
wide area network	WAN

18.4.9   Tips for Translations

Many user guides are translated. To facilitate translations, pay attention to words, phrases and sentences. Keeping alert to the nuances and idiosyncrasies of English can help avoid misinterpretation and translation errors and reduce translation costs.

Writing hints

The following tips pinpoint some of the potential problem areas for translators.

- **Limit the use of acronyms. If use, write out every acronym and abbreviation at its initial use.** Knowing what the abbreviation stands for determines whether its article changes, whether the term is translated and whether the order of the letters in the acronym is changed. (This is especially helpful if the term is not the glossary.)

- **Verify that the antecedent for each pronoun is obvious.** In some languages, the words "it" and "they" have different forms, depending on the gender of the word translated. The translator must be certain of what the antecedent is or the translation will shift from being ambiguous in English to just plain wrong in the translation.
- **Avoid the use of "there is/are," "here is/are," it is," etc. as the subject/verb of a sentence.** These phrases have no meaning in English and lead to ambiguity in the translation.
- **Check the compound modifier phrases in your document.** Translators, who are less familiar with the topic, may have difficulty determining what adjective/adverb modifies what noun/verb. Phrases like "real time processing," can be classified by using a hyphen, "real-time processing."
- **Always use complete sentences.**
- **Do not omit the word "that," to start restrictive or defining clauses.**
- **Rewrite any slang or jargon.** These terms are difficult to translate and to understand for non-native English speakers.
- **Do not expect the translator to know if your use of the "/" symbol means "and," "or," "and/or" or something else.**
- **Be sure to use the words "if" and "when," "which" and "that" and "can" and "may" correctly.**
- **Do not use humor, especially puns or "cute" words and phrases in your documentation.** These techniques have strong regional bias and do not translate into another language. Watch out for cultural bias in your examples and symbols. A smiley face or birthday cake may have little or no meaning or a different meaning outside North America.
- **Limit verb forms.** Do not use compound structures, gerunds or subjunctive structure.
- **Minimize the use of passive voice.** Do not use passive voice in procedures.

Illustration hints

- **Graphics should be specific enough to convey the message,** but avoid illustration product features that vary from country to country (for example, electric plugs, connections).

- **Avoid images of hands unless add clarity to illustration.** The meanings of hand gestures vary from culture to culture -- even the use of a female versus male looking hand has cultural nuances.
- **Do not use symbols or icons to merely save space or for fun.** Use only those that are universally accepted and recognized or have gone through testing to avoid ambiguity and misinterpretation.

18.5   Manual Tips

From your fifth grade teacher to your technical writing professor, you learned how to write. The information in this section serves as an abridged refresher course to the writing knowledge you already possess. You will also find a few "dos and dont's" when it comes to graphics.

18.5.1   The Right and Wrong of the Graphical Element

Graphics have tremendous power; they can often make the difference between just a "user" manual and a "used" manual. If created right, a graphical element is the first thing a reader notices on a page -- may even be the only thing a reader notices.

Like the perfect sentence, a graphical element must be created, revised, tested and revised again. Like written information, a graphical element may either give information or simply be noise that gets in the way of the real message. A graphic may be just noise if:

- It is the wrong graphic for the message
- The color is wrong or there is too much color
- The graphic contains too much detail
- It is placed in the wrong location
- It is a photograph that should have been cropped for emphasis
- It is a photograph that should have been a line drawing
- It is just visual clutter -- has no meaning and is just taking up space.

Graphics should make an impact. Design graphics to make a single point, which should then be immediately clear to the reader upon viewing the graphic. This point should not be blurred by the use of color. Color, by itself, is powerful and often blurs the point of the graphic.

If the graphic escapes from the demons color and over-design, it must also win the battle of location. It is often said in sales that location is everything. This is also true in graphical design. Often you will see "refer to the figure on page 30 and you are reading from page 12." The graphic is obviously in the wrong location. Try to locate graphics within two pages of its citing.

Studies show that the absolutely best location of a graphic for impact is the upper left corner of a page. For technical writing, the best location is in the same location as where the written text would have been placed.

Sometimes, the graphical element or illustration complements the written text. Today, the trend is for the graphical element or illustration to replace the written text.

If you are not a graphic artist or technical illustrator or have one working with you to create a manual, the best advice in working with graphics is to keep it simple. Remember:

- Graphics are powerful; use them to present the most important and difficult information
- Graphics are useful; use the different graphical elements to portray the different types of information in the most succinct and clear way
- Graphics can be noisy; delete the extraneous detail
- Photos are famous for noise; use that cropping tool
- Graphics are like technical writing; you do not need to be artistic to get the point across.

On the subject of color, it is preferred over and generates a more positive attitude than black and white materials. Color in and of itself does not make the material more effective. Use color to focus attention. Color is also more effective than black and white in search tasks. Color has also been shown to improve retention when used as a coding device or an integral part of the content to be used.

18.5.2 Which is Right?

Debates exist today on the best way to write certain phrases and sentences and even words. Years ago, everyone wrote "data are;" today that battle is over and you see "data is" more often than not. The following represents one side of the battlefield.

> **data is versus data are** - in a technical manual data is generally viewed as a group so either way is acceptable; just be consistent.
> **media is versus media are** - either way is acceptable; just be consistent.
> **fewer versus less** - fewer refers to number; less modifies a noun.
> **between versus among** - use between when there are two; use among when there are more than two.
> **numerous versus many** - numerous refers to an exact, maybe unknown, number; many refers to a large indefinite number.

18.5.3 Rules to Live By

- The most important rule is to know and to write to your audience.
- Organize by task -- so users can follow the manual based on what they are trying to do.
- Accept constructive criticism gracefully -- be willing to rewrite.
- Write short sentences; generally less than 15 words.
- Use active voice.
- Use parallel construction.
- Use positive rather than negative words. For example:
    Positive - Remember to use the shutdown steps.
    Negative - Do not forget to use the shutdown steps.
- Make sure the subject and verb agree.

Keep it simple

You are trying to get a point across. You are trying to provide information in the clearest, most easy-to-find way. You are not going to impress anyone by using two or three words when one will work.

Words to avoid	Substitutes
accordingly	so
applicable	apply to
assistance	help
utilize	use
in order to	to
in regard to	about
provided that	if
whether or not	whether
with the result that	so that
in the near future	soon
facilitate	ease
considerable	much
consequently	so
compensate	pay
due to the fact that	because
prioritize	rank
in the event that	if
has the ability	can
quantify	measure
at this point in time	now

Proofreading

The ugly job that no writer wants to do. The difficult job when you are the writer as well as the proofreader. Proofreading your own writing is difficult.

References

Albers, J., *Interaction of Color*. Yale University Press, 1975.

Backinger, C. and P. Kingsley, "Write it Right," U.S. Department of Health and Human Resources, Food and Drug Administration, 1993.

Benson, P.H. "Designing Documents: Illustration, Instruction and collaboration," *InterCom*, July, 1997.

Bias, R.G., Mayhew, D.J., (eds) *Cost-Justifying Usability*. Academic Press, 1994.

Brockman, J., *Writing Better Computer User Documentation*. John Wiley & Sons, 1990.

Cady, D. *Bulletproof Documentation*. New York: McGraw Hill, 1996.

Greenbaum, T.L., *The Handbook of Focus Group Research: Revised and Expanded Edition*. Lexington Books, 1993.

Hackos, J, and J. Redish, *User and Task Analysis for Interface Design*. Wiley, 1998.

Hoft, N., *International Technical Communication*. Wiley, 1995.

Horton, W., *Illustrating Computer Documentation*. John Wiley and Sons, 1991.

Horton, W., *The Icon Book*. Wiley, 1994.

Horton, W., *Designing and Writing Online Documentation*. Wiley, 1994.

"Prepare your documents for better translation," printed in the STC newsletter, *Intercom* 1996.

Schoff, G, Robinson, P., *Writing and designing manuals.* Lewis publishers, 1991.

Schriver, K. *Dynamics in Document Design.* John Wiley & Sons, 1997.

Smart, K.L. and K. Sewright, "Documentation Value," *InterCom*, July, 1997.

Frequently asked questions on questionnaires:
            http://www.UCC.IE/hfrg/resources/qfaq1.html

Archive of graphic design discussions:
            http://www.nothingness.org/graphicsweb/digests/>

Note: Internet sites change. Sites were checked and running at time of writing.

Chapter 19

Translation: "It's A Small World After All"

Margaret Rickard – Datex-Ohmeda, Inc.
Madison, Wisconsin

Fact or fiction -- many companies today find themselves in a market where 50 percent or more of their profit comes from countries other than the United States. The answer -- most definitely a fact, and this segment of the market continues to grow in volume and complexity every day.

As mentioned in Chapter 18, there are 101 places where something could go wrong when creating a user manual; international markets compound the challenge. There are several hurdles to jump when localizing a product and documentation. One of the hurdles, "knowing the user," is the first step toward good user manuals and localization. This challenge is daunting when you need to understand users that are thousands of miles away and experience a life quite different from your own. Another high hurdle is the expense involved in localization and translation.

While this chapter addresses these challenges and others along the road to a localized and translated user manual, the emphasis is on translation.

- Defining localization and translation
- Importance of good English
- Translation process
- Symbols and graphics
- Choosing translators.

19.1   Defining Translation and Localization

Many people believe translation and localization mean the same thing. But they do not. Translation is but a phase of localization. Localization, building and customizing a product to a specific market, starts during the user research phase and translation occurs later in the development cycle. A caveat here is that awareness of translation requirements must occur early in development so field lengths are adequate, the software code design facilitates translation, and hardware requirements are considered.

The degree of localization or translation of a product depends on market and legal requirements. These requirements vary by company and by products within a company.

The market requirements focus on whether or not there is enough business within a specific market to warrant localization or translation expense. Some companies develop formulas to determine the return on investment for these costs. Another driving force behind market requirement is what the competitors are doing.

Legal requirements drive the translation and localization of many products. The development of the European Council (EC) requirement that products sold into these countries must have the CE mark is the impetus for many companies to start translating their products.

Many regulations require that a product be translated into the native language of the countries into which they are to be sold. The degree of translation required varies by country. Some countries require the translation of all manuals; others require only installation and basic operating instructions. Some countries require that the software also be translated. Of course, you should translate all product safety information.

19.1.1   Localization

Localization is the process of designing and producing a product for the global market. Localization involves designing and adapting the product to suit the requirements, language, conventions and marketing culture of the locale in which the product is to be sold. This locale is often different from that of the main market for which the product is developed. While localization most often includes translation, especially in today's global economy, it may not. Localization may include:

- Translating some or all parts of the user information for the product
- Developing the product to meet needs of the market or specific markets
- Adding information to support specific market needs or options to meet those needs
- Adding or modifying the user information to meet regulatory requirements
- Building cultural differences into the product or modifying the product to account for cultural differences
- Adding options or modifying the product to meet market and/or regulatory requirements.

19.1.2   Translation

Translation is the process of putting all or part of the user information into the native language of the target market. Translation is more than just placing text in the native language of the target country; it involves linguistic and cultural differences. The complexity of translation deepens with the knowledge that differences occur within countries that have similar linguistics and cultures.

The United States and the United Kingdom share the English language. Yet each country brings differences to the English language. Many words mean the same but are spelled differently: gray - grey, color - colour, utilize - utilise. Similar functions also have different names, such as zip code in the United States and post code in the United Kingdom. For translation to succeed, one must pay attention to these details.

19.2   The Importance of Good English

The usefulness and success of the translations directly relate to how well the English text is written. Well-written information is useful for your customers regardless of the country in which they work. This well organized and written information often needs to be changed, removed, replaced or added to address the needs of specific locales.

Clear writing with short sentences, active verbs, and unambiguous and culture-free words facilitates good translation. The sentences, paragraphs and step-by- step instructions you write must first be understood by the translator, and then through the translations, by the end user.

19.2.1 Checklist of What to Look For

Many of the guidelines needed to present clear and unambiguous text is covered in Chapter 18. Here is a check list of what do look for:

Terminology

- Be consistent -- develop a terminology list
- Do not use jargon
- Do not create new words
- Avoid using acronyms
- Avoid using words with multiple meanings
- Develop a glossary
- Develop a conventions table; for example, what press and select mean
- Do not abbreviate
- Avoid mnemonics; if you have to use them, define them the first time they are used.

Cultural issues

- Avoid cultural-specific examples; be sensitive to cultural differences
- Be careful about local conventions, such as measurement, day/month/year, time, monetary values and time zones

- Be careful with color; if in doubt, contact the specific country representative (The International Standards Organization [ISO] developed specifications on the use of color on computer displays)
- Use care when describing local devices, such as keyboards, power cords, and fuses.

Regulatory and Legal

- Check with your legal or regulatory department regarding the requirements for the target markets
- Make sure the safety information is included and tested
- Make sure the trademarks, copyright, patent notices, warranties, references to user and manufacturers responsibilities and safety labels are included and correct
- Make sure the international business requirements are included, such as service information numbers, addresses,and product and parts ordering information.

Writing

- Follow grammar rules
- Avoid using auxiliary verbs like can, may, might, should
- Be careful with conjunctions; it is often unclear how much text is included in the phrase
- Remember that transitive verbs take an object
- Remember to include the articles *a, an* and *the* and the words *is* and *of*
- Be friendly; but not too friendly, as in some cultures this may be interpreted as condescending
- Write short sentences -- recommend an average of 12-15 words
- Avoid verbosity
- Write gender-free text
- Be careful when using metaphors and humor -- humor can be confusing or even offensive to other countries, and the metaphor might not have international applicability
- Be aware of punctuation differences, such as hyphenation.

Most languages (except for Asian-character based languages) incorporate hyphenation. For example, the German language likes to combine smaller words into long words and hyphenation can change the spelling. The traditional spelling of ballet theater "Ballettheater" becomes "Ballet-the-eater" if it breaks across two lines.

19.2.2   Technology and translation

Machine translations or machine-aided translation software packages have come a long way. For a translation to be effective, however, human interaction is required. There are many machine translation packages available. One such tool is called "Author's Structured Simplified English Tool" (ASSET). If you are interested in this type of translation, check out the Internet or visit the exhibition hall at a Society for Technical Communication (STC) conference.

Machine translation or translation memory systems need a lot of input in the beginning from the writer and editor. The system needs to learn your industry's terminology and your company's style and accepted phraseology. The system needs to learn how you instruct the users. Do you say "Press the Enter key" or "Press Enter?"

Another way to take advantage of technology in the translation process is the use of controlled or simplified English packages. Working similarly to the grammar package in Word™, these packages check for approved words and verbs. Simplified English (SE), based on good English practices, limits the use of flowery, non-specific language. For example, if the writer writes "To utilize the Stop function,..." the SE checker flags the word "utilize" and suggests the word "use." You can usually customize these SE packages to meet the requirements of your industry and company.

Most word processing packages include a grammar checking package. Even the most qualified and experienced writer benefits from taking a minute or two to run these checks. The results should reflect your department's guidelines, such as Flesch Reading Ease, Flesch Kincaid Grade Level or Bormuth Grade Level. These tests keep you honest in terms of words per sentence and active versus passive structure.

19.3   The Translation Process

Translations, like manual development, must result from a well-defined process. This process supports the awareness of and planning for translation must happen early in the manual development process. The writers and graphic personnel meet early in the process to identify areas where they can reuse existing text and illustrations. See figure 19-1.

The translation process is a process within a process -- the manual development and product localization processes. The translation process needs cooperation from several departments. For this cooperation to happen, involve the appropriate departments in developing the process. This way everyone knows what needs to be done, when and by whom.

Example translation process

Responsibility	Steps
1. Translation requester	Notify translation coordinator a minimum of 30 days prior to start of project. Provide information like target languages, approximate format and desired completion date. Verify the code strings and messages.
2. Translation coordinator	Identify translation resources, establish schedule and cost estimates. Assemble reference material for translators.
3. Translation requester	Insure English version has received appropriate approvals.
4. Translation requester	Provide Translation coordinator with hard and/or soft copy of approved materials for translation.

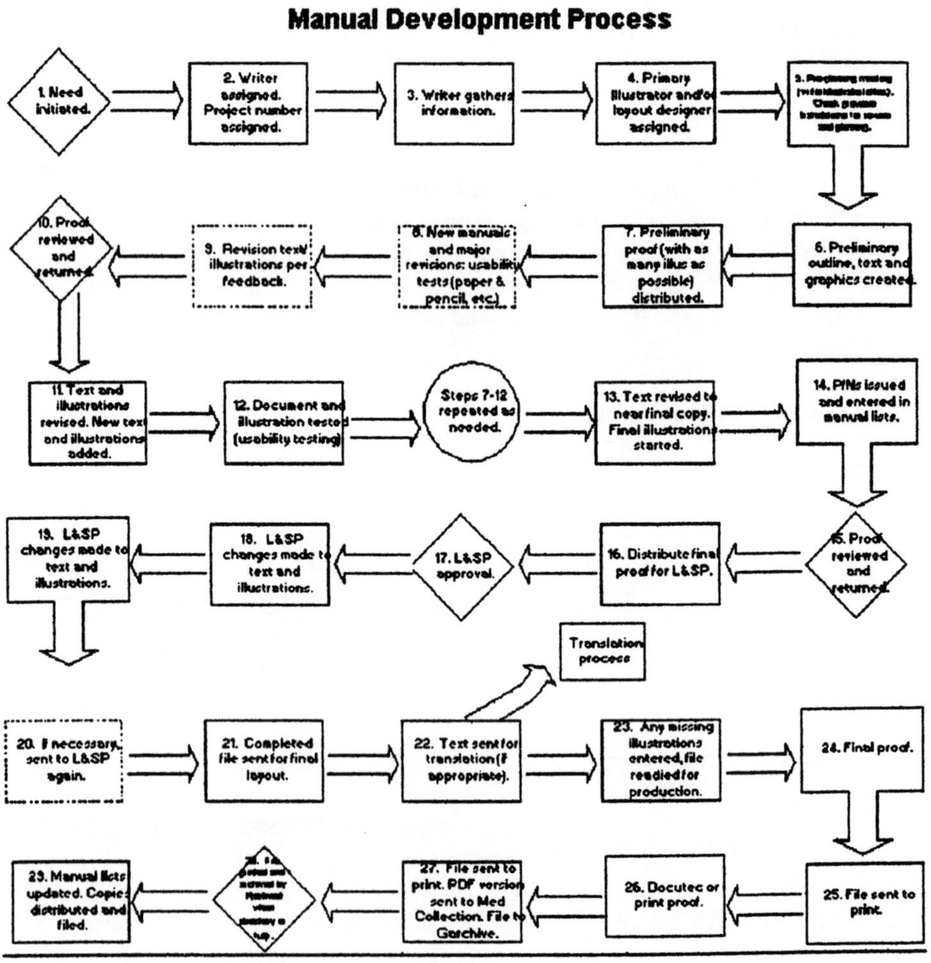

Manual Development Process

Figure 19-1 Translation as part of the manual development process.

Responsibility	Steps
5. Translation coordinator	Send translation materials and schedule to translator. Notify in-country reviewers. Track project. Provide technical support as needed to translators and reviewers.
6. Translator	Translate electronic file. Send completed translation, schedule and approval forms to reviewers. Notify Translation coordinator when materials are forwarded for review.
7. Reviewer	Verify materials for technical and cultural accuracy. Return materials to translator with signed approval form.
8. Translator	If necessary, make any changes or corrections noted by the reviewer.
9. Translation coordinator	Send copy of approval form to Quality Control or Regulatory. Send translated materials to appropriate department to prepare for printing.
10. Translator requester	Proof the final formatting of materials. Coordinate any revisions with the appropriate department. Validate user-accessible software translations in accordance with software development processes. Release materials.

Responsibility	Steps
11. Translation Coordinator	Notify reviewer and project manager that material is ready.
12. Others	Print, archive and supply as required.

19.4   Symbols and Graphics

The market for medical products is growing more global every day. Selling globally brings with it translation issues. Translations are costly and time consuming.

The best way to hold down translation cost is to look at each written word to make sure it adds value to the information – the fewer the words, the lower the translation costs. Many companies are using more symbols and graphics to create manuals and product information that require less translation. In addition to clear, concise writing, the use of symbols and graphics work together to create more readable, less expensive to translate documents. Remember "A picture is worth a thousand words," but if you end up translating, that picture saves you those words in every language you translate.

Manuals are using more and more illustrations and photographs. The trend is to use more graphics and to complement these graphics with minimal text or to replace text with graphics. This move toward more graphical documentation saves on translation costs. To optimize on these savings, use development tools and software packages that support the transfer of these illustrations into layout and word processing programs used in-house and by your translators around the world or your translation house.

The American National Standards Institute (ANSI) and the International Standards Organization (ISO) require certain symbols and colors for different functions and levels of warnings. There are cultural differences, but the U.S., Canada and other Western countries are quite similar in what people associate with symbols and colors. Noticeable differences come into play when dealing with Eastern countries.

Symbols and icons, and to a lesser degree, graphics help create internationally accepted products but they must be easily recognizable or identifiable by the products' markets. Icons and graphics can communicate messages more effectively, create the perception of international product, lower the costs of translation, and if done right, replace terms or ideas that may be difficult to translate.

Like many things in life, there is a time and place to use graphics, symbols or icons. Use them:

- To pictorially show a complex function or concept
- When an object or function must be reliably and or quickly understood
- To make the manuals more user-friendly
- To differentiate between visually different buttons
- To show location
- For critical distinction.

As mentioned in Chapter 18, words and pictures work best when they complement each other; for example,

- To depict complex functions that an icon or graphic alone can not describe
- When a picture or verbal description alone is still to vague
- When communicating to such a diverse audience that one may not understand just the picture or description.

Studies show that a picture takes less time to process than a string of words, but only if the picture is quickly and reliably understood by all target audiences.

19.4.1 Basic Guidelines

- Use illustration tools that are accepted and used in the different locales and by your translators
- Place labels far enough from the illustration to accommodate the alphabet of all languages -- callouts often solve this problem

- Keep illustrations simple
- If using symbols or icons that are not industry approved, test them in your specific markets
- Do not limit illustration text by placing text in boxes
- Identify and define all symbols and icons
- Keep graphics, icons and symbols simple
- Use internationally accepted symbols and icons whenever possible
- Be consistent in color, shapes, and context
- Avoid culture-specific metaphors and design elements
- Do not include text within a symbol or icon
- If symbol or icon can not safely represent a function or idea, use words
- Be careful when using gestures- these carry specific cultural nuances
- Create gender-free and culture-free people (unisex/universal graphics).

19.4.2 Different Strategies for Different Countries

Style of learning varies both by country and by individual. While it may be an insurmountable task to accommodate the learning style of everyone in your target audience, be aware of the differences and design and write accordingly. Some examples, include:

- Americans want text that is short and straight to the point
- Germans prefer details and lots of information
- Americans like informality
- The French lean toward formal and authoritative
- The Japanese place emphasis on accuracy
- The Chinese favor stressing the basic principles where the readers infer the details
- Some people learn best through visual stimuli
- Some people learn best through textual stimuli
- Some people learn best through auditory stimuli
- Many people prefer the exploratory method of hands-on trial and error.

Good graphics, icons and the use of symbols create a more culture-free manual. Text often carries more baggage like emotion and tone. Below are some tips for creating unisex/universal drawings.

- Use simple, abstract representations when drawing people -- hair, coloring, facial structure should not be identifiable
- Simplify clothing -- omit buttons, seams and other details that may represent one culture over another
- Avoid hand gestures
- Be careful with color.

19.5   The Importance of Glossaries

Glossaries provide consistency within a manual set and across the different product lines. Glossaries provide important and useful information to product development teams, writers and translators.

A glossary can be as simple as just listing functions and their definitions. A well-developed glossary also includes phrases like "To save the selection, press Enter." Before you start translation of the glossary, make sure everyone approves the English text. As you add a language or product, add the appropriate information to the glossary table.

Function	Phrase	Definition	Spanish	French
Bag ventilation		Manually bag the system	*Spanish text*	*French text*
	Turn the control knob	This is how you select a function or parameter	*Spanish text*	*French text*

A glossary helps

- Writers maintain consistency in writing phrases and selecting terminology.

- Software programmers maintain function consistency across products.
- Translators as a tool in translating the manuals and software.

This glossary also becomes an important tool in reducing translation costs. As the glossary grows and the writers and programmers reuse the phrases and functions, less and less of the manual and software will require translation.

19.6 Choosing a Translator

Who should do the translations? Choosing a translator is a time-consuming job -- one you should take seriously.

19.6.1 Basic Requirements for a Translator

There are several key traits to look for in translators.

- Are they native speakers? Though debated, it is best if they reside in the local country.
- Basic knowledge of the field. This knowledge is imperative if translating for a medical device. It's recommended that for a neurological device, the translator be a clinician in that field; the same for anesthesiology, cardiology, etc. To inform the translators on products specifics, send them product materials like brochures and previous manuals.
- Do they know English? Many manuals are written in English regardless of the country of origin. For the translator to correctly translate, they must be fluent in English.
- Do they have decent writing skills? Often a translator writes minimal text to localize paragraphs and software or hardware requirements, such as power.
- Are they familiar or experienced in the software packages used to create the manuals? Do they have these packages?
- Can you trust them to meet schedules?
- Can they effectively communicate with the translator coordinator and the reviewers?

19.6.2   How to Get the Job Done

There are basically four ways translations can be done.

1. In-house (you can do some or all in-house)
2. A translation company
3. A network of translators; usually one or two per language
4. Local subsidiaries or distributors.

In-house translators

Volume is key if you decide to bring your translators in-house. If you have enough translations to keep the translator(s) busy, bringing them in-house may be the way to go. You may choose to do only the high volume languages in-house and contract out the others.

Advantages

- Translator is close to product development
- Translator can develop hands-on knowledge of products
- Translator can improve consistency of translation across products.

Disadvantages

- May lose culture-specific knowledge over time
- Depending on volume of work, may not be cost effective
- May be hard to find translator, who is also a good writer, that is from the target countries.

Translation company

The globalization of the market place created a boom in the translation and localization industry. New companies start up every day, and older, existing companies continue to grow their services. If you are in a hurry, don't have the resources in-house, and have an unlimited budget, you can quickly get the job done through a translation company.

Advantages

- Experience
- Often provide project coordination
- Large network of translators.

Disadvantage

- Often more expensive (average 50% more than individual translators)
- Don't always have translators specific to your industry
- Translators not always located in target country.

Develop a network of translators

Developing a network of translators takes time and energy. Building a relationship of mutual trust reaps large rewards in the translation business.

Advantages

- About half as expensive as translation companies
- You control who is doing the translation
- One time investment in developing network.

Disadvantages

- Takes a lot of work to develop network
- Requires resources to perform project coordination.

Use subsidiaries and local company representatives

No one should know your companies' products than your subsidiaries and local company representatives. No one should have more at stake if translation into the native language is not complete. Sometimes, however, local representatives may work for more than one company, which can complicate issues and priorities.

Advantages

- Product knowledge
- Interested in good translation
- Capability of handling internally or externally, depending on need and resources.

Disadvantages

- Inability to allocated time or resources
- Conflicting priorities
- Difficulty in meeting deadlines.

19.6.3   Which Way to Go

You can probably meet your translation needs through any of the four methods described in section 19.4.2. You may find that a combination of methods works best for your company's situation.

If your company is small and does not have resources for coordinating the translation effort, then using a translation company or the subsidiaries might be the answer. If, however, you have someone who could take on the responsibilities of a translation coordinator, your company would benefit from the development of a translation network. Companies often believe the cost savings from using individual translators is worth the effort.

Determine your needs, assess your personnel resources and examine your budget. Look at these three items carefully to choose the method best for you.

19.6.4   What Translators Need

For translators to successfully translate your materials, they need certain things.

- Glossaries -- translators need glossaries of functions, terminology, specific phrases used in your product and the accompanying documentation. Glossaries are critical to the translation's success and are often the first thing a translator asks for.
- Product literature -- translators need to know about the product. The more they know, the better the translation.
- Existing translated materials -- translators use these materials to cut and paste existing words and phrases. They also use these materials to learn about the product and to assess the writing style.
- Help or reference person -- translators need a single contact person. They need to know they can call this person with any questions they may about the product or the billing process.
- Appropriate software -- translators need to work from the same programs in which the materials are created. It is usually in your best interests if you help them with this.

19.7   It's a Small World

This chapter explained the basics of translating your product materials. The world is getting smaller every day. The marketing department needs to assess the markets and determine whether the return on the investment for translations and localization for a specific country make sense.

Some companies place the costs for translations in each product's budget. Other companies have one big translation budget where projects are chosen and priorities are set. Either way, the cost of translation needs to be in someone's budget; otherwise they often are late, hastily scheduled or do not get done at all.

As noted earlier in this chapter, regulations and specific country requirements drive the need for translations in today's market. Translating and localizing a product makes sense from a fiscal and corporate responsibility and accountability standpoint. The employee who can help their company set up an efficient and cost-effective translation process, is indeed an employee to be valued.

References

Courtney, A.M., *Chinese Population Stereotypes: Color Associations, Human Factors*, 28(1), 97-99. 1986.

Hoft, N., *International Technical Communication*. Wiley, 1995.

Horton, W., *Illustrating Computer Documentation*. New York: John Wiley and Sons, Inc., 1991.

Horton, W., *The Icon Book*. New York: Wiley, 1994.

Jones, S., C. Kennelly, C. Mueller, M. Sweezy, B. Thomas, and L. Velez, *Developing International User Information*. Digital Equipment Corporation, 1992.

http://www.bucknell.edu/~rbeard/diction.html (This page has links to over 400 dictionaries of over 130 different languages).

Chapter 20

Liability

Richard C. Fries, PE, CRE – Datex-Ohmeda, Inc.
Madison, Wisconsin

Law can be defined as the collection of rules and regulations by which society is governed. The law regulates social conduct in a formal binding way while it reflects society's needs, attitudes, and principles. Law is a dynamic concept that lives, grows, and changes. It can be described as a composite of court decisions, regulations, and sanctioned procedures, by which laws are applied and disputes adjudicated.

The three most common theories of liability for which a manufacturer may be held liable for personal injury caused by its product are negligence, strict liability, and breach of warranty. These are referred to as common-law causes of action, which are distinct from causes of action based on federal or state statutory law. Although within the last decade federal legislative action that would create a uniform federal product liability law has been proposed and debated, no such law exists today. Thus, such litigation is governed by the laws of each state.

These three doctrines are called "theories of recovery" because an injured person cannot recover damages against a defendant unless he alleges and proves, through use of one or more of these theories, that the defendant owed him a legal duty and that the defendant breached that duty, thereby causing the plaintiff's injuries. Although each is conceptually distinct, similarities exist between them. Indeed, two or more theories are asserted in many product defect suits.

20.1   Negligence

Since much of medical malpractice litigation relies on negligence theory, it is important to clearly establish the elements of that cause of action. Negligence may be defined as conduct which falls below the standard established by law for the protection of others against unreasonable risk of harm. There are four major elements of the negligence action:

- that a person or business owes a duty of care to another
- that the applicable standard for carrying out the duty was breached
- that as proximate cause of the breach of duty a compensable injury resulted
- that there be compensable damages or injury to the plaintiff.

The burden is on the plaintiff to establish each and every element of the negligence action.

The basic idea of negligence law is that one should have to pay for injuries that he or she causes when acting below the standard of care of a reasonable, prudent person participating in the activity in question. This standard of conduct relates to a belief that centers on potential victims: that people have a right to be protected from unreasonable risks of harm. A fundamental aspect of the negligence standard of care resides in the concept of foreseeability.

A plaintiff in a product liability action grounded in negligence, then, must establish a breach of the manufacturer's or seller's duty to exercise reasonable care in the manufacture and preparation of a product. The manufacturer in particular must be certain that the product is free of any potentially dangerous defect that might become dangerous upon the happening of a reasonably anticipated emergency. The obligation to exercise reasonable care has been expanded to include reasonable care in the inspection or testing of the product, the design of the product, or the giving of warnings concerning the use of the product.

A manufacturer must exercise reasonable care even though he is but a link in the production chain that results in a finished product. For example, a manufacturer of a product which is designed to be a component part of another manufactured product is bound by the standard of reasonable care. Similarly, a manufacturer of a finished product which incorporates component parts fabricated elsewhere has the same legal obligation.

A seller of a product, on the other hand, is normally held to a less stringent standard of care than a manufacturer. The lesser standard is also applied to distributors, wholesalers, or other middlemen in the marketing chain. This rule pertains because a seller or middleman is viewed as simply a channel through which the product reaches the consumer.

In general, the duty owed at any particular time varies with the degree of risk involved in a product. The concept of reasonable care is not static, but changes with the circumstances of the individual case. The care must be commensurate with the risk of harm involved. Thus, manufacturers or sellers of certain hazardous products must exercise a greater degree of care in their operations than manufacturers or sellers of other less dangerous products.

20.2   Strict Liability

Unlike the negligence suit, in which the focus is on the defendant's conduct, in a strict liability suit, the focus is on the product itself. The formulation of strict liability states that one who sells any product in a defective condition unreasonably dangerous to the user or consumer or to his property is subject to liability for physical harm thereby caused to the ultimate user or consumer or to his property if the seller is engaged in the business of selling such a product, and it is expected to and does reach the user or consumer without substantial change to the condition in which it is sold. Therefore, the critical focus in a strict liability case is on whether the product is defective and unreasonably dangerous. A common standard applied in medical device cases to reach that determination is the risk/benefit analysis - that is, whether the benefits of the device outweigh the risks attendant with its use.

The result of strict liability is that manufacturers, distributors, and retailers are liable for the injuries caused by defects in their products, even though the defect may not be shown to be the result of any negligence in the design or manufacture of the product. Moreover, under strict liability, the manufacturer cannot assert any of the various defenses available to him in a warranty action.

Strict liability means that a manufacturer may be held liable even though he has exercised all possible care in the preparation and sale of this product. The sole necessity for manufacturer liability is the existence of a defect in the product and a causal connection between this defect and the injury which resulted from the use of the product.

20.3   Breach of Warranty

A warranty action is contractual rather than tortious in nature. Its basis lies in the representations, either express or implied, which a manufacturer or a seller makes about its product.

A third cause of action that may be asserted by a plaintiff is breach of warranty. There are three types of breaches of warranty that may be alleged:

- breach of the implied warranty of merchantability
- breach of the implied warranty of fitness for a particular purpose
- breach of an express warranty.

20.3.1 Implied Warranties

Some warranties accompany the sale of an article without any express conduct on the part of the seller. These implied warranties are labeled the warranties of merchantability and of fitness for a particular purpose.

A warranty that goods shall be merchantable is implied in a contract for their sale, if the seller is a merchant who commonly deals with such goods. At a minimum, merchantable goods must:

- pass without objection in the trade under the contract description
- be fit for the ordinary purposes for which they are used
- be within the variations permitted by the sales agreement, of even kind, quality, and quantity within each unit and among all units involved
- be adequately contained, packaged, and labeled as the sales agreement may require
- conform to the promises or affirmations of fact made on the container or label.

The implied warranty of fitness for a particular purpose arises when a buyer makes known to the seller the particular purpose for which the goods are to be used, and the buyer, relying on the seller's skill or judgement, receives goods which are warranted to be sufficient for that purpose.

20.3.2   Exclusion of Warranties

The law has always recognized that sellers may explicitly limit their liability upon a contract of sale by including disclaimers of any warranties under the contract. The Uniform Commercial Code embodies this principle and provides that any disclaimer, exclusion, or modification is permissible under certain guidelines. However, a disclaimer is not valid if it deceives the buyer.

These warranty causes of action do not offer any advantages for the injured plaintiff that cannot be obtained by resort to negligence and strict liability claims and, in fact, pose greater hurdles to recovery. Thus, although a breach of warranty claim is often pled in the plaintiff's complaint, it is seldom relied on at trial as the basis for recovery.

20.4   Defects

The term "defect" is used to describe generically the kinds and
definitions of things that courts find to be actionably wrong with products when
they leave the seller's hands. In the decisions, however, the courts sometimes
distinguish between defectiveness and unreasonable danger. Other
considerations in determining defectiveness are:

- consumer expectations
- presumed seller knowledge
- risk-benefit balancing
- state of the art
- unavoidably unsafe products.

A common and perhaps the prevailing definition of product
unsatisfactoriness is that of "unreasonable danger." This has been defined as
the article sold must be dangerous to an extent beyond that which would be
contemplated by the ordinary consumer who purchases it, with the ordinary
knowledge common to the community as to its characteristics.

Another test of defectiveness sometimes used is that of presumed seller
knowledge: would the seller be negligent in placing a product on the market if
he had knowledge of its harmful or dangerous condition? This definition
contains a standard of strict liability, as well as one of defectiveness, since it
assumes the seller's knowledge of a product's condition even though there may
be no such knowledge or reason to know.

Sometimes a risk-benefit analysis is used to determine defectiveness,
particularly in design cases. The issue is phrased in terms of whether the cost
of making a safer product is greater or less than the risk or danger from the
product in its present condition. If the cost of making the change is greater
than the risk created by not making the change, then the benefit or utility of
keeping the product as is outweighs the risk and the product is not defective. If
on the other hand, the cost is less than the risk then the benefit or utility of not
making the change is outweighed by the risk and the product in its unchanged
condition is defective.

Risk-benefit or risk-burden balancing involves questions concerning
state of the art, since the burden of eliminating a danger may be greater than

the risk of that danger if the danger cannot be eliminated. State of the art is similar to the unavoidably unsafe defense where absence of the knowledge or ability to eliminate a danger is assumed for purposes of determining if a product is unavoidably unsafe. "State of the art" is defined as the state of scientific and technological knowledge available to the manufacturer at the time the product was placed in the market.

Determining defectiveness is one of the more difficult problems in products liability, particularly in design litigation. There are three types of product defects:

- manufacturing or production defects
- design defects
- defective warnings or instructions.

The issue implicates questions of the proper scope of the strict liability doctrine, and the overlapping definitions of physical and conceptual views of defectiveness.

Manufacturing defects can rarely be established on the basis of direct evidence. Rather, a plaintiff who alleges the existence of a manufacturing defect in the product must usually resort to the use of circumstantial evidence in order to prove that the product was defective. Such evidence may take the form of occurrence of other similar injuries resulting from use of the product, complaints received about the performance of the product, defectiveness of other units of the product, faulty methods of production, testing or analysis of the product, elimination of other causes of the accident, and comparison with similar products.

A manufacturer has a duty to design his product so as to prevent any foreseeable risk of harm to the user or patient. A product which is defectively designed can be distinguished from a product containing a manufacturing defect. While the latter involves some aberration or negligence in the manufacturing process, the former encompasses improper planning in connection with the preparation of the product. Failure to exercise reasonable care in the design of a product is negligence. A product which is designed in a way which makes it unreasonably dangerous will subject the manufacturer to strict liability. A design defect, in contrast to a manufacturing defect, is the result of the manufacturer's conscious decision to design the product in a certain manner.

Product liability cases alleging unsafe design may be divided into three basic categories:

- cases involving concealed dangers
- cases involving a failure to provide appropriate safety features
- cases involving construction materials of inadequate strength.

A product has a concealed danger when its design fails to disclose a danger inherent in the product which is not obvious to the ordinary user.

Some writers treat warning defects as a type of design defect. One reason for doing this is that a warning inadequacy, like a design inadequacy, is usually a characteristic of a whole line of products, while a production or manufacturing flaw is usually random and atypical of the product.

20.5   Failure to Warn of Dangers

An increasingly large portion of product liability litigation concerns the manufacturer's or seller's duty to warn of actual or potential dangers involved in the use of the product. Although the duty to warn may arise under all three theories of product liability, as mentioned above, most warnings cases rely on negligence principles as the basis for the decision. The general rule is that a manufacturer or seller who has knowledge of the dangerous character of the product has a duty to warn users of this danger. Thus, failure to warn where a reasonable man would do so is negligence.

20.6   Plaintiff's Conduct

A manufacturer or seller may defend a product liability action by demonstrating that the plaintiff either engaged in negligent conduct that was a contributing factor to his injury, or used a product when it was obvious that a danger existed and thereby assumed the risk of his injury. Another type of misconduct which may defeat recovery is when the plaintiff misuses the product by utilizing it in a manner not anticipated by the manufacturer. The applicability of these defenses in any given product suit is dependent upon the theory or theories of recovery which are asserted by the plaintiff.

20.7   Defendant's Conduct

Compliance with certain standards by a manufacturer may provide that party with a complete defense if the product leaves the manufacturer's or seller's possession or control and when it is a substantial or proximate cause of the plaintiff's injury. Exceptions to this rule include alterations or modifications made with the manufacturer's or seller's consent, or according to manufacturer's/seller's instructions.

20.8   Defendant-Related Issues

When a medical device proves to be defective, potential liability is created for many parties who may have been associated with the device. Of all the parties involved, the injured patient is least able to bear the financial consequences. To place the financial obligation upon the proper parties, the courts must consider the entire history of the product involved, often from the time the design concept was spawned until the instant the injury occurred. The first parties encountered in this process are the designers, manufacturers, distributors, and sellers of the product.

Physicians and hospitals are subject to liability through medical malpractice actions for their negligence, whether or not a defective product is involved. Where such a product is involved, the doctor or hospital may be liable for:

- negligent misuse of the product
- negligent selection of the product
- failure to inspect or test the product
- using the product with knowledge of its defect.

20.9   Manufacturer's and Physician's Responsibilities

Manufacturers of medical devices have a duty with regard to manufacture, design, warnings, and labeling. A manufacturer is required to exercise that degree of care which a reasonable, prudent manufacturer would use under the same or similar conditions. A manufacturer's failure to comply with the standard in the industry, including failing to warn or give adequate instructions, may result in a finding of liability against the manufacturer.

With regard to medical devices, a manufacturer must take reasonable steps to warn physicians of dangers of which it is aware or reasonably should be aware where the danger would not be obvious to the ordinary competent physician dispensing a particular device. The responsibility for the prudent use of the medical device is with a physician. A surgeon who undertakes to perform a surgical procedure has the responsibility to act reasonably.

It is therefore required of the manufacturer to make a full disclosure of all known side effects and problems with a particular medical device by use of appropriate warnings given to physicians. The physician is to act as the learned intermediary between the manufacturer and the patient and transmit appropriate information to the patient. The manufacturer, however, must provide the physician with the information in order that he can pass it on to the patient.

In addition, the manufacturer's warnings must indicate the scope of potential danger from the use of a medical device and the risks of its use. This is particularly important where there is "off label use" (the practice of using a product approved for one application in a different application) by a physician.

The manufacturer's warnings must detail the scope of potential danger from the use of a medical device, including the risks of misuse. The warnings must alert a reasonably competent physician to the dangers of not using a product as instructed. It would seem then the manufacturer may be held liable for failing to disclose the range of possible consequences of the use of a medical device if it has knowledge that the particular device is being used "off label."

The duty of a manufacturer and physician for use of a medical device will be based upon the state of knowledge at the time of the use. The physician therefore has a responsibility to be aware of the manufacturer's warnings as he considers the patient's condition. This dual responsibility is especially relevant in deciding what particular medical device to use. Physician judgement and an analysis of the standard of care in the community should predominate the court's analysis in determining liability for possible misuses of the device.

A concern arises if the surgeon has received instruction as to the specific device from a manufacturer outside an investigative device exemption (IDE) clinical trail approved by the FDA. In such circumstances, plaintiffs will maintain that the manufacturer and physician conspired to promote a product that is unsafe for "off label use."

20.10   Conclusion

Product liability will undoubtedly continue to be a controversial field of law, because it cuts across so many fundamental issues of our society. It will also remain a stimulating field of study and practice, since it combines a healthy mixture of the practical and theoretical. The subject will certainly continue to change, both by statutory and by common law modification.

Product liability implicates many of the basic values of our society. It is a test of the ability of private industry to accommodate competitiveness and safety. It tests the fairness and the workability of the tort system of recovery, and of the jury system as a method of resolving disputes.

References

Boardman, Thomas A. and Thomas Dipasquale, "Product Liability Implications of Regulatory Compliance or Non-Compliance," in *The Medical Device Industry - Science, Technology, and Regulation in a Competitive Environment*. New York: Marcel Dekker, Inc., 1990.

Boumil, Marcia Mobilia and Clifford E. Elias, *The Law of Medical Liability in a Nutshell.* St. Paul, MN: West Publishing Co., 1995.

Buchholz, Scott D., "Defending Pedicle Screw Litigation," in *For the Defense.* Volume 38, Number 3, March, 1996.

Gingerich, Duane, Medical Product Liability: A Comprehensive Guide and Sourcebook. New York: F & S Press, 1981.

Kanoti, George A. "Ethics, Medicine, and the Law," in *Legal Aspects of Medicine.* New York: Springer-Verlag, 1989.

Phillips, Jerry J., *Products Liability in a Nutshell.* 4th edition, St. Paul, MN: West Publishing Co., 1993.

Shapo, Marshall S., *Products Liability and the Search for Justice.* Durham, NC: Carolina Academic Press, 1993.

Chapter 21

Intellectual Property

Richard C. Fries, PE, CRE – Datex-Ohmeda, Inc.
Madison, Wisconsin

Intellectual Property is a generic term used to describe the products of the human intellect that have economic value. Intellectual property is "property" because a body of laws has been created over the last 200 years that gives owners of such works legal rights similar in some respects to those given to owners of real estate or tangible personal property. Intellectual property may be owned, bought, and sold the same as other types of property.

There are four separate bodies of law that may be used to protect intellectual property. These are patent law, copyright law, trademark law, and trade secret law. Each of these bodies of law may be used to protect different aspects of intellectual property, although there is a great deal of overlap among them.

21.1   Patents

A patent is an official document, issued by the U.S. government or another government, that describes an invention and confers on the inventors a monopoly over the use of the invention. The monopoly allows the patent owner to go to court to stop others from making, selling, or using the invention without the patent owner's permission.

Generally, an invention is any device or process that is based on an original idea conceived by one or more inventors and is useful in getting something done or solving a problem. An invention may also be a non-functional unique design or a plant. But when the word "invention" is used out in the real world, it almost always means a device or process. Many inventions, while extremely clever, do not qualify for patents, primarily because they are not considered to be sufficiently innovative in light of previous developments. The fact that an invention is not patentable does not mean necessarily that it has no value for its owner.

There are three types of patents that can be created: utility, design, and plant patents. Table 21-1 compares the three type of patents and the monopoly each type grants to the author.

21.1.1   What Qualifies as a Patent

An invention must meet several basic legal tests in order to qualify as a patent. These include:

- patentable subject matter
- usefulness
- novelty
- nonobviousness
- an improvement over an existing invention
- a design.

Type of Patent	Length of Monopoly (years)
Utility	20
Design	14
Plant	20

Table 21-1 Patent Monopolies

21.1.1.1 Patentable Subject Matter

The most fundamental qualification for a patent is that the invention consist of patentable subject matter. The patent laws define patentable subject matter as inventions that are one of the following:

- a process or method

- a machine or apparatus

- an article of manufacture

- a composition of matter

- an improvement of an invention in any of these classes.

21.1.1.2 Usefulness

Almost always, an invention must be useful in some way to qualify for a patent. Fortunately, this is almost never a problem, since virtually everything can be used for something.

21.1.1.3 Novelty

As a general rule, no invention will receive a patent unless it is different in some important way from previous inventions and developments in the field, both patented and unpatented. To use legal jargon, the invention must be novel over the prior art. As part of deciding whether an invention is novel, the U.S. patent law system focuses on two issues: when the patent application is filed, and when the invention was first conceived.

21.1.1.4 Nonobviousness

In addition to being novel, an invention must have a quality that is referred to as "nonobviousness." This means that the invention would have been surprising or unexpected to someone who is familiar with the field of the invention. And in deciding whether an invention is nonobvious, the United States Patent and Trademark Office (PTO) may consider all previous developments (prior art) that existed when the invention was conceived. Obviousness is a quality that is difficult to define, but supposedly a patent examiner knows when they see it.

As a general rule, an invention is considered nonobvious when it does one of the following:

- solves a problem that people in the field have been trying to solve for some time
- does something significantly quicker that was previously possible
- performs a function that could not be performed before.

21.1.1.5 Improvement of an Existing Invention

Earlier we noted that to qualify for a patent, an invention must fit into at least one of the statutory classes of matter entitle to a patent - a process, a machine, a manufacture, a composition of matter, or an improvement of any of these. As a practical matter, this statutory class is not very important since even an improvement on an invention in one of the other statutory classes will also qualify as an actual invention in that class. In other words, an invention will be considered as patentable subject matter as long as it fits within at least one of the other four statutory classes - whether or not it is viewed as an improvement or an original invention.

21.1.1.6 A Design

Design patents are granted to new, original and ornamental designs that are a part of articles of manufacture. Articles of manufacture are in turn defined as anything made by the hands of humans. In the past, design patents have been granted to items such as truck fenders, chairs, fabric, athletic shoes, toys, tools and artificial hip joints.

The key to understanding this type of patent is the fact that a patentable design is required to be primarily ornamental and an integral part of an item made by humans.

A design patent provides a 14-year monopoly to industrial designs that have no functional use. That is, contrary to the usefulness rule discussed above, designs covered by design patents must be purely ornamental. The further anomaly of design patents is that while the design itself must be primarily ornamental, as opposed to primarily functional, it must at the same time be embodied in something people-made. Design patents are easy to apply for, as they do not require much written description. The require drawings for the design, a short description of each figure or drawing, and one claim that says little more than the inventor claims the ornamental design depicted on the attached drawings. In addition the design patent is less expensive to apply for than a utility patent, lasts for 14 rather than 20 years, and requires no maintenance fees.

21.1.2   The Patent Process

The patent process consists of the following steps:

- note all problems caused by equipment, supplies, or nonexisting devices when performing a task
- focus on the problem every time you perform the task or use the item

- concentrate on solutions
- keep a detailed, dated diary of problems and solutions; include drawings and sketches
- record the benefits and usefulness of your idea
- evaluate the marketability of your idea. It if does not have a wide application, it may be more advantageous to abandon the idea and focus on another
- do not discuss your idea with anyone except one person you trust who will maintain confidentially.
- prepare an application with a patent attorney
- have a search done, first a computer search, then a hand search.

Purchase a composition book with bound pages for keeping your notes. Start each entry with the date, and include all details of problem identification and solutions. Use drawings or sketches of your idea. Never remove any pages. If you do not like an entry or have made a mistake, simply make an X through the entry or write "error". Sign all entries and have a witness sign and date them as frequently as possible. Your witness should be someone you trust who understands your idea and will maintain confidentiality.

The patent document contains:

- a title for the invention and the names and addresses of the inventors
- details of the patent search made by the PTO
- an abstract that concisely describes the key aspects of the invention
- drawings or flowcharts of the invention
- very precise definitions of the invention covered by the patent (called the patent claims)
- a brief summary of the invention.

Taken together, the various parts of the patent document provide a complete disclosure of every important aspect of the covered invention. When a U.S. patent is issued, all the information in the patent is readily accessible to the public in the PTO and in patent libraries across the U.S. and through on-line patent database services.

U.S. patents are obtained by submitting to the PTO a patent application and an application fee. Once the application is received, the PTO assigns it to an examiner who is supposed to be knowledgeable in the technology underlying the invention. The patent examiner is responsible for deciding whether the invention qualifies for a patent, and assuming it does, what the scope of the patent should be. Usually, back and forth communications - called patent prosecution - occur between the applicant and the examiner regarding these issues. Clearly the most serious and hard-to-fix issue is whether the invention qualifies for a patent.

Eventually, if all of the examiner's objections are overcome by the applicant, the invention is approved for a patent. A patent issue fee is paid and the applicant receives an official copy of the patent deed. Three additional fees must be paid over the life of the patent to keep it in effect.

21.1.3 Patent Claims

Patent claims are the part of the patent application that precisely delimits the scope of the invention - where it begins and where it ends. Perhaps it will help you understand what patent claims do, if you analogize them to real estate deeds. A deed typically includes a description of the parcel's parameters precise enough to map the exact boundaries of the plot of land in question, which in turn, can be used as the basis of a legal action to toss out any trespassers.

With patents, the idea is to similarly draw in the patent claims a clear line around the property of the inventor so that any infringer can be identified and dealt with. Patent claims have an additional purpose. Because of the precise way in which they are worded, claims also are used to decide whether, in light of previous developments, the invention is patentable in the first place.

Unfortunately, to accomplish these purposes, all patent claims are set forth in an odd, stylized format. But the format has a big benefit. It makes it possible to examine any patent application or patent granted by the PTO and get a pretty good idea about what the invention covered by the patent consists of. While the stylized patent claim language and format have the advantage of lending a degree of precision to a field that badly needs it, there is an obvious and substantial downside to the use of the arcane patentspeak. Mastering it amounts to climbing a fairly steep learning curve.

It is when you set out to understand a patent claim that the rest of the patent becomes crucially important. The patent's narrative description of the invention - set out in the patent specification - with all or many of the invention's possible uses, and the accompanying drawings or flowcharts, usually provide enough information in combination to understand any particular claim. And of course, the more patent claims you examine, the more adept you will become in deciphering them.

21.1.4   Protecting Your Rights as an Inventor

If two inventors apply for a patent around the same time, the patent will be awarded to the inventor who came up with the invention first. This may or may not be the inventor who was first to file a patent application. For this reason, it is vital that one carefully document the inventive activities. If two or more pending patent applications by different inventors claim the same invention, the PTO will ask the inventors to establish the date each of them first conceived the invention and the ways in which they then showed diligence in "reducing the invention to practice."

Inventors can reduce the invention to practice in two ways: 1) by making a working model - a prototype - which works as the idea of the invention dictates it should or 2) by constructively reducing it to practice - that is, by describing the invention in sufficient detail for someone else to build it - in a document that is then filed as a patent application with the PTO.

The inventor who conceived the invention first will be awarded the patent if he or she also showed diligence in either building the invention or filing a patent application. If the inventor who was second to conceive the invention was the first one to reduce it to practice - for instance by filing a patent application - that inventor may end up with the patent.

It is often the quality of the inventor's documentation (dated, written in a notebook, showing the conception of the invention and the steps that were taken to reduce the invention to practice) that determines which invention ends up with the patent.

You especially should be aware that you can unintentionally forfeit your right to obtain patent protection. This can happen if you disclose your invention to others, such as a company interested in the invention, and then do not file an application within one year from that disclosure date. The same one year period applies if you offer your invention, or a product made by your invention, for sale. You must file your patent application in the United States within one year from any offer of sale.

Even more confusing is the fact that most other countries do not allow this one year grace period. Any public disclosure before you file your first application will prevent you from obtaining patent protection in nearly every country other than the United States.

21.1.5   Patent Infringement

Patent infringement occurs when someone makes, uses, or sells a patented invention without the patent owner's permission. Defining infringement is one thing, but knowing when it occurs in the real world is something else. Even with common technologies, it can be difficult for experienced patent attorneys to tell whether patents have been infringed.

There are multiple steps in deciding whether infringement of a patent has occurred:

- identify the patent's independent apparatus and method claims
- break these apparati and method claims into their elements
- compare these elements with the alleged infringing device or process and decide whether the claim has all of the elements that constitute the alleged infringing device or process. If so, the patent has probably been infringed. If not, proceed to the next step.
- if the elements the alleged infringing device or process are somewhat different than the elements of the patent claim, ask if they are the same in structure, function, and result. If yes, you probably have infringement. Note that

for infringement to occur, only one claim in the patent
needs to be infringed.

A patent's independent claims are those upon which usually one or
more claims immediately following depend. A patent's broadest claims are
those with the fewest words and that therefore provide the broadest patent
coverage. The patent's broadest claims are its independent claims. As a
general rule, if you find infringement of one of the broadest claims, all the
other patent's claims that depend on that claim are infringed. Conversely, if
you don't find infringement by comparison with a broad claim, then you won't
find infringement of claims which depend on it. Although an infringement is
declared on a claim-by-claim basis, generally it will be declared that the patent
itself is infringed.

In apparatus (machine) claims, the elements are usually
conceptualized as the a), b), c), etc., parts of the apparatus that are listed,
interrelated, and described in detail following the word "comprising" at the end
of the preamble of the claim. Elements in method (process) claims are the
steps of the method and sub-parts of those steps.

If each and every element of the patent's broadest claims are in the
infringing device, the patent is probably infringed. The reason you start by
analyzing the broadest claim is that by definition, that claim has the fewest
elements and it is therefore easier to find infringements.

Even if infringement can't be found on the basis of the literal language
in the claims, the courts may still find infringement if the alleged infringing
device's elements are equivalent to the patent claims in structure, function, and
result. Known as the Doctrine of Equivalents, this rule is difficult to apply in
practice.

21.2   Copyrights

A copyright is a legal device that provides the creator of a work of
authorship the right to control how the work is used. If someone wrongfully
uses material covered by a copyright, the copyright owner can sue and obtain
compensation for any losses suffered, as well as an injunction requiring the
copyright infringer to stop the infringing activity.

A copyright is a type of tangible property. It belongs to its owner and the courts can be asked to intervene if anyone uses it without permission. Like other forms of property, a copyright may be sold by its owner, or otherwise exploited by the owner for economic benefit.

The Copyright Act of 1976 grants creators many intangible, exclusive rights over their work, including reproduction rights - the right to make copies of a protected work; distribution rights - the right to sell or otherwise distribute copies to the public; the right to create adaptations - the right to prepare new works based on the protected work; performance and display rights - the right to perform a protected work or display a work in public.

Copyright protects all varieties of original works of authorship, including:

- literary works
- motion pictures, videos, and other audiovisual works
- photographs, sculpture, and graphic works
- sound recordings
- pantomimes and choreographic works
- architectural works.

21.2.1   What Can Be Copyrighted?

Not every work of authorship receives copyright protection. A program or other work is protected only if it satisfies all three of the following requirements:

- fixation
- originality
- minimal creativity.

The work must be fixed in a tangible medium of expression. Any stable medium from which the work can be read back or heard, either directly or with the aid of a machine or device, is acceptable.

Copyright protection begins the instant you fix your work. There is no waiting period and it is not necessary to register the copyright. Copyright protects both completed and unfinished works, as well as works that are widely distributed to the public or never distributed at all.

A work is protected by copyright only if, and to the extent, it is original. But this does not mean that copyright protection is limited to works that are novel - that is new to the world. For copyright purposes, a work is "original" if at least a part of the work owes its origin to the author. A work's quality, ingenuity, aesthetic merit, or uniqueness is not considered.

A minimal amount of creativity over and above the independent creation requirement is necessary for copyright protection. Works completely lacking creativity are denied copyright protection even if they have been independently created. However, the amount of creativity required is very slight.

In the past, some courts held that copyright protected works that may have lacked originality and or creativity if a substantial amount of work was involved in their creation. Recent court cases have outlawed this "sweat of the brow" theory. It is now clear that the amount of work put in to create a work of authorship has absolutely no bearing on the degree of copyright protection it will receive. Copyright only protects fixed, original, minimally creative expressions, not hard work.

Perhaps the greatest difficulty with copyrights is determining just what aspects of any given work are protected. All works of authorship contain elements that are protected by copyright and elements that are not protected. Unfortunately, there is no system available to precisely identify which aspects of a given work are protected. The only time we ever obtain a definitive answer as to how much any particular work is protected is when it becomes the subject of a copyright infringement lawsuit. However, there are two tenets which may help in determining what is protected and what is not. The first tenet states that a copyright only protects "expressions," not ideas, systems, or processes. Tenet two states the scope of copyright protection is proportional to the range of expression available. Let us look at both in detail.

Copyright only protects the tangible expression of an idea, system or process - not the idea, system or process itself. Copyright law does not protect ideas, procedures, processes, systems, mathematical principles, formulas, algorithms, methods of operation, concepts, facts and discoveries. Remember, copyright is designed to aid the advancement of knowledge. If the copyright law gave a person a legal monopoly over ideas, the progress of knowledge would be impeded rather than helped.

The scope of copyright protection is proportional to the range of expression available. The copyright law only protects original works of authorship. Part of the essence of original authorship is the making of choices. Any work of authorship is the end result of a whole series of choices made by its creator. For example, the author of a novel expressing the idea of love must choose the novel's plot, characters, locale and the actual words used to express the story. The author of such a novel has a nearly limitless array of choices available. However, the choices available to the creators of many works of authorship are severely limited. In these cases, the idea or ideas underlying the work and the way they are expressed by the author are deemed to "merge". The result is that the author's expression is either treated as if it were in the public domain or protected only against virtually verbatim or "slavish" copying.

21.2.2   The Copyright Process

21.2.2.1 Copyright Notice

Before 1989, all published works had to contain a copyright notice, (the "©" symbol followed by the publication date and copyright owner's name) to be protected by copyright. This is no longer necessary. Use of copyright notices is now optional in the United States. Even so, it is always a good idea to include a copyright notice on all work distributed to the public so that potential infringers will be informed of the underlying claim to copyright ownership. In addition, copyright protection is not available in some 20 foreign countries unless a work contains a copyright notice.

There are strict technical requirements as to what a copyright notice must contain. A valid copyright must contain three elements:

- *the copyright symbol* - use the familiar "©" symbol, i.e., the lower case letter "c" completely surrounded by a circle. The word "Copyright" or the abbreviation "Copr." are also acceptable in the United States, but not in many foreign countries. So if your work might be distributed outside the U.S., always use the "©" symbol.

- *the year in which the work was published* - you only need to include the year the work was first published.
- *the name of the copyright owner* - the owner is 1) the author or authors of the work, 2) the legal owner of a work made for hire, or 3) the person or entity to whom all the author's exclusive copyright rights have been transferred.

Although the three elements of a copyright notice need not appear in a particular order, it is common to list the copyright symbol, followed by the date and owners.

According to Copyright Office regulations, the copyright notice must be placed so as not be concealed from an ordinary user's view upon reasonable examination. A proper copyright notice should be included on all manuals and promotional materials. Notices on written works are usually placed on the title page or the page immediately following the title page.

21.2.2.2 Copyright Registration

Copyright registration is a legal formality by which a copyright owner makes a public record in the U.S. Copyright Office in Washington, DC of some basic information about a protected work, such as the title of the work, who wrote it and when, and who owns the copyright. It is not necessary to register to create or establish a copyright.

Copyright registration is a relatively easy process. You must fill out the appropriate pre-printed application form, pay an application fee, and mail the application and fee to the Copyright Office in Washington, DC along with two copies of the work being registered.

21.2.3   Copyright Duration

One of the advantages of copyright protection is that it lasts a very long time. The copyright in a protectable work created after 1977 by an individual creator lasts for the life of the creator plus an additional 50 years. If there is more than one creator, the life plus 50 term is measured from the date the last creator dies. The copyright in works created by employees for their employers last for 75 years from the date of publication, or 100 years from the date of creation, whichever occurs first.

21.2.4   Protecting Your Copyright Rights

The exclusive rights granted by the Copyright Act initially belong to a work's author. There are four ways to become an author:

- an individual may independently author a work
- an employer may pay an employee to create the work, in which case, the employer is the author under the work made for hire rule
- a person or business entity may specially commission an independent contractor to create the work under a written work made for hire contract, in which case, the commissioning party becomes the author
- two or more individuals or entities may collaborate to become joint authors.

The initial copyright owner of a work is free to transfer some or all copyright rights to other people or businesses, who will then be entitled to exercise the rights transferred.

21.2.5   Infringement

Copyright infringement occurs when a person other than the copyright owner exploits one or more of the copyright owner's exclusive rights without the owner's permission. A copyright owner who wins an infringement suit may stop any further infringement, obtain damages from the infringer and recover other monetary losses. This means, in effect, that a copyright owner can make a copyright infringer restore the author to the same economic position they would have been in had the infringement never occurred.

Copyright infringement is usually proven by showing that the alleged infringer had access to the copyright owner's work and that the protected expression in the two works is substantially similar. In recent years, the courts have held that the person who claims his work was infringed upon must subject his work to a rigorous filtering process to find out which elements of the work are and are not protected by copyright. In other words, the plaintiff must filter out from his work ideas, elements dictated by efficiency or external factors, or taken from the public domain. After this filtration process is completed, there may or may not be any protectable expression left.

21.3   Trademarks

A trademark is a work, name, symbol, or a combination used by a manufacturer to identify its goods and distinguish them from others. Trademark rights continue indefinitely as long as the mark is not abandoned and it is properly used.

A federal trademark registration is maintained by filing a declaration of use during the sixth year after its registration and by renewal every twenty years, as long as the mark is still in use. The federal law provides that non-use of a mark for two consecutive years is ordinarily considered abandonment, and the first subsequent user of the mark can claim exclusive trademark rights. Trademarks, therefore, must be protected or they will be lost. They must be distinguished in print form from other words and must appear in a distinctive manner. Trademarks should be followed by a notice of their status. If it has been registered in the U.S. Patent Office, the registration notice "®" or "Reg. U.S. Pat Off," should be used. Neither should be used however, if the trademark has not been registered, but the superscripted letter "TM" should follow the mark, or an asterisk can be used to refer to a footnote starting "a trademark of xxx." The label compliance manager should remember that trademarks are proper adjectives and must be accompanied by the generic name for the product they identify. Trademarks are not to be used as possessives, not in the plural form.

A trademark is any visual mark that accompanies a particular tangible product, or line of goods, and serves to identify and distinguish it from products sold by others and it indicates its source. A trademark may consist of letters, words, names, phrases, slogans, numbers, colors, symbols, designs, or shapes.

As a general rule, to be protected from unauthorized use by others, a trademark must be distinctive in some way.

The word "trademark" is also a generic term used to describe the entire broad body of state and federal law that covers how businesses distinguish their products and services from the competition. Each state has its own set of laws establishing when and how trademarks can be protected. There is also a federal trademark law, called the Lanham Act, which applies in all fifty states. Generally, state trademark laws are relied upon for marks used only within one particular state, while the Lanham Act is used to protect marks for products that are sold in more than one state or across territorial or national borders.

21.3.1   Selecting a Trademark

Not all trademarks are treated equally by the law. The best trademarks are "distinctive" - that is, they stand out in a customer's mind because they are inherently memorable. The more distinctive the trademark is, the stronger it will be and the more legal protection it will receive. Less distinctive marks are "weak" and may be entitled to little or no legal protection.

Generally, selecting a mark begins with brainstorming for general ideas. After several possible marks have been selected, the next step is often to use formal or informal market research techniques to see how the potential marks will be accepted by customers. Next, a "trademark search" is conducted. This means that an attempt is made to discover whether the same or similar marks are already in use.

21.3.1.1 What is a Distinctive Trademark?

A trademark should be created that is distinctive rather than descriptive. A trademark is "distinctive" if it is capable of distinguishing the product to which it is attached from competing products. Certain types of marks are deemed to be inherently distinctive and are automatically entitled to maximum protection. Others are viewed as not inherently distinctive and can be protected only if they acquire "secondary meaning" through use.

Arbitrary, fanciful or coined marks are deemed to be inherently distinctive and are therefore very strong marks. These are words and/or symbols that have absolutely no meaning in the particular trade or industry prior to their adoption by a particular manufacturer for use with its goods or services. After use and promotion, these marks are instantly identified with a particular company and product, and the exclusive right to use the mark is easily asserted against potential infringers.

Fanciful or arbitrary marks consist of common words used in an unexpected or arbitrary way so that their normal meaning has nothing to do with the nature of the product or service they identify. Some examples would be APPLE COMPUTER and PEACHTREE SOFTWARE.

Coined words are words made up solely to serve as trademarks, such as ZEOS or INTEL.

Suggestive marks are also inherently distinctive. A suggestive mark indirectly describes the product it identifies but stays away from literal descriptiveness. That is, the consumer must engage in a mental process to associate the mark with the product it identifies. For example, WORDPERFECTand VISICALC are suggestive marks.

Descriptive marks are not considered to be inherently distinctive. They are generally viewed by the courts as weak and thus not deserving of much, if any, judicial protection unless they acquire a "secondary meaning" - that is, become associated with a product in the public's mind through long and continuous use. There are three types of descriptive marks: 1) marks that directly describe the nature or characteristics of the product they identify (for example, QUICK MAIL), 2) marks that describe the geographic location from which the product emanates (for example, OREGON SOFTWARE), 3) marks consisting primarily of a person's last name (for example, NORTON'S UTILITIES). A mark that is in continuous and exclusive use by its owner for a five year period is presumed to have acquired secondary meaning and qualifies for registration as a distinctive mark.

A generic mark is a word(s) or symbol that is commonly used to describe an entire category or class of products or services, rather than to distinguish one product or service from another. Generic marks are in the public domain and cannot be registered or enforced under the trademark laws. Some examples of generic marks include "computer," "mouse," and "RAM." A term formerly protestable as a trademark may lose such protection if it becomes generic. This often occurs when a mark is assimilated into common use to such an extent that it becomes the general term describing an entire product category. Examples would be ESCALATOR and XEROX.

21.3.2   The Trademark Process

A trademark is registered by filing an application with the PTO in Washington, DC. Registration is not mandatory. Under both federal and state law, a company may obtain trademark rights in the states in which the mark is actually used. However, federal registration provides many important benefits including:

- the mark's owner is presumed to have the exclusive right to use the mark nationwide
- everyone in the country is presumed to know that the mark is already taken
- the trademark owner obtains the right to put an "®" after the mark
- anyone who begins using a confusingly similar mark after the mark has been registered will be deemed a willful infringer.
- the trademark owner obtains the right to make the mark "incontestable" by keeping it in continuous use for five years.

To qualify for federal trademark registration, a mark must meet several requirements. The mark must:

- actually be used in commerce
- be sufficiently distinctive to reasonably operate as a product identifier
- not be confusingly similar to an existing, federally registered trademark.

A mark you think will be good for your product could already be in use by someone else. If your mark is confusingly similar to one already in use, its owner may be able to sue you for trademark infringement and get you to change it and even pay damages. Obviously, you do not want to spend time and money marketing and advertising a new mark only to discover that it infringes on another preexisting mark and must be changed. To avoid this, state and federal trademark searches should be conducted to attempt to discover if there are any existing similar marks. You can conduct a trademark search yourself, either manually or with the aid of computer databases. You may also pay a professional search firm to do so.

21.3.3   Intent to Use Registration

If you seriously intend to use a trademark on a product in the near future, you can reserve the right to use the mark by filing an intent to use registration. If the mark is approved, you have six months to actually use the mark on a product sold to the public. If necessary, this period may be increased by six-month intervals up to 24 months if you have a good explanation for the delay. No one else may use the mark during this interim period. You should promptly file an intent to use registration as soon as you have definitely selected a trademark for a forthcoming product.

21.3.4   Protecting Your Trademark Rights

The owner of a valid trademark has the exclusive right to use the mark on its products. Depending on the strength of the mark and whether and where it has been registered, the trademark owner may be able to bring a court action to prevent others from using the same or similar marks on competing or related products.

Trademark infringement occurs when an alleged infringer uses a mark that is likely to cause consumers to confuse the infringer's products with the trademark owner's products. A mark need not be identical to one already in use to infringe upon the owner's rights. If the proposed mark is similar enough to the earlier mark to risk confusing the average consumer, its use will constitute infringement.

Determining whether an average consumer might be confused is the key to deciding whether infringement exists. The determination depends primarily on whether the products or services involved are related, and, if so, whether the marks are sufficiently similar to create a likelihood of consumer confusion.

If a trademark owner is able to convince a court that infringement has occurred, she may be able to get the court to order the infringer to stop using the infringing mark and to pay monetary damages. Depending on whether the mark was registered, such damages may consist of the amount of the trademark owner's losses caused by the infringement or the infringer's profits. In cases of willful infringement, the courts may double or triple the damages award.

A trademark owner must be assertive in enforcing its exclusive rights. Each time a mark is infringed upon, it loses strength and distinctiveness and may eventually die by becoming generic.

21.4   Trade Secrets

Trade secrecy is basically a do-it-yourself form of intellectual property protection. It is based on the simple idea that by keeping valuable information secret, one can prevent competitors from learning about and using it. Trade secrecy is by far the oldest form of intellectual property, dating back at least to ancient Rome. It is useful now as it was then.

A trade secret is any formula, pattern, physical device, idea, process, compilation of information or other information that 1) is not generally known by a company's competitors, 2) provides a business with a competitive advantage, and 3) is treated in a way that can reasonably be expected to prevent the public or competitors from learning about it, absent improper acquisition or theft.

Trade secrets may be used to:

- protect ideas that offer a business a competitive advantage
- keep competitors from knowing that a program is under development and from learning its functional attributes
- protect source code, software development tools, design definitions and specifications, manuals, and other documentation

- protect valuable business information such as marketing plans, cost and price information and customer lists.

Unlike copyrights and patents, whose existence is provided and governed by federal law that applies in all fifty states, trade secrecy is not codified in any federal statute. Instead, it is made up of individual state laws. Nevertheless, the protection afforded to trade secrets is much the same in every state. This is partly because some 26 states have based their trade secrecy laws on the Uniform Trade Secrecy Act, a model trade secrecy law designed by legal scholars.

21.4.1   What Qualifies for Trade Secrecy

Information that is public knowledge or generally known cannot be trade secret. Things that everybody knows cannot provide anyone with a competitive advantage. However, information comprising a trade secret need not be novel or unique. All that is required is that the information not be generally known by people who could profit from its disclosure and use.

21.4.2   Trade Secrecy Authorship

Only the person that owns a trade secret has the right to seek relief in court if someone else improperly acquires or discloses the trade secret. Only the trade secret owner may grant others a license to use the secret.

As a general rule, any trade secrets developed by an employee in the course of employment belongs to the employer. However, trade secrets developed by an employee on their own time and with their own equipment can sometimes belong to the employee. To avoid possible disputes, it is a very good idea for employers to have all the employees who may develop new technology sign an employee agreement that assigns in advance all trade secrets developed by the employee during their employment to the company.

21.4.3   How Trade Secrets Are Lost

A trade secret is lost if either the product in which it is embodied is made widely available to the public through sales and displays on an unrestricted basis, or the secret can be discovered by reverse engineering or inspection.

21.4.4   Duration of Trade Secrets

Trade secrets have no definite term. A trade secret continues to exist as long as the requirements for trade secret protection remain in effect. In other words, as long as secrecy is maintained, the secret does not become generally known in the industry and the secret continues to provide a competitive advantage. It will be protected.

21.4.5   Protecting Your Trade Secret Rights

A trade secret owner has the legal right to prevent the following two groups of people from using and benefitting from its trade secrets or disclosing them to other without the owner's permission:

- people who are bound by a duty of confidentiality not to disclose or use the information
- people who steal or otherwise acquire the trade secret through improper means.

A trade secret owner's rights are limited to the two restricted groups of people discussed above. In this respect, a trade secret owner's rights are much more limited than those of a copyright owner or patent holder.

A trade secret owner may enforce their rights by bringing a trade secret infringement action in court. Such suits may be used to:

- prevent another person or business from using the trade secret without proper authorization
- collect damages for the economic injury suffered as a result of the trade secret's improper acquisition and use.

All persons responsible for the improper acquisition and all those who benefitted from the acquisition are typically named as defendants in trade secret infringement actions. To prevail in a trade secret infringement suit, the plaintiff must show that the information alleged to be secret is actually a trade secret. In addition, the plaintiff must show that the information was either improperly acquired by the defendant or improperly disclosed, or likely to be so, by the defendant.

There are two important limits on trade secret protection. It does not prevent others from discovering a trade secret through reverse engineering, nor does it apply to persons who independently create or discover the same information.

21.4.6   A Trade Secrecy Program

The first step in any trade secret protection program is to identify exactly what information and material is a company trade secret. It makes no difference in what form a trade secret is embodied. Trade secrets may be stored on computer hard disks or floppies, written down, or exist only in employees' memories.

Once a trade secret has been established, the protection program should include the following steps:

- maintain physical security
- enforce computer security
- mark confidential documents "Confidential"
- use non-disclosure agreements.

21.4.7   Use of Trade Secrecy with Copyrights and Patents

Trade secrecy is a vitally important protection for any medical device, but because of its limitations listed above, it should be used in conjunction with copyright and, in some cases, patent protection.

21.4.7.1 Trade Secrets and Patents

The federal patent laws provide the owner of a patentable invention with far greater protection than that available under trade secrecy laws. Trade secret protection is not lost when a patent is applied for. The Patent Office keeps patent applications secret unless or until a patent is granted. However, once a patent is granted and an issue feed paid, the patent becomes public record. Then all the information disclosed in the patent application is no longer a trade secret. This is so even if the patent is later challenged in court and invalidated.

If, for example, a software program is patented, the software patent applies only to certain isolated elements of the program. The remainder need not be disclosed in the patent and can remain a trade secret.

21.4.7.2 Trade Secrets and Copyrights

Trade secrecy and copyright are not incompatible. To the contrary, they are typically used in tandem to provide the maximum legal protection available.

References

American Intellectual Property Law Association, *How to Protect and Benefit From Your Ideas*. Arlington, VA: American Intellectual Property Law Association Inc., 1988.

Banner & Allegretti, *An Overview of Changes to U.S. Patent and Trademark Office Rules and Procedures Effective June 8, 1995*. Chicago: Banner & Allegretti, Ltd., 1995.

Fishman, Stephen, *Software Development - A Legal Guide*. Berkeley, California: Nolo Press, 1994.

Fries, Richard C., *Reliable Design of Medical Devices*. New York: Marcel Dekker, Inc., 1997.

Noonan, William D., "Patenting Medical Technology," in *The Journal of Legal Medicine*. Volume 11, Number 3, September, 1990.

Rebar, Linda A., "The Nurse as Inventor - Obtain a Patent and Benefit from Your Ideas," in *AORN Journal*, Volume 53, Number 2, February, 1991.

Sherman, Max, "Developing a Labeling Compliance Program," in *The Medical Device Industry*. New York: Marcel Dekker Inc., 1990.

U.S. Department of Commerce, *General Information Concerning Patents*. Washington, DC: U.S. Government Printing Office, 1993.

Section 4

Verification and Validation

Chapter 22

Testing

Lisa Henn – Datex-Ohmeda, Inc.
Madison, Wisconsin

Testing is a vital and integral element in the successful design and release of a medical device. Regulatory bodies require it, but the manufacturer would be wise to embrace it in any event. A proactive and thorough testing program can find previously overlooked weak areas of the product prior to release. It provides a check of the designer's expectations of the product, a comparison of theory to reality. Either the manufacturer finds the product's weaknesses, or the customers and competitors will.

The subject of product testing is too vast to cover adequately in detail in only one chapter. Consequently, this chapter provides an overview of the testing process, assuming only a general technical background, with references to provide greater depth. It should be noted that the bulk of this chapter text is devoted to the setup of the test. So it is in actual testing. Adequate preparation simplifies the analysis, reporting, and justification of the work.

22.1 Purposes

"Would you tell me, please, which way I ought to walk from here?"

> *"That depends a good deal on where you want to get to," said the Cat.*
> *"I don't much care where," said Alice.*
> *"Then it doesn't matter which way you walk," said the Cat.*
> *"--so long as I get somewhere," Alice added as an explanation.*
> *"Oh, you're sure to do that," said the Cat, "if you only walk long enough!"*
> *--Lewis Carroll, Alice in Wonderland*

Without a goal for a test, the experimenter would certainly reach the end of the test, but not reach meaningful conclusions. The tester must know what the end goal is in order to take a testing approach that will achieve it. It is essential for the tester to have in mind the purpose for the proposed test.

Testing is performed for several purposes:

1. Verification--ensuring that the product meets the specification.
2. Validation--ensuring that the product meets the customer's expectations. This is not the same as verification.
3. Evaluation--exploration of the product's or component's capabilities. The designer's first focus is naturally on the short-term performance--will the component be at all suitable for use? Consideration of long-term performance is essential to a successful design as well, as it is part of the customer's expectations. Even if the device is a disposable one, it might sit on the shelf for a length of time.
4. Rectification--the correction of issues that surface. The issues arise in the course of other activities, which include:

    i) Testing of the larger system.
    ii) Paper analyses, such as Failure Modes, Effects, and Criticality Analyses (FMECA) and Fault Tree Analyses (FTA). Both these techniques link culprit components to manifested problems. The FMECA starts from the bottom up, from the specific component's failure mode, to the effect and its

criticality. The FMECA approach is exemplified by the verse by George Herbert: "For want of a nail the shoe is lost, for want of a shoe the horse is lost, for want of a horse the rider is lost." (*Jacula Prudentum*, no. 499) By comparison, the FTA is a top-down approach, starting with the manifested fault. The techniques help the design team ferret out all potential issues with the device. Preventative measures identified by the techniques should be tested for effectiveness.

iii) Production--issues arising from this arena are generally unexpected variation in the components (lot-to-lot, process drift, etc.) or difficulties in actual execution of the design. Using testing to address this latter area is a last-resort effort; the problem is solved better by considering design for manufacturing and design for assembly principles during the actual design of the product. Finally, prior to testing of the proposed solutions, it may be necessary to determine how sensitive the component is to the variation.

iv) Field--this can encompass nearly anything, including unintended applications of the product, unexpected amount of usage of the product, aging effects, local environmental conditions, and interactions with other components or chemicals. As with issues arising from production, it may be necessary to probe for the extent of the sensitivity in addition to the testing of any proposed solutions.

22.2 Proper Setup

22.2.1 Specific Outcome

It is essential to have a specific focus in mind when performing the test. Consider an evaluation test. The evaluator should have a list, incorporated into the test report, of the descriptors to be detailed by the test. Examples include the following: "to assess the extent, in percentage or in absolute measure, of the sensor reading's drift over the temperature or humidity or altitude range required by the product," "to verify that the proposed correction algorithm reduces error in the flow produced by the valve to within X% of the command," "to determine the average flow and standard deviation produced by the sample of pumps at the proposed voltage," and "to determine which among temperature, humidity, inlet pressure, and volumetric flow alter the sensor's output curve from its characteristic shape." In this last case a quantitative measure of change from the characteristic shape should also be defined. Note in these examples the specificity of issue and of information gathered.

Sometimes the question to be answered can be quantified into a hypothesis test. A hypothesis test compares the numeric outcome of the test against an assertion, termed the "null hypothesis". The null hypothesis is the default condition, the assumption of the state of things unless proven otherwise. It is generally in the form "the current sample produces a value not significantly different from that in previous cases." An example is "the average length of the specimen samples is no different than the length of previously produced specimens." The actual difference between the average length in the sample set is subtracted from the average length in the population, and that difference is compared to the variation typically expected in the population. If the difference exceeds what one would expect from the population, then the null hypothesis is rejected. One would conclude that a change such as a process improvement has occurred.

If the difference does not exceed what one would expect from the population, then the null hypothesis cannot be rejected. It is then said that there is insufficient evidence by which to reject the null hypothesis. That is not to say that the change attempted had no effect whatsoever on the specimen, just that it was not noticeable in comparison with the usual population variation. The null hypothesis would be maintained in such a case because it would not be clear that a benefit would accrue in expending the energy in changing practice. This is the same philosophy employed by the U.S. trial system: the defendant is considered not guilty until proven otherwise. In both cases, with insufficient evidence to warrant taking action, it is better to leave well enough alone.

In determining whether a measured value is significant, the measured value is converted to a standard scale. One example of a standard scale would be a normalized value, as described by Strait (1989) or any other statistics book. This converted value is compared to how a sample from the reference population would fare on the same standard scale. Values of a population fitting the normal distribution are included in the appendix. If, for example, the test value is more extreme than the values that 99% of samples from the reference population would have, then an argument could be made that the test case is significantly different from what one would expect through usual variation in the population. If the test value is more extreme than only 50% of the reference population, the conclusion is not nearly so certain. The threshold for rejecting the null hypothesis--90%, 95%, 99%--is a question of judgment of the risks and benefits involved.

When determining a threshold for rejection, the analyst should consider the two ways in which a test value can differ from a population mean. First, the test value can be a certain absolute distance away from the mean, in either the positive or negative direction. An example would be, "the average of the daily high temperatures this month is within 5° of the historic average." For a case such as this one, the Two-Tail Test is desired. The Two-Tail Test considers the fraction of the population that is farther away from the mean than the either the positive or negative value of the test sample. It considers the area in both the left-hand "tail" and the right-hand "tail" in a distribution curve. If one is comparing the test result of 3 against a mean of 2 using a two-tail test, then the more extreme fraction of the population would be larger than +3 or smaller than -3.

The other way in which the test value can differ from the mean is as an offset in a particular direction from the mean. An example of this second case would be, "the average of the daily high temperatures for this month is no more than 5° colder than the historic average." For this test, the One-Tail Test is used. A one-tail test might be used to determine if a population of pegs is going to be, in general, larger than a particular hole diameter. The test in that example would evaluate the area in the right-hand tail; that area would represent the fraction of the population of peg that are too big.

Choosing a one-tail test over a two-tail test is not determined by the specific numeric threshold chosen. Rather, the choice impacts how the areas read from the tables are interpreted. For example, suppose the experimenter would want the test sample average daily high temperature to be more extreme than 95% of the historic averages before concluding that the difference is significant. In other words, the experimenter is willing to accept that up to 5% of the population would be more extreme than the test value and would still reject the null hypothesis. If the hypothesis being tested is that the test sample is *within* 5° of the historic average, then the experimenter would want to find the tail area to be less than 2.5% of the total population before rejecting the hypothesis. Half the 5% area would be in the "hotter" extreme and half the area would be in the "colder" extreme. If the hypothesis is that the test sample is no more than 5° *colder,* then the experimenter would reject the hypothesis when the tail had 5% of the population or less. The entire 5% area would be in the "colder" tail.

Even if it is found that 99% of samples from the reference population would have values less extreme than the test value, there is still risk that the null hypothesis will be rejected erroneously. After all, 1% of the population would be expected to have values more extreme than the test value. This risk of rejecting the null hypothesis when it is true is called the Type I Error, or α error. Its counterpart is the Type II Error, or β error, the chance that one does not reject the null hypothesis when it is false. Most standard tests focus on the Type I error. The question of which type of error is more important depends on the perspective. For example, consider the pre-employment drug screening test. The null hypothesis is that the value from testing the sample, an indicator of the level of suspected illegal substances in the sample, is no different than the value that would be expected in the general population. The candidate wants the lab to minimize the Type I error, whereas the employer wants it to focus on Type II error.

When using a threshold of, for example, 95%, some writers may state that a difference is "significant at the 0.05 level." By this they mean that only 5% of samples from the population would be expected to have values more extreme than that of the test case, and they judge the difference exhibited by the test case to be significantly different from variation exhibited by samples from the reference population. The 95% value is called the "confidence interval." The term "confidence interval" is also used in reporting a test value, as in, "the resistance value exhibited by these resistors lies in the 95% confidence interval of 98 to 102 ohms." Specifically, the phrase encompasses the following concept: if a test were to be repeated over and over with a reference population, 95% of the observed values would lie in the interval. The endpoints of the interval are also called the "confidence limits."

Most introductory statistics texts, such as Strait (1989), describe a variety of tests in which the reference population is assumed to be normally distributed. The various examples demonstrate how to put the test value into standardized form, called the "test statistic," and then compare it against the standard normal table. Examples with small sample sizes and with unknown population variance are given too, using the Student t table and test statistic.

Table 22-1 provides an example of a hypothesis test. Two sets of a particular product, 30 in each set, were tested for output value. The first set had been processed in the usual manner. The second set had been processed in a proposed manner. The null hypothesis is "there is no difference in output values between the two sets." If the difference is not significant, the proposed process could be used.

To compare the two arithmetic averages, or means, the following test statistic is used:

$$Z = \bar{X}_1 - \bar{X}_2 - d / \bar{O}(\varsigma_1^2/n_1 + \varsigma_2^2/n_2)$$

Set 1			Set 2		
Unit #	Value	Rank	Unit #	Value	Rank
1-1	2.22	53.5	2-1	1.99	16
1-2	2.04	25.5	2-2	2.08	33.5
1-3	1.99	16	2-3	2.13	38.5
1-4	2.26	58.5	2-4	2.13	38.5
1-5	2.26	58.5	2-5	2.04	25.5
1-6	1.90	6	2-6	2.04	25.5
1-7	2.08	33.5	2-7	1.95	11
1-8	2.22	53.5	2-8	2.08	33.5
1-9	2.17	45.5	2-9	1.99	16
1-10	2.26	58.5	2-10	1.90	6
1-11	2.17	45.5	2-11	2.17	45.5
1-12	2.04	25.5	2-12	2.17	45.5
1-13	2.22	53.5	2-13	2.22	53.5
1-14	2.08	33.5	2-14	2.22	53.5
1-15	2.08	33.5	2-15	1.99	16
1-16	1.95	11	2-16	1.90	6
1-17	2.05	29	2-17	2.26	58.5
1-18	2.03	22	2-18	1.95	11
1-19	1.95	11	2-19	2.08	33.5
1-20	2.13	38.5	2-20	1.88	3.5
1-21	2.22	53.5	2-21	1.91	7
1-22	2.14	41.5	2-22	2.17	45.5
1-23	2.00	19.5	2-23	1.99	16
1-24	2.00	19.5	2-24	2.17	45.5
1-25	2.19	50	2-25	1.88	3.5
1-26	1.86	1	2-26	2.05	29
1-27	2.18	49	2-27	2.05	29
1-28	1.95	11	2-28	2.03	22
1-29	2.13	38.5	2-29	1.86	2
1-30	2.03	22	2-30	2.14	41.5
Average: 2.09, Ranks Sum: 1017.5			Average: 2.05, Ranks Sum: 811.5		
Standard Deviation: 0.11			Standard Deviation: 0.11		

Table 22-1 Comparison of Means Example.

In this case, d, the difference between the two means, $\bar{X}_1$ and $\bar{X}_2$, is zero. The standard deviations are σ_1 and σ_2, and the sample sizes n_1 and n_2 are both 30.

The calculated z value will be compared to the area on the normal distribution table. If the sample size were smaller, it would be necessary to compare the test statistic to the Student t table instead. The Student t table corrects for small sample size. Strait (1989) reports that the normal table is approximately correct for sample sizes larger than 15. The normal table, then, is adequate in this case.

For this example, the Z value is 1.41. The table value corresponding to this Z value is 0.4207. If pairs of samples both from the same population were compared to each other, the differences would be less than what was exhibited in this example about 84% of the time. It is judged that there is insufficient evidence to claim that these two samples have means which are significantly different.

Perhaps the experimentalist wishes to test the null hypothesis that "there is no difference in the variances of the two test groups." The variance is, of course, the square of the standard deviation. The ratio of the standard deviations is calculated in the following test statistic:

$$F_{\alpha,\, v1,\, v2} = S_1{}^2/S_2{}^2$$

in which v_1 and v_2 are the degrees of freedom for the two sample sets and α is the familiar Type I error tolerance. The number of degrees of freedom for each sample set in this case is equal to the number of data points minus one, 29.

In this example, the test statistic is equal to unity. A statistics book such as Strait (1989) contains an F-table which can be referenced. The table value for $F_{29,\, 29}$ is approximately 1.87 for $\alpha = 0.05$ and 2.44 for $\alpha = 0.01$. It can be judged, then, that there is insufficient evidence with which to conclude that a significant difference exists between the two variances.

Some hypothesis tests can be made without the assumption of the normal distribution. They are based on transforming the information from the sample, the distribution of which isn't known, into another variable, the distribution of which is known. Consider this hypothesis: "The proportion of red, white, blue, black, green, and metallic cars at the local outlet of a car rental firm is the same as are owned nationwide." The number of each of red, white, blue, black, green, and metallic cars to be expected if the nationwide fleet were as small as the local fleet are calculated, and compared against the numbers found in the local fleet. The chi-squared distribution is used with the appropriate test statistic, and the null hypothesis evaluated. Specifically, the test statistic for this example would be as follows:

$$\times \ \frac{(\text{Cars of this color from the local fleet-Cars of this color if drawn from national fleet})^2}{\text{Cars of this color if drawn from national fleet}}$$

This statistic has the chi-squared distribution. This sum is compared to the c^2_k value from a standard table, such as the one found in the appendix. The subscript k is called the degrees of freedom. It is equal to $m - t - 1$, where m is the number of colors and t is the number of parameters used in the process of setting up the test. To compare the number of cars in the local fleet to what should be expected from the national fleet, no extra parameters are required, so it would be equal to 0 in this case. Strait (1989) includes examples in which intermediate parameters are calculated.

To expand upon this example, values for car colors in a local rental fleet, as well as those of cars owned nationwide, were invented and displayed with their test statistic in Table 22-2.

The resultant test value of 8.82 is compared against values in the c^2_{k} values in the table in the back of this book. The degrees of freedom k is equal to $6 - 0 - 1 = 5$. It can be seen by examining the table that α would need to be smaller than 0.10, or 10%, before the table value would be smaller than the test value. It would be reasonable to conclude that there is insufficient evidence to justify claiming that the local car rental fleet had a color distribution significantly different from what was seen nationwide.

Now suppose instead that only the most popular colors--red, white, and black--are considered. Table 22-3 shows the appropriate calculations. For this case, there are only two degrees of freedom. The test value falls between the $\alpha = 0.10$ and $\alpha = 0.05$ columns on the table. Some experimenters might find that α value small enough to justify calling the difference in car color distribution significant, despite the fact that the calculated χ^2 value is smaller than in the Table 22-2 example.

In this case, no assumption was made concerning the type of distribution appropriate for the national fleet. Indeed, the quantification of cars-by-color is not even a continuous function. This chi-squared test allows an assessment to be made without a distributional assumption.

This technique, as well as caveats to its use, is discussed more fully in references such as Strait (1989) (see "non-parametric test of distribution" or "goodness-of-fit test" using the chi-squared distribution). D'Agostino and Stephens (1986) devotes a chapter to the technique, and it is also touched upon in Box, Hunter, and Hunter (1978).

Color of Car	Cars Owned Nationwide (Millions)	Fraction of Nat'l Total	If Nat'l Were Local Size (N)	Actual Local Fleet (A)	$\frac{(A-N)^2}{N}$
red	47.3	0.227	70	81	1.73
white	40.9	0.197	61	72	1.98
blue	26.5	0.127	39	29	2.56
black	53.1	0.255	79	66	2.14
green	17.4	0.084	26	24	0.15
metallic	22.7	0.109	34	37	0.26
Sum	208	0.999	309	309	8.82

Table 22-2 Car Color Comparison Example

Another non-parametric test, that is, a test that does not assume a particular distribution, is the Sign Test. The Sign Test works by comparing the sample data against a standard. If the particular datum is greater than the standard, it counts as a success (a "+"). If the datum is less than the standard, it counts as a failure (a "-"). If the datum is equal to the standard, it is not counted. An example would be: "the null hypothesis is that the difference between the means of the two samples is no more than three." The data in the two samples would be compared pair-by-pair against the value of three, and appropriate +'s and -'s assigned.

This type of assessment gives results that fit a Bernoulli distribution. The Bernoulli distribution governs tests that have only two outcomes: up or down, yea or nay, heads or tails. Coin flips can be evaluated with the Bernoulli distribution. The Sign Test reshapes the data to fit into a Bernoulli assessment, allowing one to test the null hypothesis without knowing what the underlying distribution is. The caveat is that the Sign Test assumes that the mean and the median are the same for the underlying population. Several Sign Tests are described in Strait (1989).

An even more versatile non-parametric test of two means is the Mann-Whitney-Wilcoxon Rank-Sum Test, also described in Strait (1989). The two samples are put together into ascending order. The sum of the individual ranks from each sample can be transformed into variables which are actually normally distributed. The null hypothesis can then be evaluated in the usual manner. The sample sizes must be larger than eight to employ this test.

Color of Car	Cars Owned Nationwide (Millions)	Fraction of Nat'l Total	If Nat'l Were Local Size (N)	Actual Local Fleet (A)	$\frac{(A-N)^2}{N}$
red	47.3	0.335	73	81	0.88
white	40.9	0.29	64	72	2.25
black	53.1	0.377	83	66	3.48
Sum	141.3	1	220	219	6.61

Table 22-3 Color of Cars Example

The example in Table 22-1 includes information by which to make a Mann-Whitney-Wilcoxon Rank-Sum Test as well. The two samples were ranked together from lowest to highest. In cases of multiple instances of the same value, each occurrence is given the mid-point rank--the average of the ranks that the occurrences would have had if they had been unique numbers. For example, the two occurrences of 1.88 would have had ranks of 3 and 4, but are instead both assigned the rank of 3.5. The following intermediate value is calculated:

$$I = R - (n(n+1)/2)$$

in which R is the sum of the ranks for one of the sets and n is the number of sample points from that set.

The normalized test statistic is then calculated:

$$z = \frac{I - \frac{(n_1 n_2)}{2}}{\sqrt{\frac{n_1 n_2 (n_1 + n_2 + 1)}{12}}}$$

The null hypothesis being tested is that the two means are the same. The alternative, assumed if the null hypothesis is rejected, is that the mean of the sample for which R was calculated is more extreme than the mean for the other sample.

Taking sample set 1, R is shown in Table 22-1 to be 1017.5, I is calculated as 552.5, and z is 1.52. Approximately 87% of samples taken from the same population would be expected to have Z values smaller than in this case. This is a result similar to what was found with the normal distribution comparison of the means. Calculations with the set 2 data would have yielded the same result. Finally, note that the equation given for the intermediate value is invalid at small sample sizes.

22.2.2 Cast A Wide Net

The value that a testing program adds to a manufacturer's business practice lies in the reexamination of the design and of the assumptions concerning its capabilities. Crucial to realizing that benefit is the sufficiency of data. In order to know, rather than to surmise, that the product meets expectations, it is vital to verify product performance in as many contexts as possible.

The first aspect of variety to consider is the number of factors that can affect the component's outputs of interest. Included in the term "factor" is not only an expected input, such as voltage, but also environmental conditions. Laboratory conditions are often well-regulated with minimal variation. No factor should be taken for granted when contemplating product performance in the field. How can each factor, such as voltage or temperature, vary? Over what range can it vary? Are there any special circumstances? For example, there may be a single country or region of the world in which local regulations or customs dictate special environmental conditions or processes applied to the product. How will the product fare in such an instance?

It is tempting to argue in the absence of any safety issue that such a case represents a diminishingly small fraction of the total customer base and thus an unlikely scenario that need not be addressed. At least three arguments counter this position. First, a pragmatic one: those responsible for promoting the product would likely claim that each and every customer is important to the company. The expectation to address such a case, then, exists. Second, a fiscal one: it is not necessary for a large fraction of the customer base to request legal remedy to have a significant financial impact; a small number will do. Finally, a philosophical one: most, if not all, workers are dedicated to producing the best work that they can, and to serving the public good. For engineers, these maxims are enumerated in codes of ethics promulgated by various professional societies. Paying attention to the unusual case serves that customer and these ends.

A technique to identify significant factors from among all the others is Design of Experiments. Design of Experiments provides a structure whereby many factors can be varied over a minimal number of tests. It is not necessary to test each factor at, say, five levels in order to estimate the magnitude of the factor's effect. Only two levels are used, high and low, for each factor. For example, suppose a test is proposed evaluating three factors. A full factorial design appears in Table 22-4. The pattern is standard. The order in which the tests are run has been randomized, as shown in the second column. This practice will be discussed later.

Outcomes are measured, and the results from all the tests are compounded. Not only are the significant factors identified, but significant interactions between factors can be identified, depending on the specific set of designed experiments run. The possibility of interactions is not always considered in initial design work, and often is forgotten later, but can nonetheless be significant to the ultimate performance of the product.

If this study were to be made traditionally, each of the three factors might be set to five levels while the other two are held at constant values. A battery of fifteen tests would be required, and it would not yield information on the interactions. The reason why interactions can be measured in the Design of Experiments technique with a little more than half the tests is the fact that all combinations of low and high with each factor are present. Looking at the last two rows of the table, it can be seen that Factor 3 is varied while Factors 1 and 2 are held steady, at the high value. But the first two rows also incorporate change in Factor 3, but with Factors 1 and 2 held at the low value. All the cases in which Factors 1 and 2 vary together (A to G, B to H) can be collected and compared with the outcomes when Factors 1 and 2 move in opposite directions (C to E, D to F). In this way the interaction of Factors 1 and 2 can be measured. The estimates of all significant factor effects and all significant interaction effects can be collected into a mathematical model or equation of the outcome under study.

A ninth test might be added to this design, in which all three factors are set to the midpoint of their respective low-to-high range. The purpose of this ninth test is to give an indication of the curvature that might be present in the model. The presence of curvature might indicate a new avenue of testing.

In addition to the benefit of insight into interactions, the Design of Experiments technique provides direction on how to improve the design, and allows the tester a quick assessment of an improvement suggested by the test results. Box, Hunter, and Hunter (1978) is an excellent, detailed, and practical reference for this approach.

It is also important to test a large number of samples. How many samples are adequate? The cynical answer is "more than are available for the test." Brush (1988) gives a book of charts that allow the reader to calculate the sample size required for tests against the normal distribution for given levels of Type I and Type II errors.

Test Designator	Run Number	Factor 1 Value	Factor 2 Value	Factor 3 Value
A	8	low	low	low
B	2	low	low	high
C	7	low	high	low
D	1	low	high	high
E	5	high	low	low
F	6	high	low	high
G	3	high	high	low
H	4	high	high	high

Table 22-4 Three Factor, Full-Factorial Test Design

Some tests focus on the failures of the test specimens. Failure times are often modeled with a distribution called the Weibull distribution, described in Nelson (1990), O'Connor (1991), Meeker and Escobar (1998) and many other references. For tests in which the objective is to establish a Weibull scale parameter, sometimes termed a "life" parameter, Abernethy (1996) provides a table and Nelson (1985) provides a formula by which the minimum sample size can be determined given a proposed testing time. Both items presume knowledge of the Weibull shape parameter. Without knowledge of the appropriate shape parameter, it will need to be estimated from in-house information or from judgment. In some cases, both testing time and sample size are, to some extent, at the discretion of the tester.

It should be kept in mind that components often vary in substantive characteristics from one lot to another, and even within a lot. Incorporating a large sample size helps to capture this source of variation in the test. The samples should represent the variation that could occur from the supplier. The tester should seek samples from different production lots, made on different shifts, at different sites, by different workers, at different times. That one cannot see these differences affecting the performance of the component is precisely the point. Including as much variation as possible, including unsuspected variation in supply, reveals sensitivity of the product to what was regarded as a harmless factor. The design can then be made more robust. In the absence of proof through testing, any significant differences will wend their way into the final product, and ultimately generate mysteries in the field. Solving the mysteries will require tracing through the supply records and still more testing to ferret out the heretofore unknown sensitivity. A proposed redress is likely to be more expensive than buying the extra samples would have been in the first place.

22.2.3 Records

Proper, detailed records provide important support in a testing effort. Detailed records made before and during a test assist with the analysis and later reproduction of the results. The test setup should be described completely-- dimensions, equipment used, placement in the lab, and so forth. Photographs are well suited for this purpose. The environmental conditions of the test should be noted. If those conditions shift significantly, that fact too should be noted. The estimation of "significant" is a matter of judgment, however. The reason for noting these things is to have the information at hand in the event that the test results do not conform to expectations. This information may point to an external factor that influenced the test.

If data are recorded by hand, the test sheets should be retained. In the course of subsequent analysis, some points may appear anomalous. While all transcriptions into analysis packages such as spreadsheets should be proofread, it is nevertheless possible that a transcription error would occur, even after such a check. With the original sheets, the datum in question can be verified. Naturally, this does not eliminate the possibility of the datum having been recorded erroneously in the first place.

Legal considerations influence record practices for laboratory notebooks as well. The use of a bound notebook for preliminary work helps to establish that the record is complete, though its use also precludes tightening the presentation of the information. Sometimes a computer printout might be taped into a notebook. Such pages should be taped down, with an "X" across the underlying page. The work should be signed and dated by the worker, and a witness should sign, too. If the work is a page taped into the notebook, the signature should be partly on the printout page and partly on the notebook page. These directives assist in the defense of a company's patents. It may be important to establish the time frame in which something was invented.

Signatures by both the worker and the witness are required by regulatory bodies as well. FDA also provides for electronic signatures of records in FDA (1997). Considerable attention is given to the security of the signature. While a physical signature cannot be reproduced easily and undetectably, security of electronic signatures is more elusive. It is easier to reproduce an electronic signature, and harder to detect the fraud. Among specific requirements included in FDA (1997) for electronic signatures are the following:

- it should be unique to the individual
- it should be retired from the company with the individual

- it should be non-transferable
- it should not be possible to excise the signature from the signed document by electronic means

As of this writing, popular electronic packages do not seem to be well-suited to accommodating secure electronic signatures.

Finally, in all documents, the writer should be as concise, clear, and thorough as possible. It is difficult to anticipate which documents will be important to a company's later legal advocacy, either for patents or other cases, so the writer should always document the work well. Moreover, having good documentation is good common sense, as it helps future workers build on the work.

22.2.4 Other Considerations

If the test consists of several runs, as with the Design of Experiments technique, the runs should be randomized. Doing so helps to encompass any other unforeseen factors. If the runs are organized to run so that a known factor is increased with each successive run, an unforeseen factor, which might also increase as time goes by, could be correlated with the increase in the known factor. The observed effect might be due to the unforeseen factor, but because of the order in which the tests were run, the effect may well be attributed to the planned, known factor. An erroneous conclusion would result. Randomizing the runs scrambles the change in known factor versus time and versus other conditions of the test, such as relative placement on the fixture. Any observed effect, then, can more properly be attributed to the known factor itself.

Many tests involve electronic acquisition of the data. Several considerations affect such acquisition. First is the question of how often the data should be recorded. If an analysis of the frequency content of the signal is to be made with a Fast Fourier Transform (FFT) calculation, the algorithm requires that the signal be sampled at least twice as fast as the highest frequency that is believed to be in the signal. If the time history of the signal is to be plotted, this sample rate will not resolve much detail in the highest frequency component. For a time domain plot, at least ten times the frequency produces a better visual result. Balancing that guideline is the resolution of the output device. It is not necessary to acquire tens of thousands of points if the entire signal is to be plotted on one sheet of paper. Even if the device can produce 1200 dots per inch, the printer is not likely to be able to produce the captured detail over the entire time range. Nothing would be gained for the extra expenditure of time and disk space. A smaller time range would be necessary to make use of the information.

Another aspect to keep in mind is the limits of the data acquisition system. In particular, there is a difference between "precision" and "accuracy." Precision refers to how repeatable a measurement is for an instrument. It can also refer to the number of digits presented by a computer. Accuracy refers to how close the measured value is to the true value. An instrument might repeatedly read 4.98375 volts, and be consistently off by a volt. Precision is several darts in the same locale; accuracy is the bullseye. Precision is not accuracy; a long string of numbers is not necessarily impressive.

Some tests call for acceleration factors in order to minimize the time spent acquiring the data. Implicit in any such action is the assumption that the output, or rate of change of the output, is linearly proportional to the value that would be produced had the test been run without acceleration. It is vital to reexamine this assumption and ensure it has a solid basis for the specific test in question. Be wary of glib "rules of thumb," handed down across industries and through technological revolutions, generalized beyond their original scope. They may no longer have factual foundations, if they ever did. They are not "better than nothing," for they give test plans associated with them a misleading aura of a theoretical foundation for the acceleration factor. The best acceleration factors are those derived from the behavior of similar products or from the product in question itself. A preliminary estimate can be made based on the physics and chemistry of the situation, as well as on past performance. The test can be structured to confirm the estimate by running some units at the unaccelerated condition and fewer units at the progressively more extreme accelerating conditions. Nelson (1990) is an excellent book on the subject of accelerated testing, as are the last chapters of Meeker and Escobar (1998).

If time and other constraints permit, repetitions of the test, or replicates, should be run. Replicates provide a confirmation of the original test result. They can also allow a rough calculation of the variability in the parameter being measured from test to test.

Finally, the test should be reviewed for built-in assumptions. These assumptions will shape the outcome of the test, explicitly or implicitly, so each one should be challenged for validity. It is important to understand the weak areas of the proposed work in order to appreciate the limitations of the results. That the results are limited is not fatal; it is merely an aspect of the work. By taking the time to review the assumptions of the proposed test, the tester gains the opportunity to improve the test design. The test should not begin until the tester feels that the dependencies of the test design on a priori assumptions is minimized.

22.3 Running the Test

If the test has been set up properly, the running of the test will be straightforward, almost anti-climactic. To ensure the successful outcome, the tester should do several things when running the test. First, verify the test setup. If this seems excessive, consider the apocryphal comment from the senior engineer to the junior engineer: "There's never time to do it right, but there's always time to do it over." Second, conduct a trial run. Sometimes a condition that has not been considered will manifest itself in the first run of the test. One learns how to run the test by running the test. A trial run accommodates the learning curve. Finally, record all anomalies. As stated before, to yield the most information out of the test, it is important to capture as many sources of variability as possible. Randomizing the runs will help compensate for any other unforeseen factors, but there may yet be a spurious event that affects the outcome of the test. By recording them when they happen, the information concerning them is retained for the analysis stage. Without the record, the tester must depend on the short-term memory to help explain surprising test results. Human memory is sometimes subjective, so this dependence is riskier than making a record of the event.

22.4 Analyzing the Outcome

The first, best way to analyze the data is to look at a picture of it--plot the data. If possible, include error bars to indicate the uncertainty in the measurement device, to put the plotted values into context. Plot markers on the actual test points unless they are so numerous that the overlapping markers obscure the actual plotting positions. Some plotting packages will automatically scale the axes to the range of the plot. This helps to show detail in the data, but can sometimes exaggerate small changes. Look at the data on a full and meaningful scale as well. The changes that appear large on the automatic plot may appear more like minor noise in the second plot. It may also be instructive to plot the data by hand. Depending on the user-interface of the software package, that may in fact be easier anyway. Taking the time to plot the data by hand also provides time to consider the data at greater length.

The analyst should review several aspects of a completed plot. First, what are the global features of the plot? Is there a response at all? Is it of the expected magnitude? What about trends? Next, are there any unusual points? When and where do they occur? Is there a correlation that points to a possible causality for the unusual point?

Two caveats should be highlighted at this juncture. First, a point that looks unusual may not actually be unusual. The deviation the point shows from the general trend may be within expectation from either the uncertainty of the measurement device or variation that could be expected from the underlying population of similar points. As an example, a local news telecast reported "recently winning" and "recently losing" lottery numbers; they were numbers that had occurred the most and least frequently in recent samples. No estimate of the variance to be expected was reported. The proposition that a particular number would be more likely to yield winnings is nonsense; each number has an equal probability of being selected, and the process is monitored by the government and independently audited. Without the uncertainty estimate, the report could be interpreted to indicate that some numbers have a significance that isn't actually there. Including error bars or confidence intervals on the plot helps temper the assessment of unusual points. Second, correlation is not causality. An absurd example would be to note the correlation between the ringing of an alarm clock and the rising of the sun, and then to conclude that the clock's ring causes the sun to rise. The logical extension of that conclusion would be that the time of dawn could be altered by changing the clock setting. Similarly, while it is instructive to identify factors that correlate with the incidence of an unusual point, care should be taken that these factors are not labeled causes without appropriate investigation and justification.

Another possible analysis is to determine the frequency content of the data. This is often done through a Fast Fourier Transform (FFT) of the data. As mentioned earlier, it is necessary to sample the data at a rate at least twice that of the highest frequency of interest. The FFT assumes that the sample of the data taken is repeated infinitely in both directions in time. Because the record is merely a sample of the entire data stream, it is not actually complete. In fact, depending on when the sample begins and ends, there may be a significant discontinuity between the end of the signal and the beginning of its repeat. Such a discontinuity introduces errors into the FFT calculation. A way to compensate for these errors is to multiply the output signal by a window. The window has a value of unity in the center of the signal and tapers off to zero at the beginning and end of the signal. The window, then, forces the endpoints of the signal to be nearly continuous, at a value of approximately zero.

Bendat and Piersol (1986) and Oppenheim and Schafer (1975) both provide extensive information on this type of signal analysis. Bendat and Piersol (1986) is theoretical. Because Oppenheim and Schafer (1975) focuses on digital signals and discretized signals, it is of more immediate help for a particular test.

A model, or equation, of the measured output as a function of one or more input factors may be fit to the data. One technique for fitting a model is through linear or curvilinear regression. The regression techniques find the parameters for the given order polynomial that minimize the distance between each data point and the model. That distance is called the residual. The Design of Experiments technique also provides for fitting a model to the data, and residuals can be calculated for the data and the resulting model.

If a model is fitted, it is instructive to plot the residuals. The residuals should be evenly distributed about the abscissa; there should be the same number of positive differences as negative ones. A variety of magnitude should be represented, and they should be randomly distributed along the abscissa. Look for patterns in the data, termed "trends"; there should not be any. If there are, that indicates that the model is becoming increasingly unsuitable in the range of the trend, or that another factor is significant to the output of the system.

Another technique useful in the analysis of test results is the Analysis of Variance (ANOVA). It is employed with the Design of Experiments technique, and is also printed with some curve-fitting programs. The variance associated with each source of variation, the residuals of the model, the applied factors, and any other major grouping of the data are calculated. Then the ratios of the sources of variation to the residual variation are calculated. These ratios are used in an F-test for significance (see Box, Hunter, and Hunter (1978) for more details).

The data in all its representations should be used to review the premises of the test, the assumptions of the governing phenomena, and the expectations of the outcome. If an error was made, the data should indicate where the discrepancy lies. Such indicators should be pursued until the behavior of the system is understood. It may require retests, or new tests, but the leads should be pursued to their ends.

22.5 Limits to Analysis

The results of analysis can only produce so much information. The techniques are limited, and the assumptions enabling their use are limited as well.

First, data acquisition devices have limited accuracies, sometimes less than their reported precision. Reports from subsequent calculations with this data should not list additional digits behind the decimal point. The fact that the computer can calculate the digits does not necessarily signify any meaning. In addition, if two data each with uncertainties are combined, the resulting uncertainty should be assessed. One method to do this is to consider the extremes of the values, compute the result, and estimate the uncertainty from the result. For example, suppose a force of 1.00 ± 0.05 Newton is applied to a beam of length 0.500 ± 0.005 m. What is the resulting moment? The moment is the product of the two. One could expect the product to range from $0.95 \times 0.495 = 0.47$ N-m to $1.05 \times 0.505 = 0.53$ N-m, that is, 0.50 ± 0.03 N-m. Another approach is to compute the geometric mean of the standard deviations for each measurement. That approach assumes that the distribution of expected measurements from the devices is normal.

If the analyst is writing computer code to process the data, it is particularly important to be aware that the computer will do what it is told to do, not necessarily what the analyst intends it to do. The same attention to precision of the numbers in hand calculations applies in reporting computed results. Error in a lower digit can propagate to higher digits, particularly after many computations, so it is important that calculations be made with larger precision data types, and that constants such as π be represented with as many digits as possible. These concepts of numerical analysis take on greater importance as the number of computations required for the analysis increases. More information can be found in Burden and Faires (1989).

Also, many analyses involving the assumption of a distribution involve plotting the data on probability paper. The paper's ordinate is spaced unevenly such that data from a population fitting that particular distribution will lie on a straight line. From the resulting straight line, parameters of the distribution can be estimated. When the sample set is small, though, the data can be surprisingly non-linear, even if the distributional assumption is sound. Hahn and Shapiro (1967) and Daniel and Wood (1980) both provide instructive examples of small samples drawn from the normal distribution plotted on normal distribution paper. Even a sample size of 20 of mathematically generated points can produce odd shapes on the paper. With minor uncertainties in the measurement, the straightness of a line can indeed be suspect. This factor is another reason why the experimentalist should seek to include as many samples as possible in the test. Even with a sufficient number of data points, the analyst should not expect a perfectly straight line.

The ability of a model to predict product behavior is naturally dependent on the model being appropriate in the first place, and that includes the selection of the distribution. The normal distribution is widely known and widely employed. It is symmetric about a central tendency. If a variable is to be modeled as normally distributed, it should have the property that it is equally likely to assume a value above the arithmetic mean as one below it. Other distributions describe other situations. Certain components, for example, are inspected for flaws. In the case in which there is a minimum flaw size that can be detected, the smallest extreme value function would be more appropriate, because flaws larger than the detection threshold would be removed from the population. Nelson (1990) and O'Connor (1991) review common distributions and give some examples of appropriate applications of them. Meeker and Escobar (1998) do as well, and also include the parent distributions of which the popular distributions are special cases.

Finally, models can only really speak to the data to which they were fit. Often, though, there is interest in behavior outside the range of input data. This is particularly true with accelerated tests. Generally speaking, the closer the estimate is to the range of the actual data, that is, the shorter the extrapolation, the more accurate will be the prediction. Models cannot be used over the entire abscissa range.

22.6 Conclusion

The process of testing a component or product can yield a bounty of information. It is necessary to set up the test carefully, thoroughly considering all possibly relevant factors. The tester should take little for granted, challenging assumptions and presented maxims, as well as reviewing the quality of the test at all stages. The subsequent analysis can yield much information, but the tester should be aware of limitations to this information. Above all, the experimenter should have a clear idea of what information is to result from the test, in order to be successful in achieving that goal.

References

Abernethy, Robert B. *The New Weibull Handbook.* 2nd ed. North Palm Beach, FL: By the author, 1996.

Bendat, Julius S., and Allan G. Piersol. *Random Data: Analysis and Measurement Procedures.* 2nd ed. New York: John Wiley & Sons, 1986.

Box, George E.P., William G. Hunter, and J. Stuart Hunter. *Statistics for Experimenters.* New York: John Wiley & Sons, 1978.

Brush, Gary. *How to Choose the Proper Sample Size.* Vol. 12, *The ASQC Basic References in Quality Control: Statistical Techniques.* Milwaukee, WI: ASQC Quality Press, 1988.

Burden, Richard L., and J. Douglas Faires. *Numerical Analysis.* 4th ed. Boston: PWS-Kent Publishing Co., 1989.

D'Agostino, Ralph B. and Michael A. Stephens. *Goodness-of-Fit Techniques.* New York: Marcel Dekker, Inc., 1986.

Daniel, Cuthbert and Fred S. Wood. *Fitting Equations to Data: Computer Analysis of Multifactor Data.* 2nd ed. New York: John Wiley & Sons, 1980.

Food and Drug Administration. "FR FDA 03/20/97 F62 FR 13423: Electronic Records; Electronic Signatures." Washington, DC: U.S. Department of Health and Human Services, Food and Drug Administration, 1997.

Hahn, Gerald J. and Samuel S. Shapiro. *Statistical Models in Engineering.* New York: John Wiley & Sons, 1967.

Meeker, William Q., and Luis A. Escobar. *Statistical Methods for Reliability Data.* New York: John Wiley & Sons, 1998.

Natrella, Mary Gibbons. *Experimental Statistics.* Washington, DC: U.S. Department of Commerce, National Bureau of Standards (National Institute of Science and Technology): For sale by the Supt. of Documents, U.S. Government Printing Office, 1976.

Nelson, Wayne. "Weibull Analysis of Reliability Data with Few or No Failures," *Journal of Quality Technology,* 17, no. 3 (July, 1985): p.140-146.

Nelson, Wayne. *Accelerated Testing: Statistical Models, Test Plans, and Data Analyses.* New York: John Wiley & Sons, 1990.

O'Connor, Patrick. *Practical Reliability Engineering.* 3rd ed. New York: John Wiley & Sons, 1991.

Oppenheim, Alan V., and Ronald W. Schafer. *Digital Signal Processing.* Englewood Cliffs, NJ: Prentice-Hall, Inc., 1975.

Strait, Peggy Tang. *A First Course in Probability and Statistics with Applications.* 2nd ed. Orlando, FL: Harcourt Brace Journovich, 1989.

Chapter 23

Overview of Verification and Validation for Embedded Software in Medical Systems

Andre Bloesch – Datex-Ohmeda, Inc.
Madison, Wisconsin

This chapter is devoted to an overview of Verification and Validation (V&V) for embedded software in medical devices. In this chapter, we will briefly discuss verification and validation concepts such as planning, test development, and test execution.

23.1   Verification and Validation Planning

The key to success in verification and validation is planning. Verification and validation planning encompasses the entire development life cycle, from requirements generation to product release. The initial planning of V&V is documented in a Software Verification and Validation Plan (SVVP). The SVVP describes the verification and validation life cycle, gives an overview of verification and validation, describes the verification and validation life cycle activities, defines the verification and validation documentation, and discusses the verification and validation administrative procedures. An excellent guideline for verification and validation planning can be found in IEEE Std 1012-1986, with an explication of Std 1012-1986 found in IEEE Std 1059-1993.

23.1.1   Verification and Validation Life Cycle

An SVVP lays out the framework from which the verification and validation activities proceed. IEEE 1012-1986 is very detailed about development life cycle and the verification and validation products that are generated at each phase. Specifically, the standard calls out the following phases:

- Concept phase
- Requirements phase
- Design phase
- Implementation phase
- Test phase
- Installation phase
- Operation and maintenance phase.

In industry, it is more typical for software verification and validation to follow a simpler model, as shown in the Figure 23-1.

This model is simpler in that it focuses verification and validation activities on the software that is generated, rather than output of every phase of development. Another document, called the Software Quality Assurance Plan (SQAP), is used to cover other verification and validation aspects of product development, like software requirements reviews, hazard and risk analysis, and design reviews.

Using the model as shown in Figure 23-1, Software Validation Testing covers validation of the software product by testing against the requirements generated in the requirements generation phase. Software Validation is analogous to black box testing. Integration Testing covers verification of features defined from the requirements generation phase, the concept/high level

Typical Software Development Model

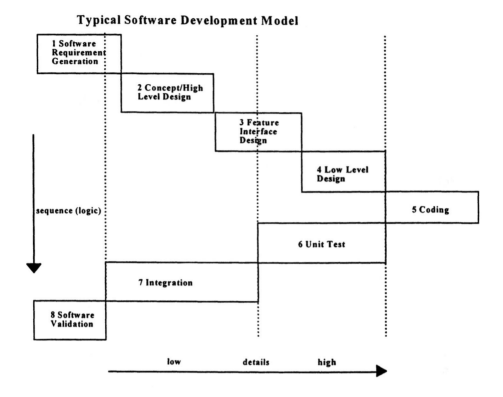

Figure 23-1   Typical software development model.

design phase, and the feature interface design phase. Integration Testing tests the collection of software modules, where the software modules are joined together to provide a product feature or higher level of functionality. Finally, Unit Testing covers verification at the lowest level, which includes feature interface design phase and the low-level design phase. Unit Testing typically covers the verification of smaller collections of software modules.

23.1.2   Verification and Validation Overview

The verification and validation overview describes much of the project management details that must be addressed in order to perform the verification and validation functions. This includes the verification and validation organization, a schedule, resources, responsibilities, and any special tools, techniques, and methodologies.

The organization describes who is responsible for carrying out the various verification and validation efforts. In practice, this section is used to describe who will be responsible for maintaining the laboratory, who will manage the validation testing, who will manage verification testing, and who is responsible for anomaly resolution.

Verification and validation scheduling is very important for planning activities in order to support the overall product schedule. Oftentimes, a higher level schedule is entered into the Software Verification and Validation Plan, and a detailed scheduled is maintained separately from the Software Verification and Validation Plan. This is generally due to different software applications for generating a schedule and for generating documentation.

The resources section describes all the equipment, software and hardware, required to perform verification and validation activities. A subsection should also be included on the validation of using any software tools, where the software tool is used as part of the verification and validation process. Per the FDA's regulations (FDA, Quality System Regulation, 21 CFR Part 820, June 1, 1997), any device used in a company's quality system must be validated. A test fixture or a customized software application clearly falls under this definition. Thus, it is necessary to validate the software tool.

23.1.3   Verification and Validation Life Cycle Activities

In the SVVP, this section typically includes the Criteria, Inputs/Outputs, Reviews, Testing Approach, and Training for each verification and validation phase. The Criteria describes the goal that each phase is defined to achieve. The Inputs/Outputs phase defines what things are needed as inputs into the phase and what the product of each phase are.

It is also helpful to add a subsection on the general functionality that will be tested. The IEEE standard does not call this out. However, adding this subsection is helpful to reviewers of the Software Verification and Validation Plan. It provides information on what functionality is planned to be tested.

23.1.4   Verification and Validation Documentation

Each verification and validation phase has its activities and documentation that is associated with it. For Unit, Integration, and Software Validation test phases, typically there are test plans, test procedures, and test results/reports.

For Software Validation, there are usually some additional documents. The Software Validation group typically has a requirements-to-test cross reference. The cross reference ensure that all the requirements defined in the SRS are covered in some test. It is also helpful in the cross reference document to include a test-to-requirement cross reference. This backwards reference helps to ensure that a requirement has adequate coverage. The Software Validation group also generates a procedure response document. The procedure response document serves as a means to close out any issues or comments that occurred on during an official validation pass. Finally, the Software Validation group has been responsible for writing a final report, called the Software Verification and Validation Report (SVVR). The SVVR summarizes the activities from all the previous verification and validation phases.

23.1.5   Verification and Validation Administrative Procedures

The verification and validation administrative procedures section provides additional guidance on how the verification and validation will be conducted. IEEE Std 1012-1986 defines this section as including anomaly reporting/resolution, task iteration policy, deviation policy, control procedures, and standards/practices/conventions.

It is also useful to include a section metrics. IEEE Std 730.1-1989, IEEE Standard for Software Quality Assurance Plans, includes metrics as part of a SQAP. The following subsections describe in more detail anomaly reporting, metrics collection and reporting, and provide some additional topics that are important to verification and validation.

23.1.6   Anomaly Reporting and Resolution

One result of verification and validation is the generation of anomalies found during testing. A process for reporting anomalies must be in place to record anomalies. Some places have used a lab notebook to document anomalies. More frequently, a PC based database program is used to log and store anomalies electronically. See Figure 23-2 below for an example of an anomaly form.

A process must also be in place for resolution of anomalies found against the product software. This can be a committee of people responsible for the product or simply the Software Test Coordinator working with the primary software developer. The responsible parties determine the risk of each anomaly.

23.1.7   Validation Metrics

There are several aspects of verification and validation in which it is helpful to generate metrics. The first and most obvious one is anomaly metrics. Provided are two primary metrics charts: Open Anomalies, sorted by severity, and Anomaly History. These charts are shown below in Figures 23-3 and 23-4. These charts help the development group prioritize the analysis and correction of anomalies. The charts also provide visibility to upper level management about the project status.

The second aspect of test metrics are those involving test development. These metrics are used to monitor the test development process and to monitor overall test parameters for all projects. Monitoring the test development process ensures that the test development is proceeding according to schedule. An example is shown in Figure 23-5.

The metric for monitoring of overall test parameters, shown in the Figure 23-6 below, provides a unique view of all the important test criteria in

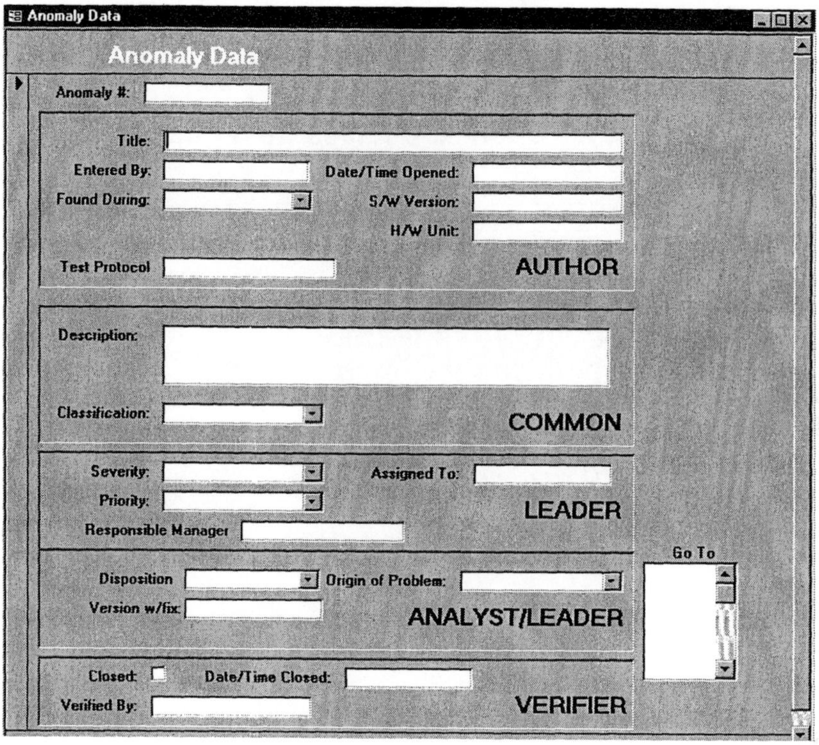

Figure 23-2   Anomaly form.

the test development process. This allows the test management to compare and contrast the projects, reflecting on what tools and techniques worked best.

23.1.7.1 Configuration Management

Just as it is important to maintain a configuration for product development code, it is equally important to practice configuration management on test protocols. Configuration of test materials includes:

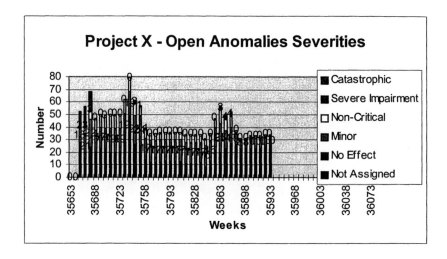

Figure 23-3   Metric chart showing open anomalies sorted by severity.

- script libraries
- test scripts
- manual protocol
- test results
- test plans and procedures
- test system design.

23.1.7.2 Protocol Templates

To make the development of tests more uniform and efficient, it is recommended to have templates for the test protocol. If test scripts are written, then a set of development guidelines is suggested. An example of a template for test file a header and manual protocol is shown in figure 23-7. The header contains fields that are important to the test development team, like file name, title, author, date last modified. Below the header is a list of requirements that the test will attempt to verify.

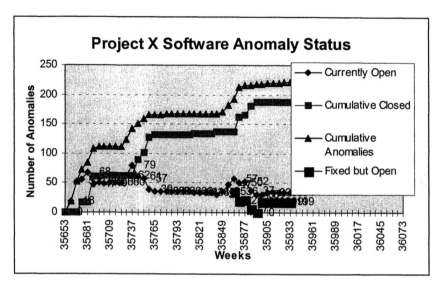

Figure 23-4   Anomaly history.

23.1.7.3 Test Execution

Section discusses approaches used when executing manual protocol and automated scripts.

23.1.7.4 Process Improvement

No test process is perfect. There are always ways to improve the test development process to do things more efficiently. Thus, some time should be set aside to review the current processes that are in place. If the test team is large enough, a process team may be created to address processes and process changes in the test group. Discussions should occur between test team members to determine those processes that worked well and those that did not.

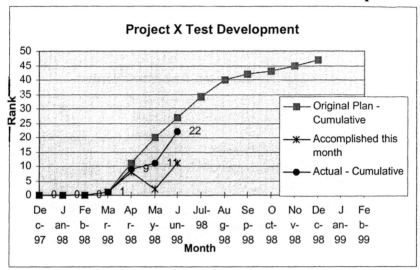

Figure 23-5   Monitoring the test development process.

23.2   Test Development

23.2.1   Requirements Analysis and Allocating Requirements

Today, it is assumed that a Software Requirements Specification (SRS) is written. The SRS describes the behavior and functionality of the software in the medical device. The SRS should get its inputs from the following sources:

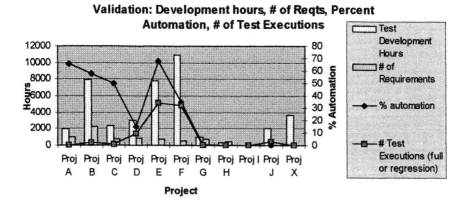

Figure 23-6   Monitoring overall test parameters.

- Derivation of the product specification
- Control procedures from the Risk and Hazard analyses
- Regulatory requirements, such as Safety Relevant Computing.

A large part of the verification and validation effort will concentrate on proving that these software requirements are fulfilled. Therefore, the requirements in the Software Requirements Specification must be enumerated to permit proper allocation to the different test phases and the specific tests.

The initial analysis of the Software Requirements Specification involves determining where best to test a particular requirement. Where a requirement gets tested is often based on the capabilities of the test fixture used in Validation. Usually, most requirements can be tested at the Validation level. The balance of the requirements then gets tested during Integration or Unit testing. In general, a requirement that has external stimulus (to the Central Processing Unit (CPU)) and ability to monitor externally are done at the Validation level. Exceptions to this are conditions that might require very specific timing, and that timing is calculated internally to the CPU.

Filename:	
Revision Number:	
Revision Date:	
Purpose:	
Code Reuse:	
Origination Date:	
Method Design:	
Script Design:	
Company:	
Company Address1:	
Company Address2:	
Copyright:	
Change Log		
Version 1		
User:	Date:	Time:
Updated In :		
Changes:		
Version 2		
User:	Date:	Time:
Updated In :		
Changes:		
Requirements		
Methodology		
Setup:		
Overview of the Task:		
Specific Test Steps:		
Equipment Used:		
Manufacturer:	Model Number:	Serial Number:

Figure 23-7   Test file template.

Requirements that are tested during Integration or Unit testing are typically ones that cannot be tested sufficiently during Validation testing. A good example of a requirement tested during Integration or Unit testing is testing a "software watchdog error" requirement. In this case, the software is monitoring itself, and there is no external means to cause the fault.

The second step of the requirements analysis phase is to determine how best to group the requirements into tests. One approach to doing this that is relatively straightforward is to create tests based on sections in the Software Requirements Specification. Typically, a section in an SRS will almost fully describe a feature. By following the Software Requirements Specification format, the tests then get developed by feature, which is a logical approach. Of course, there are going to be requirements in the Software Requirements Specification where this approach will not apply. In this case, further analysis will need to be done to assess if additional tests should be created, or if one of these "special" requirements can be allocated into those tests which follow the Software Requirements Specification.

As mentioned at the beginning of this section, control procedures from the risk and hazard analysis should be written into the Software Requirements Specification. If this is done, then those risk/hazard requirements will simply be analyzed and allocated to tests just like all other requirements.

A final aspect of requirements allocation to test is storing the allocation matrix. It is simple enough to keep the matrix in a spreadsheet or an electronic document. However, it can also be stored in a database. The advantage of storing it in a database is that a user can track test development, and can also generate numerous reports.

23.2.2   Test Fixture

Whether a test fixture will need to be built will depend on several factors:

- The nature of the medical device
- The equipment needed to adequately validate the medical device

- Development schedule
- The commitment of the company to developing automated testing.

The subsections below will give an overview of an approach to build a test system.

23.2.2.1 Determination of Need - Specifying Test Fixture Features

Assuming that a test fixture is needed, the next step is determining exactly what is needed. It may be that all is required is some lab equipment like an oscilloscope or a multi-meter. But if the testing will include automated testing, then further analysis must be done. A test system for performing automated software testing involves being able to simulate the inputs to the CPU, and also monitor the outputs. The test system should be able to perform many tasks, and that implies some sort of programmability.

Inputs into the CPU come in many varieties. There can be keyboard, keypad, mouse, serial, knob turns, Ethernet, analog, and digital inputs. In addition, some of these inputs may have variability to them, such as waveform input. Thus, designing a test system may involve writing sophisticated simulation to provide adequate input to the target.

A way to limit the amount of inputs and simulation required is to consider an interface that allows the real external signals pass directly through to the CPU. The test system would then control whether the signal coming into the CPU is real simulated.

Output types from the CPU can also be numerous. They can include analog, digital, serial, Ethernet, printer, and graphical outputs.

Whatever inputs are simulated and whatever outputs are monitored should be written into a test system specification. The test system specification should be written to a level that allows an engineer to design it.

23.2.2.2 Designing a Test Fixture

From the test system requirements, a test design can be developed. The design should account for instumenting the Unit-Under-Test (UUT) as well as provide an environment for test development. During the design phase, some experiments may need to be run to determine whether some technologies are feasible for use.

The test system design should be documented and put under configuration management.

23.2.2.3 Building the Test Fixture

After the test system design is complete, the fixture can be built.

23.2.2.4 Validating the Test Fixture

Per the FDA's regulations, any device used in a company's quality system must be validated. A test fixture clearly falls under this definition. Thus, it is necessary to validate the test fixture. The test fixture is validated before it is put into service. It is later re-validated at regularly scheduled intervals or when the test fixture has changed.

The validation of the must cover the intended use of the test system. The FDA guidelines state that the "quality system" must have written requirements. Test protocol is written to cover the test fixture requirements. Usually, a well written user's manual can serve the purpose of a requirements document. The test developer then writes protocol to cover the functionality described in the user's manual.

23.2.3 Testing Phases and Approaches

23.2.3.1 Unit Testing

Unit testing is the testing performed on a smallest amount of code. What comprises a "unit" is often the subject of lengthy discussion and debate.

However a unit is defined, the intent of unit testing is to ensure that the lowest level software modules get tested.

There are several approaches to doing unit test, such as Branch Path Analysis or Module Interface Testing. In Branch Path Analysis, the developer uses a development tool to step through each path within a unit. In Module interface testing, the developer tests the unit from a "black box" perspective. Thus, the unit only gets tested by varying the inputs into the software unit.

The type of unit testing required depends on many factors. In medical devices, the detailed Branch Path Analysis testing is usually done against software units that are considered to be critical to the safety of the patient or the user. Other lesser critical software units can justifiably be tested using the less thorough Module Interface testing.

23.2.3.2 Integration Testing

Integration testing has several definitions. The first definition covers the integration two or more software units together. A broader definition of Integration testing covers the integration of physical subsystems (each having their own embedded software) to ensure that they work together.

Either type of integration testing brings separately developed entities together to ensure they work together. The type of testing usually performed at these levels involves writing protocols to exercise the interface.

23.2.3.3 Validation Testing

Validation testing is the process of proving the product meets the product specification. It can also mean going the extra step and trying to make sure that the product does not do what it is not supposed to do. Thus, several approaches to testing are employed to exercise the software product. These approaches are discussed below.

23.2.3.3.1 Requirements Based Testing

Requirements based testing is the primary approach used to validate software. Essentially, the requirements from the Software Requirements Specification are analyzed and allocated to specific tests. Different approaches to testing, such as threshold testing or boundary testing, are used to develop these tests. The test steps are the sequential actions which must be taken to prove the requirement has been met.

23.2.3.3.2 Threshold Testing

Threshold testing is the process of proving that an event will occur when a specified parameter exceeds a certain value. A good example of this is in a medical device is an alarm, such as a low battery alarm. If the device is running on a battery, and the voltage level in the battery falls below a threshold level, then an alarm is enunciated. In these types of tests, a tolerance band is placed around the threshold level. The tolerance is determined by the requirements in the Software Requirements Specification and may also be influenced by the accuracy of the test system. The test is then designed to vary the battery voltage to cross through the threshold and montior that the alarm is tripped within the tolerance band.

Once the alarm has been tripped, the next part of the threshold test is to vary the parameter, in this case the battery voltage, in the reverse direction to ensure that the alarm no longer enunciates.

23.2.3.3.3 Boundary Testing

Boundary testing is the exercise of testing a parameter at the its limits and to try to exceed those limits. A good example of this might be a measured value of O_2, which is defined as not to exceed 110%. (An O_2 reading can exceed 100% if the O_2 sensor is out of calibration or calibrated incorrectly). The test would then be designed to prove that 110% O_2 could be displayed. Additionally, the test would then see how the device would react if the measured O_2 value exceeded 110%.

23.2.3.3.4 Stress Testing

Stress testing is the process of subjecting the unit under test to a bombardment of random inputs, oftentimes keypad presses or knob turns, to try to cause a software failure. This can be done manually, or done with an automated test system.

Manual stress testing and automated stress testing each have their own advantages. The advantage of doing manual stress testing is that the tester can test a certain aspect of the device and observe anomalous behavior in other areas of the device. The advantage of automated stress testing is that the test system can provide inputs into the device much faster than a human tester.

23.2.3.3.5 Volume Testing

Volume testing is the process of exercising the unit under test for an extended period of time. In our medical applications, we have found that running a volume test for a 72-hour period can uncover problems not found elsewhere.

Volume testing is almost always done with an automated test system. Volume testing doesn't necessarily use random fast slam bang key presses like stress testing. Volume testing uses a logical approach to testing all the paths in a software program. Once the device is in a certain state, probabilistic algorithms like Probability Density Function (PDF) are used to determine the next state.

23.2.3.3.6 Scenario Testing

Scenario testing is the act of writing a test that emulates the actual use of the software from the user perspective. For example, in anesthesia machines, a test may be written to cover a clinical situation. Scenario testing is helpful because it can uncover problems in the system or can surface flaws in the overall use of the product.

23.2.3.3.7 System Testing

System testing is the testing that occurs to validate the entire medical device, not just the software that is embedded in the device. Depending on how a test station is instrumented for software testing, there can be significant overlap between software and system testing. For example, software embedded in a ventilator usually requires other mechanical/electrical subsystems in order to function. It is difficult to write sophisticated simulations to trick the ventilator software into thinking that all of the other subsystems of the ventilator are present. Therefore, a software test system may resemble a complete system. It is up to the responsible parties to ensure that the degree of overlap is made known. More importantly, it is vital that everything gets tested at some point in the product development.

23.3   Test Execution and Reporting

23.3.1   Test Plan

For software validation, a test plan is written prior to executing a test pass. The test plan format follow the format defined in ANSI/IEEE Std 1012-1986. The key aspect to the plan is the description of the software change, and the tests that will be run to prove those software changes are implemented correctly. The test plan is written anytime a full validation or a regression test is run.

23.3.2   Test Configuration Form

Since it is very important to be able to repeat a test, it is therefore necessary to document the configuration of the equipment used to run a test against. This documentation is written on to a Test Configuration Form. The contents of one of these forms can vary. However, the primary fields are date, item, item serial number, and a place for the test engineer to sign their name. The Test Configuration Form becomes part of the test documentation suite.

23.3.3   Executing Manual Protocol

Executing manual protocol for a formal test involves printing out the test procedures and going through the steps in the procedures. Because these printouts are a part of the official documentation, the test engineer must sign and date the documents. If the tester finds problems during the test, he/she will document the issue on the test procedures.

It is important that the hand written notes on the paper procedures be addressed. The notes on the procedures could be problems found or procedure deviations. All of these markings need to have closure. This closure is formally documented in the Procedures Response document. The Procedures Response document is covered later in this chapter.

23.3.4   Executing Automated Protocol

Typically, executing automated protocol amounts to setting up a batch job to submit a series of tests to be run. A test engineer fills out a test configuration form to have a piece of paper to start off the test. The batch job is then run overnight and the results are analyzed the following day.

Experience has shown that occasionally a test in the batch may fail. This has usually been attributable to either timing issues or the target device feature changed but the test had not. When this happens, it is usually a practical matter to simply correct the test script and rerun it. However, in instances where correcting the test script would consume a large amount of time, it sometimes is more efficient to run that test manually to complete the test pass.

23.3.5   Test Results

Once test results get generated, they must be analyzed. The results from the automated tests are reviewed by running searches for key words that indicates if the test had problems. Additional analysis is performed by reviewing samples of the automated test results. This ensures that the tests executed as expected. Other analysis may also need to occur. An example is when a large amount of data is generated during the test, after which data reduction and analysis must be performed to assess correctness.

Test results need to be managed along with the other test documentation. The results from the manual test procedures need to be included with the other paper documentation and stored in the formalized location. The electronic results files also need to be put under configuration control. This is done with a configuration management tool or a process of backing up the files to controlled media.

23.3.6   Test Reports

23.3.6.1 Software Validation Test Report

The key items in this report is a summary of what was tested, how it was tested, any problems that were encountered, and a recommendation for release.

23.3.6.2 Requirements to Test Cross Reference

This document covers how the requirements were allocated to tests.

23.3.6.3 Procedures Response Document

As mentioned earlier, all hand written marks on the manual test procedures must be reviewed and provided a closure. The results of this closure are documented in the Procedures Response document. Typically, each mark up in a test procedure is a software problem, a procedure error, a procedure deviation, or a comment.

References

Food and Drug Administration, 21 CFR Part 820. Washington, DC: Department of Health, 1997.

Institute of Electrical and Electronic Engineers. IEEE Standard 730 – IEEE Standard for Quality Assurance Plans. New York: Institute of Electrical and Electronic Engineers, 1989.

Institute of Electrical and Electronic Engineers. IEEE Standard 829 – IEEE Recommended Practice for Software Requirements Specifications. New York: Institute of Electrical and Electronic Engineers, 1998.

Institute of Electrical and Electronic Engineers. IEEE Standard 830 – IEEE Standard for Quality Assurance Plans. New York: Institute of Electrical and Electronic Engineers, 1989.

Institute of Electrical and Electronic Engineers. IEEE Standard 1012 – IEEE Standard for Software Verification and Validation. New York: Institute of Electrical and Electronic Engineers, 1986.

Institute of Electrical and Electronic Engineers. IEEE Standard 1016 – IEEE Recommended Practice for Software Design Descriptions. New York: Institute of Electrical and Electronic Engineers, 1986.

Institute of Electrical and Electronic Engineers. IEEE Standard 1059 – IEEE Guide for Software Verification and Validation Plans. New York: Institute of Electrical and Electronic Engineers, 1993.

Chapter 24

Software Verification and Validation

Sherman Eagles – Medtronic, Inc.
Minneapolis, Minnesota

Software development consists of a series of activities that each transform a definition of the software into a less abstract definition. Each activity in the software development process transforms the definition of the software that it receives into a work product that is used by the next activity. The purpose of verification is to ensure that the output of the activity is a correct transformation of its input. As defined by the FDA's Quality System Regulation, verification is "confirmation by examination and provision of objective evidence that specified requirements have been fulfilled."

Since verification assures that the output conforms to the input, it may not detect errors in the input. A mistake in initial user requirements or an undetected mistake in an early software development activity may be carried through to the final product even though verification is accurately performed on later activities. To address this possibility, validation is used to supplement the verification activities. Validation is the process used to determine whether the final, as-built software fulfills its specific intended use for its intended users, in its intended environment on its intended platforms. The FDA definition is "establishing by objective evidence that device specifications conform with user needs and intended use(s)." Validation cannot be successful without prior verification of the software development activities.

24.1   Planning Software Verification and Validation

Verification and validation comprise a large part of the activities of software development for safety-critical medical device systems. Planning for them is as important as planning for the software design activities.

Software system verification and validation are associated with user requirements. Planning for these activities should be done as early as possible in development, as these plans may affect the design decisions that are made.

Regardless of the software development process model used, there are verification activities associated with the fundamental technical development process activities. These activities are used to verify the work products produced by each technical software development process. Additional validation activities are used to show that the system meets the user's needs. The relationship between the technical software development activities and the verification and validation activities is often represented as a V as shown in Figure 24-1 below.

The expected size and scope of the work product that is to be verified must be considered in planning the verification activity. Planning for verification also depends upon the criticality of the software product. The criticality is determined by the potential of an undetected software error to cause death or personal injury and is established by the system hazard analysis.

A verification plan identifies the software development activities and work products subject to verification, the required verification tasks for each software development activity and work product, and related resources, responsibilities, and schedule. The verification activities and tasks are selected based upon the scope, size and criticality analysis. Criteria for beginning verification are documented in the plan, as are criteria for completing the verification activity.

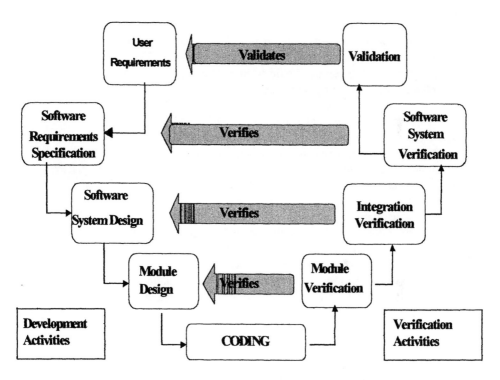

Figure 24-1   Relationship of software development and
verification and validation activities.

The degree of independence of the verification is documented in the verification plan. The degree of independence may range from the developer doing the verification, to a different developer in the same organization doing the verification, to a person in a different organization doing the verification. The different organization may have varying degrees of separation from the development organization. In the case where the verification is performed by an organization that is financially, technically and managerially independent of the development organization, it is called an Independent Verification Process. The degree of independence should be higher for software with higher potential impact on user or patient safety.

Verification strategies, techniques and tools are selected and documented in the verification plan. The means of documenting verification results and reporting errors are included in the plan. In some cases verification planning is integrated with software development project planning or quality assurance planning.

A validation plan also needs to be developed and documented. Similar to the verification plan, the validation plan must identify the items subject to validation, the validation tasks to be performed and the resources, responsibilities and schedule for validation. It should identify the degree of independence of the validation organization. The validation plan should also include a description of the modes of the software system operation and the environment in which it will be validated.

Technical strategies for validation, the pass/fail criteria, techniques, and tools are also documented in the verification plan. The means of documenting and reporting validation results are included in the plan.

24.2   Static Verification Techniques

Verification techniques can be divided into three basis types, static analysis, modeling, and dynamic testing. Static techniques are those that analyze the work product without operating it. Some static analysis techniques are manual, such as walkthroughs, reviews, inspections and software fault tree analysis. Others have been automated, such as control flow analysis and range checking. For some languages, static verification techniques have been built into compilers. There are also tools available that do static code analysis and generate complexity metrics.'

An important characteristic of static verification techniques is that they can be used to determine how the software will perform under all conditions. This contrasts with dynamic verification, which can only describe how the software performs for the actual tests that have been executed.

When static techniques are used for verification, the work product being verified must be complete and free from any known defects. Documentation of errors found and how they were addressed should be retained as evidence that the verification activity was performed.

24.2.1 Technical Reviews

There is a great deal of variation in how technical reviews are performed. When performed as a verification activity, the purpose of a technical review is to identify errors.

The basic process for a technical review is that the producer of the work product releases it to a group of peers who review it for defects. These reviewers check the product for errors, and return comments to the producer.

A frequent variation is to have a meeting after the reviewers finish their review to document the issues that were found and establish as a group if the issue is really a problem. The meeting also allows the reviewers to take responsibility as a group for the quality of the review.

24.2.2 Walkthroughs

A walkthrough is a peer review conducted as a meeting. The goal is to discover and document problems. The material is presented by the author, by "walking through" the product describing how it functions. The walkthrough approach formalizes the task of explaining the work to colleagues. The product is evaluated by the reviewers, who raise questions or issues of concern. The walkthrough provides an opportunity for an in-depth examination and expression of opinion by reviewers who qualify as experts. The emphasis is on identifying errors, resolving them is left until after the meeting.

A successful walkthrough depends upon a positive, non-threatening atmosphere. To ensure such an atmosphere exists, several guidelines are recommended:

- All work produced by a team should have a walkthrough. No team member should be exempt from having a walkthrough on their work.
- Emphasis should be placed on identifying defects.
- Walkthrough meetings should be limited to one or two hours.
- Managers should not be included in a walkthrough.
- Performance in a walkthrough should not be considered in an employee's evaluation.

24.2.3 Inspections

Inspections are similar to walkthroughs, but are more rigorous and formal. Inspections have been found to be very effective at finding defects. Inspections are performed by teams of usually three to seven people. Besides the author, there is an inspection leader and a recorder. Inspection is a peer activity, managers should not participate. The purpose of an inspection is to detect and remove defects. When done well, inspections have found up to 70% of the defects present in a software product.

Inspections use a set of documents to check the work product for errors. First there are source documents. These are the inputs to the activity that produced the product being inspected. For example if code is being inspected, the source document would be the design for that code. Other documents include standards and procedures that tell how the activity is to be performed, and checklists which are developed from frequent types of defects.

The basic steps in an inspection are:

- Planning - participants are chosen, materials gathered, the product checked for readiness for inspection, and meetings scheduled.

- Overview or kickoff meeting - the product is presented, materials distributed, roles assigned and participants generally made aware of what is expected of them.
- Individual preparation - the participants inspect the product using the rules, checklists and source materials to identify potential defects.
- Inspection meeting - the product is stepped through and the potential defects identified during the individual preparation are documented, along with any additional issues identified during the meeting.
- Rework - the author revises the product to address the defects found during the inspection.
- Follow-up - the inspection leader or other members of the inspection team follow-up to verify the defect resolution. When the rework is completed satisfactorily, the inspection is complete.

An important difference between inspections and walkthroughs is the collecting of metrics on inspections. Inspections collect data on the inspection itself, such as number of inspectors, number of hours checking the product, and number of hours of rework correcting the defects. They also collect data on the defects found in a product, such as the defect location, defect class and severity of the defect. By analyzing the data collected during inspections, the quality of the software can be controlled, as well as the quality of the inspection process.

24.2.4 Software Fault Tree Analysis

While most verification techniques try to prove that the software works correctly, and contains no errors, software fault tree analysis tries to prove that the software is not unsafe. The software fault tree analysis focuses on hazards instead of errors. It starts from the system hazard analysis, when the system hazard analysis shows that a certain software behavior can lead to a hazardous condition. Starting with the assumption of the hazardous output condition from the software, software fault tree analysis works backward through all possible paths that could produce the hazardous output. The hope is to find a logical contradiction in each path that demonstrates that the output cannot occur. If a path is found that can be followed back to an input, the software is not safe, and the design must be changed.

Software fault tree analysis does not determine whether the software is producing correct results, only whether or not specific unsafe results can be produced. In fact, unsafe results could be produced while the software is functioning correctly if the software's specifications are not correct. Thus, software fault tree analysis is one verification technique that can detect incorrect requirements if they result in an unsafe output. It is also a technique that can prove whether a design constraint in the form of "the software shall *not*" is implemented correctly. It is impossible to prove something the software shall not do by testing. It is only possible to show it by using logical contradiction, which software fault tree analysis does.

Software fault tree analysis generally takes the form of a structured walkthrough of the code, but working backward from the hazardous output rather than forward from the inputs. Only the part of the code that takes part in the safety critical functions will need to be reviewed. Software fault tree analysis forces software developers to view the code for what it does not do, instead of what it does. Software developers find this very useful in detecting errors, including some that are not related to the actual hazardous condition.

24.2.5   Formal Verification

When requirements have been specified with a formal mathematical technique that allows the system to be described unambiguously, it is theoretically possible to do proofs of correctness for the design and implementation of a system. In practice, this activity requires high cost and is very time consuming. This makes it impractical for all but the highest level of critical software. Sometimes, instead of doing a formal proof of correctness, a formal specification can be rigorously verified by establishing that the formal proof could be performed, but not actually performing it.

Another method that is used to verify formal specifications, is to prove that a system has some specific properties. This method does not prove correctness of the entire system, but only of selected requirements that are considered important. To prove specific properties, the system specification is described using propositional logic. Then particular properties, such as safety constraints, are also specified using propositional logic. The particular properties can then be proved correct with respect to the formal description of the system specifications.

24.3   Modeling Techniques

Modeling is used to investigate and analyze system characteristics before the system is implemented. This analysis allows verification of certain constraints sooner than could be determined with dynamic testing of the completed system. It is important to verify that these constraints can be met before implementation, since changing the system design after implementation is very costly.

Modeling is also used to analyze systems that are too complex to analyze either with static analysis or dynamic testing. An example is concurrent systems that have more than one point of control.

There are many different modeling techniques and tools that have been developed to analyze them. The three examples described here are used to address important system characteristics.

24.3.1   Rate Monotonic Analysis

Rate monotonic analysis is a technique for modeling real-time resource management. It is a model for prioritizing real-time scheduling of resources. This technique provides a method for assigning priorities to processes and a formula for determining whether a set of periodic processes will meet all of their deadlines. Using rate monotonic analysis allows early verification that all timing constraints on a system can be met with the proposed design.

24.3.2   Finite State Machines

A system can be represented as a finite number of states and the inputs required to move between the states. The operation of a state machine can be completely described by a state transition diagram. State transition diagrams can be analyzed for completeness, consistency and whether it is possible to get from one state to another. A problem with state machines is that very large numbers of states may be necessary to describe a complex system. This explosion of states can be handled by the use of hierarchical decomposition to provide higher level concepts.

24.3.3   Petri Nets

Petri nets address the limitations of finite state machines in specifying concurrent processes. Concurrent processes can have some unique errors that cannot be identified with methods that describe sequential processes. These errors, which can be identified with a Petri net model include:

- Two or more concurrent processes gaining simultaneous access to a shared resource
- Two concurrent processes failing to synchronize their communication
- All concurrent processes within a system waiting for other concurrent processes in the same system to complete some action so they can proceed (deadlock)
- One or more concurrent processes waiting for a resource that will not be available in an acceptable time (starvation).

24.4   Dynamic Testing Techniques

Dynamic testing executes the software and observes the results of the execution. There are two purposes for dynamic testing; one is as a way to verify the requirements of the software, and two is to find errors. To verify the requirements, tests are developed from the stated specifications to show that given expected inputs, the expected outputs are produced. Testing to find errors generally focuses on constraints that are not documented in the specifications. That is, testing to find errors looks at what the software is not supposed to do. Since what the software does not do is impossible to test completely, the tests that are most likely to find errors should be run first. This requires using a variety of techniques and strategies that will reveal the errors. A strategy is just a systematic method of creating test cases. Some strategies can be used for all types of testing and some are just useful for one type.

24.4.1   Types of Testing

Because there are different types of errors, different types of testing are performed to try to uncover them. Some types of testing are very efficient at detecting a particular type of defect, but not too good at detecting other types. Using a combination of several types of testing is the best way to find most of the errors in the software. It is often better to add an additional type of testing rather than to spend more time doing any particular type.

24.4.1.1 Functional Tests

Functional tests are those where an input is supplied and the behavior of the software is compared to the expected results. This type of testing is also called "black box" testing or "behavioral" testing because the tester does not need to understand how the software works in order to develop test cases, just what it is supposed to do. These tests focus on the requirement specifications of the system. They attempt to find incorrect or missing functions, interface errors, errors in data structures or database access, and initialization and termination errors. Functional testing generally begins by creating a model of the requirement specifications and then developing test cases from the model. Some strategies that are used for functional testing include the following.

24.4.1.1.1 Behavioral Control-Flow Testing

This strategy models the requirement specifications as a behavioral control-flow graph. The graph contains nodes, which represent a sequence of steps that are all executed together, and links, which indicates the next node that directly follows the current one. A node may have several links to following nodes, depending on the logic of the specifications. Once the model is complete, paths are chosen starting from the entry node and continuing from node to node until the exit node is reached. Then input values are chosen that will cause the path to be executed. Full coverage is obtained by selecting tests that include all of the links.

24.4.1.1.2 Data-flow Testing

Data-flow diagrams model the transformation of data as it is processed by the software. A data-flow diagram is a graph with links representing data and nodes representing functions that process the data. The data-flow diagram is created from the specifications. There will be one input data-flow for each input and one output data-flow for each output. To create test cases, start with an output data-flow and work backward through all the connected nodes to the input data-flows.

24.4.1.1.3 Transaction-flow Testing

A transaction-flow graph adds the notion of a transaction, a unit of work, that travels between the processing nodes of a system. A transaction has a type and a state, and there may be many transactions in the system at any time. A system may also have multiple types of transactions. Transactions may be created or eliminated in the system. Links in a transaction-flow graph are similar to a control-flow graph, they indicate that the transaction is processed by the second node directly after the first. Each link can have a designated number of transactions associated with it at any one time. A link that has more than one transaction represents a queue. Transaction-flow graphs combine aspects of control-flow and data-flow. Test cases are created by starting with an output transaction and working backward to the origin nodes for that output. Because transactions can be created and deleted, additional testing must address synchronization. If the transaction-flows have queues, additional tests must be devised to test the queue discipline.

24.4.1.1.4 Finite-state Testing

Testing using a finite state model is applicable to many kinds of software. As in other functional testing, it begins by creating a model of the system's behavior from the specifications. The operation of a system can be modeled as a set of states and the transitions between them. A state is the sum of the status of all of the entities in the system at a particular time. A transition occurs when an input event causes a change to the status of at least one of the entities. For functional testing, a state change must be visible from outside the system.

A finite-state model of a system can be represented as a state transition table, a matrix where there is one row for every state and one column for every input. The cell at the intersection of a row and a column contains the value for the state resulting from the transition that was initiated by the input in that column occurring while the system was in the state shown by the row. In many cases of course, the state will not change when the input occurs.

A test for a finite state model always begins at the initial state. Inputs are selected to reach some target state and then to return to the initial state. This is called a tour. Tests are added until all transitions have been tested.

24.4.1.1.5 Domain Testing

Domains are a subset of the input space of the software that are processed differently than other input values (other domains). Domains are defined by domain boundaries, usually boundary inequalities. Domain testing tries to determine if the software is correctly classifying the inputs into the correct domains. Equivalence partitioning and boundary value testing are strategies that fall under domain testing. Input values are classified and processed according to their domain. For a specification to be unambiguous, it must define a set of domains that covers the entire input space. To not be contradictory, the domains in the set must not overlap each other.

Domain testing defines two types of input values, ON point, which is a point on or as close to the boundary as possible while satisfying the conditions of the boundary, and OFF point, which is a point as near as possible to the boundary without satisfying the conditions associated with the boundary. For one dimension domains (only one input variable), domain testing requires testing one ON point and one OFF point per domain boundary (this is called 1X1 strategy). For two or more input variables, testing one ON point and one OFF point for each variable domain boundary that are as close together as possible is generally sufficient. This level of testing can miss some errors, so for safety critical requirements, more test cases are needed. If n is the number of dimensions and b is the number of boundaries, then $b(n+2)$ is the minimum number of test cases needed to verify the correctness of the domain.

24.4.1.2 Structure Tests

Structure tests are intended to exercise the internal logic or structure of
the software. This type of testing is also called "white box" or "glass box"
testing because the tester must be able to study how the code is written in order
to determine the inputs that will result in a particular path being taken through
the code. This type of testing can identify unreachable code, unintentional
infinite loops, inaccessible paths that should be accessible, exception handling
errors and some concurrency issues. Some strategies used for structure testing
include the following.

24.4.1.2.1 Basis Path Testing

Basis path testing utilizes the logical control-flow graph of the
software. The logical control-graph is constructed from the code, with each
node representing one or more procedural statements and each link
representing the flow of control between nodes. A path is the combination of
nodes and links that are traversed between the starting node and the ending
node. An independent path is one that has at least one link that is not included
in other paths. The basis set is the minimum set of independent paths that
cover all the nodes and links in the software. If all the paths in the basis set,
called the basis paths, are executed, then all of the code will have been executed
at least once, and all branch conditions will have been tested. Test cases are
created by working backward from the end node to the start node, determining
what input values are necessary to cause the path to be executed.

24.4.1.2.2 Loop Testing

Special testing can be done for loops to identify initialization errors,
indexing or incrementing errors and errors at the loop limits. For simple loops,
a small set of tests can be identified that fully test the looping. If n is the
maximum number of allowable passes through the loop, these tests will provide
adequate testing.

- Testing nominal values, one, two and m passes through
  the loop (m < n)

- Testing around the maximum, n-1, n and n+1 passes through the loop
- Testing skipping the loop entirely.

If loops are nested, each loop is tested as a simple loop, the number of tests required would increase geometrically with the number of nested loops. An approach that reduces the number of tests while still providing good testing of the loops is to test each loop as if it were a single loop while holding the other loops at a single value. Start with the innermost loop while holding the outer loops to their minimum loop counter values. Then work outward, executing all the simple loop tests for the next loop, holding outer loops to their minimum loop counter values and inner loops to typical values. Continue working outward until all loops have been tested.

24.4.1.3 Random Tests

In the previous types of testing, test cases are determined by what the tester is trying to investigate. In functional testing, it is requirement specifications, in structural testing it is the code organization. In random testing, the test cases are chosen at random from all possible inputs. By randomly sampling over the input space, some cases will be selected that would not be chosen by a tester trying to investigate a particular aspect of the software. Also, random sampling allows a statistical measure of quality to be determined. If the quality measured by random testing is not sufficient, additional effort may be necessary to re-engineer the system.

24.4.1.4 Performance Tests

Performance tests show the amount of a resource used by the software to perform some known function. Performance testing often is done to show the time used either as execution time or as wall clock time. Performance tests may also demonstrate the use of some other limited resource or device. In addition to time, another other common resource that can be tested during performance testing is memory.

Performance testing needs to be done both for normal operating conditions and also for heavy load conditions. Since some resource problems appear because the software does not release a resource after use, performance tests also need to be run after the system has been operating for some time, not just after initialization. The models created for functional testing can be used to help identify other resources that should be checked by performance testing.

Performance testing is often run repeatedly to ensure that performance doesn't degrade as additional capabilities are added to the system or as problems are corrected. It also is used to identify areas which can be improved, for instance identifying which modules are most used or which use the most time.

24.4.1.5 Stress Tests

Stress tests are intended to break the software. Stress tests overload the inputs, or otherwise execute unexpected conditions to try to reveal timing problems or interface problems. Stress tests are particularly good at finding incomplete or inaccurate specifications. Some examples of stress testing:

- In the overload case, inputs are delivered to the system faster than normal, or the inputs are larger than expected. The tests are aimed at overflowing buffers or queues in the program.
- Other overload tests use very large amounts of data to see if the program has the capacity for processing the data in a timely manner, so that other inputs are not lost.
- Stress tests also look for race conditions. In a race condition, two events can happen. In the normal case, one event will always occur first. Stress testing tries to look for incorrect behavior of the software if the second event occurs first.
- Stress tests may look at how the software behaves when there are hardware errors such as transmission errors caused by electrical interference.
- No response to messages is another typical stress test
- If the processor the software is executing on unexpectedly fails, will the software be able to restart when it is restored?
- Stress tests may also exercise the system in a degraded mode; for instance, with some device not available. The condition may result from a hardware condition, such as a printer out of

paper condition, or from overloading the device, as in trying to write to a full disk drive.

24.5   Verification Activities

Verification activities use the techniques described above to verify work products during the software development process.

24.5.1   Module Verification

Module verification is done to verify one module, the smallest unit of the software design. Module verification may include static verification techniques such as reviews or inspections and dynamic module testing. Module testing is always structural or white box testing. It focuses on logic and computational correctness.

Modules are often tested separately from other parts of the software. This allows the maximum control of the variables that might affect the operation of the module. This reduces the chance of other parts of the software masking error symptoms in the module being tested. The negative side of testing modules independently is that test software must be created to control the software being tested (a driver), and to mimic the behavior of software that is subordinate to the module being tested (stubs). This test software is required to ensure that all the interfaces to the module being tested are correct.

In addition to the interfaces to the module, basis path and loop testing are performed as part of module test. Also, algorithms should be tested for computational errors. Some of the more common computational errors include:

- Incorrect initialization
- Incorrect arithmetic precedence
- Mixed mode operation
- Precision errors.

Error handling and exception handling also are tested as part of module test. Error handling paths must terminate cleanly and give sufficient clear information to assist in determining the cause of the error.

In some cases, the overhead of driver and stub development is too high to reasonably test modules independently. In this case, the module testing is delayed until the module is integrated into the system. This reduces the overhead, since not as much driver and stub software is required, but makes the isolation of problems more difficult.

24.5.2 Integration Verification

Once the individual modules have been verified, they must be combined into a system and tested to ensure interface compatibility and no adverse effect on each other. Also some acceptable results in module testing may turn out to be unacceptable when the modules are combined. An example of this is acceptable precision errors in modules that are magnified when the modules are integrated and result in unacceptable precision in the system. Integration verification attempts to uncover errors associated with the combining of verified modules into a program structure. It uses both structural and functional testing techniques. One effective method is to use functional data-flow testing with each module as a node and the interface between each module as the data-flow.

Integration verification can be performed from the top down, from the bottom up, or from the middle out, a strategy called sandwich testing. In all strategies of integration verification, it is preferable to do the integration incrementally, combining some modules and testing them, then adding additional modules and continuing testing. Incremental integration makes it easier to isolate and correct errors.

Top-down integration verification starts by verifying the top module in a program calling tree. This requires using stubs for any modules that the top module calls. These stub modules are then replaced, one by one, with the actual module and the integrated modules tested. Of course, stubs are needed for any modules called by the "real" module when it is included. This process is repeated for all the modules called by the top module. When all of them are integrated and tested, the stub modules they call are replaced one by one with real modules. This process is repeated until all modules have been integrated.

Bottom-up integration verification starts by verifying the modules that do not call any other modules. Once verification is completed on one of these modules, a module that calls it can be integrated with the verified module and the combination tested. This process is repeated adding higher level modules until reaching the top module.

Sandwich integration verification is a combination of the top-down and bottom-up approaches. In sandwich integration verification, the verification proceeds simultaneously from the top down and the bottom up.

24.5.3   System Verification

System verification occurs when the entire software system has been implemented and integrated. The purpose of system verification is to demonstrate that the completed software system satisfies its requirement specifications.

System verification uses functional testing to verify each of the functional specifications. At a minimum, tests must be executed that show that each specified requirement has been implemented. Techniques for coverage of logical sequences of specifications should be used based on the type of software system and the critical nature of the software. Any identified safety requirements must be tested during system verification testing.

In addition to testing functionality, system verification testing includes stress tests to determine if constraints on the system have been addressed properly and performance tests to verify performance specifications.

System verification often includes tests developed for unit and integration testing. Additional tests are added to reach the required level of coverage of the software requirement specifications and to stress the system looking for defects.

In complex systems, models such as finite state machines or Petri nets may be developed to verify complex sequences of inputs or behavior of concurrent components.

24.5.4   Change Verification

When a change is made to previously verified software, the changed code must be verified to evaluate the correctness of the change. The developer that makes the change must verify that the modification does indeed correct the defect. The developer also must ensure that the modified code works correctly in all other situations.

After the modified code is integrated into the system, the change must be tested to verify that it corrects the defect. In addition, the impact of the change on other modules must be analyzed and additional tests executed to ensure that the changes did not cause a new problem elsewhere. Both the logic models used for structural testing and the requirement specification models used for functional testing should be used to try to understand what impact the changes could have beyond their local code, and to identify what tests need to be run to determine if any new problems have been created.

Regression tests are run when the software changes to provide assurance that the changes did not cause defects in the software that has previously been shown to be working correctly. Regression tests are a subset of the tests that have been previously executed. They may include both structural and functional tests that have been executed during unit, integration or system testing. Regression tests usually exercise the normal behavior of the system, but sometimes include tests for abnormal situations, when those tests have been found to detect errors. Depending on the complexity of the software, the regression tests may take hours to days to complete.

24.6   Verifying Safety

Verification that the implementation of the software satisfies the requirement specification is not sufficient to verify the safety of the software. It is necessary to verify that the implementation of the software meets the safety constraints and safety-related functional requirements.

Software fault tree analysis is a static technique that is used for safety verification. To verify that a failure mode from a system hazard analysis cannot occur in the software, software fault tree analysis traces the failure mode into the software logic as implemented in the code, and determines whether a path exists that could lead to the failure mode. If the path ends in a logical contradiction, then the failure mode cannot occur and the safety is verified. If the path is traced back to inputs that can lead to the failure mode, then the hazard can results from the software as implemented, and the logic of the software must be changed.

Dynamic testing to verify safety includes testing for any safety functionality that has been added to the software specifically to control or eliminate hazardous behavior. The identification of safety-critical portions of the software allows those parts to have more rigorous verification, both using structural testing techniques, functional testing techniques and targeted stress testing.

Both static and dynamic verification techniques may not be sufficient to verify complex systems with concurrent processing that exhibits non-deterministic behavior. In these cases, it may be necessary to use a modeling technique such as petri nets to verify that the software cannot produce hazardous outputs.

24.7   Verification Measurement

As a product containing software nears release, and its safety has been assured, there are two questions that need to be answered:

1. Is the software verification complete enough?
2. Is the software reliable enough?

For verification that was performed by static analysis, completeness is determined by whether the analysis was performed and whether there is confidence in the quality of the analysis. Records of the analysis activities and their results provide assurance that the verification was complete. For verification performed by dynamic testing, the question of completeness is harder to answer. The measure that is most often used to determine testing completeness is test coverage.

Only if there is adequate test coverage, can the second question be asked. Because measuring reliability directly would require executing a very large number of tests, reliability is usually estimated from other measures that can be directly observed.

24.7.1   Test Coverage

Test coverage is the percentage of all possible items that are tested by the set of tests being measured. Test coverage can be measured for different types of testing. For structural testing, the coverage can be determined for:

- Statements - percentage of code statements that are executed
- Branches - percentage of all possible branch paths that are executed
- Compound conditions - percentage of conditions in compound conditional branches that are executed
- Entire path - percentage of all possible paths through the code that are executed.

Statement coverage is the least rigorous, since it is possible to execute all code statements without executing both sides of every branch. Branch coverage is more rigorous, but it may be difficult to reach all branches. Compound condition coverage expands upon branch to include testing all combinations that determine the branch. Complete coverage of entire paths is almost always infeasible due to the large number of possible paths through the code.

For functional testing, the coverage measurement depends upon the technique being used to model the requirement specifications. If a behavioral control-flow model is used, the coverage measurement is the percentage of the links that are covered by the tests.

If a data-flow model is used, coverage can be measured for:

- Inputs and outputs - the percentage of outputs and the inputs required to produce them that are covered by the tests
- Nodes - the percentage of functions that process the data that are covered by the tests

- Links - percentage of the uses of the data that are covered by the tests.

For a transaction-flow model, coverage can be measured for:

- Origin/exit or birth/death - percentage of transaction entry or creation and exit or death that are covered by the tests

- Nodes - percentage of the processes that change the state of a transaction that are covered by the tests

- Links - percentage of the possible orders of processing the transactions that are covered by the tests

- Slices - percentage of the origin/exit paths or birth/death paths.

For a finite state model, coverage is measured as the percentage of the transitions that are covered by the tests.

The coverage that is considered sufficient for completely testing a software system is dependent on the type of system and the criticality of the software. The coverage that will be measured and the value that is required for testing to be considered complete should be documented in the verification plan before the testing is started.

24.7.2 Reliability Modeling

Software reliability is the probability of failure-free operation of the software for a specified time in a specified environment. Software reliability modeling tries to estimate the number of failures that will occur in a specified time period, or the time between failures. Software reliability models use defect discovery data during development to estimate reliability of the released software. There are two broad categories of software reliability models: models that use defect data from the entire development process and those that use data from the formal verification testing activities after the implementation of the software is complete.

24.7.2.1 Rayleigh Model

Study of empirical defect discovery data over the entire development life cycle has resulted in a model of defect discovery that can be described by the Rayleigh density curve. This model plots the number of defects found during a specified amount of time against the elapsed time since the beginning of the software development. If good defect data is available from the software development activities, a Rayleigh curve can be constructed and the number of remaining undiscovered defects at a particular time estimated.

24.7.2.2 Reliability Growth Models

These models of software reliability use data from post-development system verification testing. They use either the time between failure as the dependent variable and predict the mean time to the next failure, or they use the number of failures in a specified time period as the dependent variable and predict the number of remaining defects. A large number of reliability growth models have been proposed. These models have a theoretical basis, but often have restrictive assumptions. If the assumptions, test process used and data collected for a model seem to fit the software being tested, then the model may be useful to estimate the reliability of the software at release.

24.8   Software Validation

Software validation is almost always done as part of system validation. Validation tests the software from the user's perspective. It tries to exercise the software in the manner that the user would exercise it. Validation testing uses an environment as similar to the user's environment as possible. The purpose of validation testing is not to find defects. That is done in verification. The purpose of validation testing is to ensure that the software will meet the user's requirements. Any manuals that will be provided to the user are carefully tested for completeness and correctness. If there are complex user interfaces, or user interfaces where an error by the user could affect safety, usability testing may be performed to demonstrate that the user understands the interface.

24.9   Conclusion

Software verification and validation constitute a substantial part of creating a software product. They must be planned as carefully as the software design. The planning should determine what types of verification activities should be performed. Static analysis activities are most useful while the development is occurring. Dynamic structure testing is generally done by the development organization, as it requires knowledge of how the software was implemented. Dynamic functional testing has several strategies for how to verify that the requirement specification is completely and correctly implemented.

Dynamic testing may be done at the individual unit level, as the units are being integrated into a system, and after all the software implementation has been completed and integrated into a complete system. The verification plan should identify what types of testing and the entry and completion criteria.

Verifying safety requires that the safety-related requirements and safety constraints that were identified as necessary to mitigate hazard conditions are verified. Requirements for verifying safety-critical portions of the software should be included in the verification plan. Dynamic verification techniques are not enough to verify safety constraints. A static analysis of the code using a technique such as software fault tree analysis is necessary.

After the software verification demonstrates that the software correctly implements the requirement specification, the software must be validated to demonstrate that it meets the user requirements. Software verification and validation assures a safe product that will execute properly and provide the user with the desired functionality.

References

Beizer, Boris, *Black-Box Testing*. New York: John Wiley & Sons, Inc., 1995.

Cho, Chin-Kuei, *Quality Programming*. New York: John Wiley & Sons, Inc., 1987.

Deutsch, Michael S., *Software Verification and Validation.* Englewood Cliffs, New Jersey: Prentice-Hall, 1982.

Deutsch, Michael S. and Ronald R. Willis, *Software Quality Engineering - A Total Technical and Management Approach.* Englewood Cliffs, New Jersey: Prentice-Hall, 1988.

Dyer, Michael, *The Cleanroom Approach to Quality Software Development.* New York: John Wiley & Sons, Inc., 1992.

Fairley, Richard E., *Software Engineering Concepts.* New York: McGraw-Hill Book Company, 1985.

Freedman, Daniel P. and Gerald M. Weinberg, *Handbook of Walkthroughs, Inspections, and Technical Reviews - Third Edition.* New York: Dorset House Publishing, 1990.

Gilb, Tom and Dorothy Graham, *Software Inspection.* Wokingham, England: Addison-Wesley, 1993.

Jones, Capers, *Applied Software Measurement.* New York: McGraw-Hill, Inc., 1991.

Kan, Stephen H., *Metrics and Models in Software Quality Engineering.* Reading, Massachusetts: Addison Wesley Longman, Inc., 1995.

Kaner, Cem and Jack Falk and Hung Quoc Nguyen, *Testing Computer Software - Second Edition.* New York: Van Nostrand Reinhold, 1993.
Leveson, Nancy G., *Safeware.* Reading, Massachusetts: Addison-Wesley Publishing Company, 1995.

McConnell, Steve., *Rapid Development.* Redmond, Washington: Microsoft Press, 1996.

Musa, John D. and Anthony Iannino and Kazuhira Okumoto, *Software Reliability.* New York: McGraw-Hill Book Company, 1987.

Myers, Glenford J., *The Art of Software Testing.* New York: John Wiley and Sons, 1979.

Pressman, R., *Software Engineering*. New York: McGraw-Hill Book Company, 1987.

Putnam, Lawrence H. and Ware Myers, *Measures for Excellence*. Englewood Cliffs, New Jersey: P T R Prentice-Hall, Inc., 1992.

Storey, Neil, *Safety-Critical Computer Systems*. Harlow, England: Addison Wesley Longman, 1996.

Strauss, Susan H. and Robert G. Ebenau, *Software Inspection Process*. McGraw-Hill, Inc., 1994.

Chapter 25

Reliability Evaluation

Richard C. Fries, PE, CRE – Datex-Ohmeda, Inc.
Madison, Wisconsin

The heart of the product development process is the verification and validation phase. During this time, testing indicates how well the product has been designed. The parts count reliability prediction had indicated whether the design would meet the reliability goal. It indicated what parts of the circuit had the potential for high failure rate. Design and tolerance analysis had indicated whether the correct component was being used and if it had been specified properly. None of these exercises had indicated how well the components would work together, once the device became operational. To obtain this information, the device must be tested both in its intended application environment as well as in the worst case condition.

25.1   Standard Tests

Standard tests are conducted at room temperature, with no acceleration of any parameters. Standard tests are varied, dependent upon their purpose, and include:

- Cycle testing

- Typical use testing

- 10 x 10 testing.

25.1.1   Cycle Testing

Cycle testing is usually conducted on individual components, such as switches, phone jacks or cable. Testing consists of placing the component in alternating states, such as ON and OFF for a switch or IN and OUT for a phone plug, while monitoring the operation in each state. One cycle consists of one pass through each state.

Cycle testing could also consist of passing through the state of operation and non-operation of a component or device. Thus a power supply could be power-cycled, with a cycle consisting of going from zero power to maximum power and back to zero. For devices, a cycle could consist of eight hours ON and 16 hours OFF.

25.1.2   Typical Use Testing

Typical use testing consists of operation of a device as it will be operated in its typical environment. This testing is usually incorporated when conducting a reliability demonstration or for calculating a long term MTBF value.

The test unit is tested electrically and mechanically prior to testing and certain parameters are checked at periodic times, such as 2, 4, 8, 24, 48, 72, 96 and 128 hours after beginning the test and weekly thereafter. These recordings aid in determining drift or degradation in certain parameters.

25.1.3   10 x 10 Testing

Ten samples of a component or device are subjected to a test where recordings of a particular parameter are taken at 10 different time periods. A chart is created with the ten units listed in the left column and the ten recordings listed across the top (Figure 25-1). Mean and standard deviation values are calculated for each of the ten recordings and ten units.

By reading the horizontal rows of data, the repeatability of the results can be determined. By analyzing the vertical columns, the variability among the units can be measured.

25.2   Environmental Testing

Environmental testing is conducted on a device to assure its ability to withstand the environmental stresses associated with its shipping and operational life. Testing is usually conducted on the first devices built in the Manufacturing area under Manufacturing processes. Environmental testing includes:

- Operating temperature
- Storage temperature
- Thermal shock
- Humidity
- Mechanical shock
- Mechanical vibration
- Impact
- Electrostatic discharge
- Electromagnetic compatibility.

Prior to each test, the device is tested electrically and mechanically to assure it is functioning according to specification. At the conclusion of each environmental test, the device is again tested electrically and mechanically to determine if the environmental test has affected the specified operation. Any observed failures will be fixed and a decision to rerun the test made, based on the type of change made and the inherent risk.

Unit	1	2	3	4	5	6	7	8	9	10	Mean	S.D.
1	350	380	400	360	340	370	330	340	360	340	357	20
2	200	130	190	200	130	150	250	230	240	160	188	41
3	270	250	270	240	300	230	330	330	300	350	287	39
4	270	140	160	170	160	140	430	130	130	130	186	90
5	230	180	170	150	260	240	210	230	240	210	212	33
6	280	180	70	390	300	210	400	440	370	230	287	110
7	180	210	270	190	210	170	170	270	190	200	206	34
8	190	220	180	190	170	190	200	120	170	130	176	29
9	200	180	160	180	200	120	90	170	140	170	161	33
10	230	190	260	180	290	170	280	220	260	170	225	43
Mean	240	206	213	225	236	199	269	248	240	209		
S.D.	50	66	85	78	67	67	100	95	80	74		

Figure 25-1   10 X 10 test matrix. (From Fries, 1991.)

25.2.1   Operating Temperature Testing

The operating temperature test assures the device will operate according to specification at the extremes of the typical operating temperature range. The test also analyzes the internal temperatures of the device to assure none exceed the temperature limits of any components.

After the functional checkout, the device has thermocouples placed inside at locations that are predicted to be the hottest. The device is turned

ON and placed in a temperature chamber for 4 hours at each of the operating temperature limits as specified in the Product Specification or at 0° Centigrade and +55° Centigrade if no limits are specified. Between temperatures, the device should be removed from the chamber until it has reached the appropriate temperature. Thermocouple readings are recorded continuously on a chart recorder throughout the test. Where a chart recorder is not available, the readings should be taken every 30 minutes.

The unit is functionally tested after the temperature exposure. The thermocouple readings are evaluated with regard to the upper extreme of component temperatures.

25.2.2   Storage Temperature Testing

The storage temperature test assures the device will withstand the stresses of the shipping and storage environment. After the functional checkout, the device is turned OFF and placed in a temperature chamber for eight hours at each of the storage temperature limits as specified in the Product Specification or at -40° Centigrade and +65° Centigrade if no limits are specified. Between temperatures, the device should be removed from the chamber, allowed to come to room temperature and then functionally tested. The unit is functionally tested after the temperature exposure.

25.2.3   Thermal Shock Testing

The thermal shock test assures the device will withstand the stresses of alternate exposure to hot and cold temperatures. After the functional checkout, the device is turned OFF and placed in a thermal shock chamber with one chamber set at -20° Centigrade, the second chamber set at +55° Centigrade and the transition time between chambers set at less than five minutes. The minimum time spent at each temperature is one hour. The device should be cycled through a minimum of five cycles of temperature extremes. The unit is functionally tested after the temperature exposure.

25.2.4   Humidity Testing

The humidity test assures the device will withstand the stresses of exposure to a humid environment. After the functional checkout, the device is turned off and placed in a humidity chamber with the environment set to 40° Centigrade and 95% relative humidity. The chamber and accessories are so constructed that condensate will not drip on the device. The chamber shall also be transvented to the atmosphere to prevent the buildup of total pressure. The device is typically exposed for 3 days, but may be exposed a maximum of 21 days.

The unit is allowed to dry following exposure. It is then opened and examined for moisture damage. All observations are documented with photographs if possible. The unit is then functionally tested.

25.2.5   Mechanical Shock Testing

The mechanical shock test assures the device is able to withstand stresses of handling, shipping and everyday use. Devices may be tested in the packaged or unpackaged state. Devices may also be tested on a shock table where parameters are set such as in Table 25-1, to meet the anticipated environment. When using the shock table, several types of waveforms are ordinarily available, depending on the type of impact expected. The haversine waveform simulates impact with a rebound while a sawtooth waveform simulates impact with no rebound. The device may also be dropped the designated distance, from Table 25-1, on to a hard surface by measuring the height above the floor and dropping the device. One disadvantage of the drop test is the inability to adjust the shock pulse to match the surface and the rebound. With either type of test, the device is usually shocked a maximum of three times in each axis. Following testing, the device is examined for any internal damage. The device is also functionally tested.

25.2.6   Mechanical Vibration Testing

The mechanical vibration test assures the device is able to withstand the vibration stresses of handling, shipping and everyday use, especially where the device is mobile.

Weight	Greatest Dimensions (inches)	Effective Free Fall Height (inches)	Acceleration (Gs)	Pulse Duration (msec)
<100	<36	48	500	2
	>36	30	400	2
100-200	<36	30	400	2
	>36	24	350	2
200-1000	<36	24	350	2
	36 – 60	36	430	2
	>60	24	350	2
>1000		18	300	2

Table 25-1   Mechanical Shock Parameters   (From Fries, 1991.)

Devices may be tested in the packaged or unpackaged state. In the unpackaged state, holes are cut in the device for observation of the internal hardware with a strobe light or for insertion of accelerometers for measuring vibration. Accelerometers are attached to the desired components and their frequencies and amplitudes recorded on an X-Y plotter.

Vibrate the device via a frequency sweep or via random vibration. The random vibration more closely simulates the actual field environment,

although resonant frequencies and the frequencies of component damage are more easily obtained with the frequency sweep.

When using the frequency sweep, the sweep should be in accordance with the suggested parameters listed in Table 25-2. Subject the device to three sweeps in one axis at a sweep rate of 0.5 octave/minute. An octave is defined as the interval of two frequencies having a basic ratio of 2.During the sweeps, the acceleration, as listed in Table 25-2, is the maximum acceleration observed at any point on the device.

Resonant frequencies are determined either through accelerometer readings or through observation of the internal hardware. Resonances are defined as board or component movement of a minimum of twice the difference between the device and table acceleration. Severe resonance is usually accompanied by a steady drone from the resonating component. Once resonant frequencies are determined, a dwell at each resonant frequency for 15 minutes follows the frequency sweeps.

The above tests are repeated until all three orthogonal axes have been tested. The unit is examined for physical damage and functionally tested after each axis is completed.

25.2.7   Impact Testing

Impact testing assures the ability of the device to withstand the collision stresses of shipping and everyday use for mobile devices. The test simulates large, mobile devices bumping into walls or door frames while being moved.

The test is conducted by rolling a device down an inclined ramp and allowing it to slam into a solid wall or by attaching the device to an adjustable piston drive, which is set to slam the device into a solid wall with a predetermined force. The unit is functionally tested following impact.

25.2.8   Electrostatic Discharge

Electrostatic discharge testing assures the ability of the device to withstand short duration voltage transients caused by static electricity, capacitive or inductive effects and load switching. For software-controlled devices, a differentiation between hard failures, that is, failures that cause the device to become inoperable and not rebootable and soft failures, that is, failures that cause the device to become inoperable but rebootable, must be made and the acceptability of each defined, according to risk.

The device is placed on a grounded metal plane. Static discharges are delivered to the four quadrants of the plane and to appropriate places on the device, such as front panel, back panel, keyboard, etc., from a static generator or a current injector. One-shot static charges should be delivered

Locale	Format	Frequency Sweep	Acceleration
Domestic	Unpackaged	5-200-5 Hz	1.5 G
International	Unpackaged	5-300-5 Hz	2.0 G
Domestic	Packaged	5-300-5 Hz	1.5 G
International	Packaged	5-500-5 Hz	2.0 G

Table 25-2   Mechanical Vibration Parameters m (From Fries, 1991.)

directly to the device and to the air surrounding the device. Where the device is connected to accessory equipment via cables, such as analog or RS-252 cables, static discharges should be delivered in the area of the cable connections, on both pieces of equipment. All discharges should be one-shot and should begin at 2,000 volts and increase in 2,000 volt increments until the maximum of 20,000 volts is reached.   The unit is functionally tested following application of ESD.

25.2.9   Electromagnetic Compatibility

Electromagnetic Compatibility (EMC) testing is conducted to determine the maximum levels of electromagnetic emissions the device is allowed to produce and to determine the minimum levels electromagnetic interference to which the device must not be susceptible. Medical devices, especially those used in the Operating Room environment, must not interfere with the operation of other devices or have its operation interfered with by other devices through electromagnetic radiations.

It is particularly important to conduct EMC testing on products containing:

- digital circuitry, especially microprocessor-based devices
- circuits containing clock or crystal oscillators

- devices where data information is transmitted via a telemetric or radio frequency link
- monitors, used in close proximity to other devices or where they cause feedback to other devices.

Tests should be conducted in a testing laboratory containing an anechoic chamber or shielded chamber of sufficient size to adequately contain the test. The device is configured and operated in a manner that approximates its use in a medical facility. When necessary, a dummy load and/or signal simulator may be employed to duplicate actual equipment operation.

It is known that most Bovie units, especially older ones, produce radiation that is worse than that called out in any standard. Thus, as a practical approach to EMC, many companies use a Bovie unit in the vicinity of the test device to check its susceptibility. In the laboratory environment, the test device can be used in the presence of other devices to test its radiation. Subject all devices to conducted and radiated emissions and to conducted and radiated susceptibility testing. Monitor the functionality of the unit throughout the test.

A new concern in the EMC area is the use of cellular phones in the hospital. It is felt these phones put out emissions to which other devices are susceptible. The FDA is currently researching this area. It is expected that this area will be included in required EMC testing.

25.3   Accelerated Testing

The length of time available to conduct a test determines whether the test is performed in a standard or an accelerated mode. In the standard mode, tests are run at ambient temperature and typical usage parameters. The test time is the actual time of operation. In the accelerated mode, test time is reduced by varying parameters, such as temperature, voltage or frequency of cycling, above their normal levels, or performing a test, such as sudden death testing.

Accelerated testing is a shortening of the length of the test time by varying the parameters of the test. Testing can be accelerated in several ways:

- Increase the sample size
- Increase the test severity
- Use sudden death testing.

25.3.1   Increasing Sample Size

Reliability tests are accelerated by increasing the sample size, provided the life distribution does not show a wearout characteristic during the anticipated life. Test time is inversely proportional to the sample size, so that increasing the sample size reduces the test time.

Large sample size reliability test conducted to provide a high total operating time should be supported by some long duration tests if there is a reason to suspect that failure modes exist which have high times to failure.

25.3.2   Increasing Test Severity

Increasing test severity is a logical approach to reducing test time when large sample sizes cannot be used. The severity of tests may be increased by increasing the stresses acting on the test unit. These stresses can be grouped into two categories:

- Operational, such temperature and humidity
- Application, such as voltage, current, self-generated heat or self-generated mechanical stresses.

Increasing the temperature severity is the usual method of accelerating testing.

It is important, in accelerated testing, to assure that unrealistic failure modes are not introduced by the higher stresses. It is also possible that interactions may occur between separate stresses, so that the combined weakening effect is greater that would be expected from a single additive process.

When conducting accelerated testing, an essential calculation is acceleration factor, that is the parameter that indicates how much acceleration was conducted. To calculate the acceleration factor, the following equation is used:

Acceleration Factor = exp(- (EA/K)(1/TA-1/TU))

where

EA = Energy of Activation (0.5 eV)
K = Boltzman's Constant (0.0000863 eV/degree Kelvin)
TU = Use temperature in degrees Kelvin
TA = Accelerate temperature in degrees Kelvin

25.3.3   Example 25-1

Ten power supplies are tested to failure at 150° Centigrade. The units are expected to be used at 85° Centigrade. What is the minimum life (time of the first failure) at 85° Centigrade? What is the MTBF at 85° Centigrade?

The failure rates in hours are listed as:

2750	3100	3400	3800	4100
4400	4700	5100	5700	6400

Calculation of Acceleration Factor:

AE = 0.5
K = 0.0000863
TU = 85 + 273 = 358° Kelvin
TA = 150 = 273 = 423° Kelvin

Acceleration Factor = exp(- (EA/K)(1/TA-1/TU))

$$= e(- (0.5/0.0000863)(1/423 - 1/358))$$

$$= 12$$

Calculation of Minimum Life at 85° Centigrade:

Minimum life = (acceleration factor) x (failure at 85°)

$$= (12) \times (2750)$$

$$= 33,000 \text{ hours}$$

Calculation of MTBF at 150° Centigrade:

MTBF = sum of the times of operation/number of errors

$$= 2750+3100+3400+3800+4100+4400+4700+5100+5700+6400/10$$

$$= 43450/10$$

$$= 4345 \text{ hours}$$

Calculation of MTBF at 85° Centigrade:

MTBF = acceleration factor (MTBF at 150°)

$$= 12 (4345)$$

$$= 52,140 \text{ hours}$$

25.3.4   Example 25-2

Integrated circuits are to be burned-in to eliminate infant mortality failures. We want the burn-in to be equivalent to 1000 hours of operation at ambient temperature (24° Centigrade). How long do we run the units at 50° Centigrade? How long do we run the units at 100° Centigrade?

Calculation at 50° Centigrade:

$$\text{Acceleration factor} = \exp(-(EA/K)(1/TA-1/TU))$$

$$= e(-(0.5/0.0000863)(1/323 - 1/297))$$

$$= 4.8$$

Length of run time = run time at 24° /acceleration factor

$$= 1000/4.8$$

$$= 208 \text{ hours}$$

Calculation at 100° Centigrade:

$$\text{Acceleration factor} = e(-(0.5/0.0000863)(1/297 - 1/373))$$

$$= 53$$

Length of time = 1000/53

$$= 19 \text{ hours}$$

25.4   Sudden Death Testing

Sudden Death testing is a form of accelerated testing where the total test sample is arbitrarily divided into several, equally-numbered groups. All units in each group are started simultaneously. When the first unit in a group fails, the whole group is considered to have failed. Testing is stopped on the remaining unfailed units in the group as soon as the first one fails. The entire test is terminated when the first unit in the last group fails. To understand the analysis for this test, it is necessary to understand the concept of Weibull testing and plotting.

25.4.1   Weibull Testing and Plotting

Weibull paper is a logarithmic probability plotting paper constructed
with the y-axis representing the cumulative probability of failure and the x-axis
representing a time value, in hours or cycles. Data points are established from
failure data, with the failure times arranged in increasing order or value of
occurrence. Corresponding median ranks are assigned from a percent rank
table, based on the sample size. An example will illustrate the point.

25.4.1.1 Example 25-3

Six power supplies were placed on life test. The six units failed at
100, 45, 170, 340, 530 and 240 hours respectively. To plot the data, first
arrange the failure times in increasing value, as listed below. Then
determine the median ranks by using the table in Appendix 2, with N =
sample size = 6. Going to the column headed by 50.0, read the six median
ranks as below:

Failure Order Number	Life in Hours	Median Rank (%)
1	45	10.910
2	100	26.445
3	170	42.141
4	240	57.859
5	340	73.555
6	530	89.090

Figure 25-2 shows the resultant plot. The resultant line can be used to
determine the MTBF and the percent that will fail at any given time. For
$\beta = 1$, the MTBF is found by drawing a line from the 63.2% point on the y-axis
to the resultant line. Then, dropping a line from this point to the x-axis gives
the MTBF value. The MTBF is 262 hours.

To find the percentage of units that will have failed at 400 hours, draw
a vertical line from the x-axis to the resultant line. Then draw a horizontal line
from that point to the y-axis. This is the failure percentage. In this case, 80%
of all units produced will fail by 400 hours.

25.4.1.2 Confidence Limits

The confidence limits for this example can be determined in a similar fashion. For example, if the 90% confidence level for the above test were desired, the 5% and 95% ranks would be obtained from the median rank table. Since a 90% confidence level means a 10% risk level, one-half the risk level is at each extreme.

Failure Order	Life Hours	Median Rank	5% Rank	95% Rank
1	45	10.910	0.851	39.304
2	100	26.445	6.285	58.180
3	170	42.141	15.316	72.866
4	240	57.859	27.134	84.684
5	340	73.555	41.820	93.715
6	500	89.090	60.696	99.149

The data is plotted in Figure 25-3. The confidence limits on the MTBF are obtained by reading the time values at the intersections of the 63.2% line with the 5% and 95% confidence bands. In this case, m_{l2} - 110 hours and m_{u2} = 560 hours.

25.4.1.3 The Shape of Weibull Plots

The type of plot obtained contains much valuable information on the test data. The shape parameter (β) value and the shape of the curve are very important.

On some Weibull papers, a perpendicular line is drawn from the plot to a point on the paper, called the estimation point. This perpendicular line passes through a scale that indicates a β value. On other papers, a line parallel to the plot is drawn through a scale to give the β value.

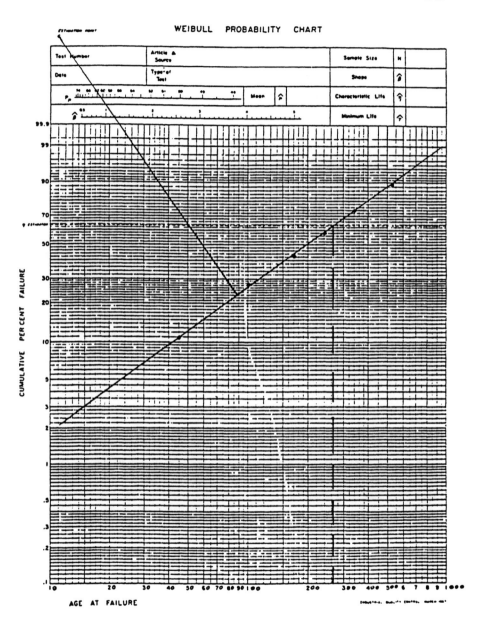

Figure 25-2   Weibull plot.   (From Fries, 1991.)

When β = 1, the failure rate is constant and the test units are in their useful life period. Where β < 1, the failure rate is decreasing with time (early life period). When β > 1, the failure rate increases with time (wearout period). In reality, the unit may be in its useful life period and indicate a β value slightly above or below 1.

Weibull plots may be of two types:

- Linear
- Curved.

Linear plots (Figure 25-4) indicate a single failure mode. The plot is used to determine the MTBF as well as the percentage of units that have failed at a particular time or number of cycles of operation. This is done by drawing a vertical line from the desired value on the x-axis to the plot and then determining the corresponding intersectional point on the y-axis.

Curved plots (Figure 25-5) are indicative of multiple failure modes. The curved plot can usually be separated into its component linear plots by fitting lines parallel to the curved portions. Once linear plots are obtained from the curved plot, information as noted in the paragraph above can be obtained.

25.5   The Sudden Death Test

Sudden Death testing consists of dividing the test sample into equal groups of samples. Each group is tested until the first failure occurs in the group. At that time, all members of the group are taken off the test. Once all groups have failed, each group is considered as one failure. The data is plotted on Weibull paper as above. This produces the sudden death line that represents the distribution of lines at the median rank for the first failure.

The median rank for the first failure for N = the number of samples in a group is determined. A horizontal line is drawn from this point on the y-axis and intersects a vertical line drawn from the sudden death line at the 50% level. A line parallel to the sudden death line is drawn at the intersection of these two lines. This is the population line that represents the distribution for all units in the test sample.

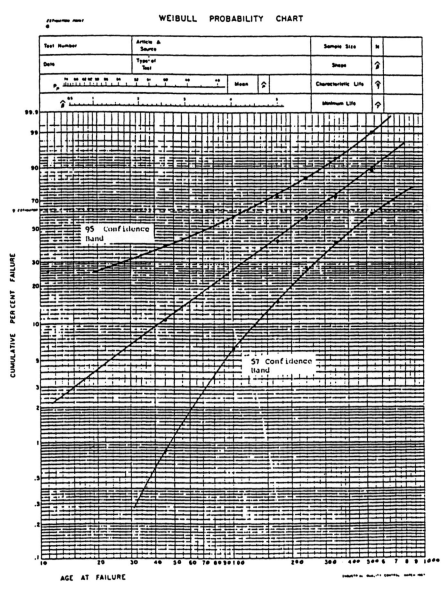

Figure 25-3 Weibull plot of confidence limits.
(From Fries, 1991.)

25.5.1   Sudden Death Example

Forty power supplies are available for testing. Randomly divide the power supplies into five groups of eight pumps each. All pumps are put on test in each group simultaneously. The testing proceeds until any pump in each group fails, at which time the testing of all pumps in that group stops.

For our example,

Group	Unit Number	Time of Failure
1	4	235 hours
2	8	315
3	3	120
4	6	85
5	2	350

To analyze the data, first arrange the failures in ascending hours to failure. The median ranks are determined from the median rank tables in Appendix 2, based on a sample size of $N = 5$, since there were only five failures.

Failure Order Number	Life in Hours	Median Rank (%)
1	85	12.95
2	120	31.38
3	235	50.00
4	315	68.62
5	350	87.06

The results are plotted on Weibull paper (Figure 25-6). The resulting line is called the sudden death line. It represents the cumulative distribution of the first failure in eight of the population of power supplies.

The median rank for the first failure in $N = 8$ is 8.30%, found by looking in the median rank table under $N = 8$ and Order Number = 1. Thus the

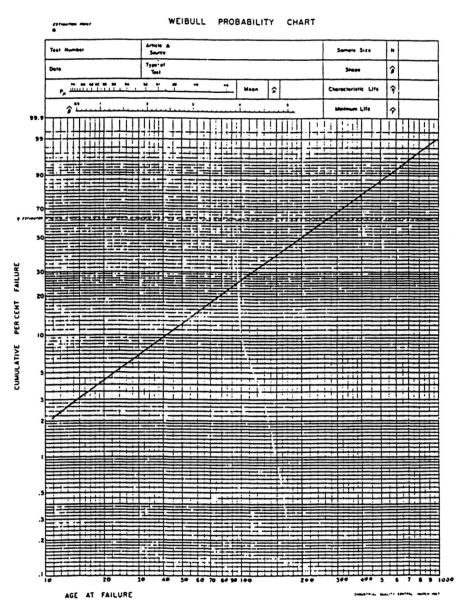

Figure 25-4   Weibull linear plot. (From Fries, 1991.)

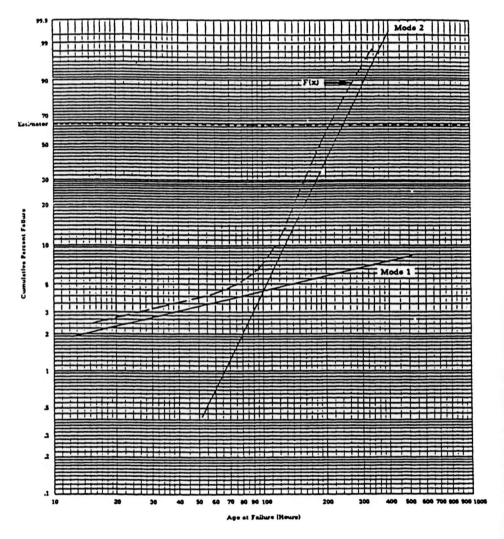

Figure 25-5   Weibull curved plot. (From Fries, 1991.)

sudden death line represents the distribution of the lines at which 8.3% of the samples are most likely to fail.

To find the population line, draw a vertical line through the intersection of the sudden death line and the horizontal line at the 50% level. Then draw a horizontal line from the 8.3% point on the y-axis until it meets this vertical line. This point is the 8.3% life point of the population. Next, draw a straight line through this point, parallel to the sudden death line, thus determining the population line (Figure 25-7). The MTBF of the population line can be determined by drawing a vertical line from the intersection of the population line and the 63.2% level and reading the corresponding life in hours. In this case, MTBF = 950 hours. Obtain the confidence limits on this result by choosing the confidence level, e.g., 90%, obtaining the corresponding ranks from the median rank table, e.g., N = 5, 5% rank and 95% rank, and plotting these to obtain the sudden death band lines. Then shift these bands vertically down by a distance equal to the vertical distance between the sudden death line and the population line. These new bands are the exact population confidence bands.

Failure Order	Life Hours	Median Rank (%)		5% Rank	95% Rank
1	85	12.95	1.02	45.07	
2	120	31.38	7.64	65.74	
3	235	50.00	18.93	81.07	
4	315	68.62	34.26	92.36	
5	350	87.06	54.93	98.98	

The bands are plotted in Figure 25-8.

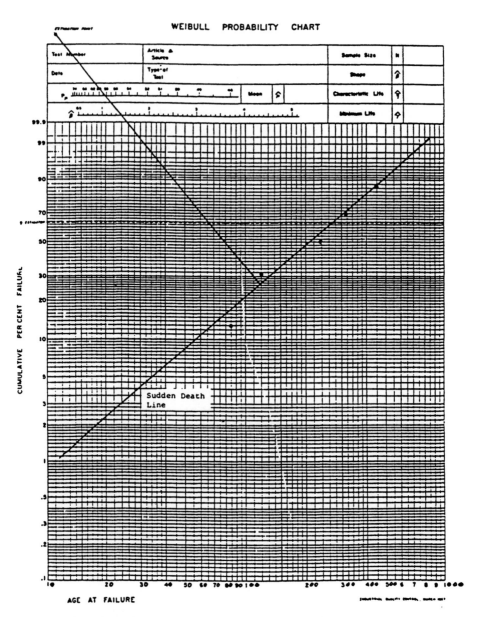

Figure 25-6   Sudden death line. (From Fries, 1991.)

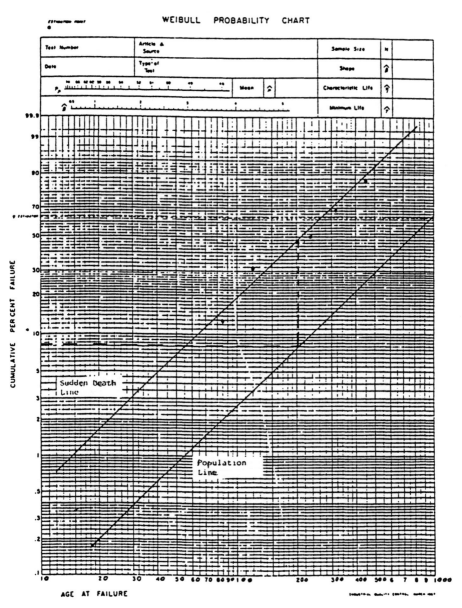

Figure 25-7   The population line. (From Fries, 1991.)

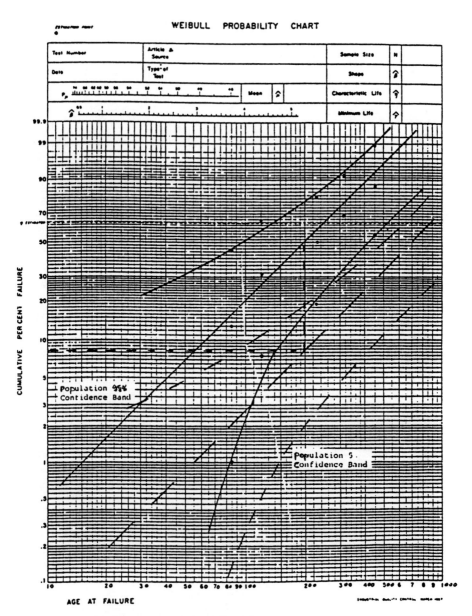

Figure 25-8   Confidence bands. (From Fries, 1991.)

References

Frankel, E. G., *Systems Reliability and Risk Analysis*. The Hague:
Martinus Nijhoff Publishers, 1984.

Fries, Richard C., *Reliability Assurance for Medical Devices, Equipment
and Software*. Buffalo Grove, IL: Interpharm Press, Inc., 1991.

Fries, Richard C., *Reliable Design of Medical Devices*. New York: Marcel
Dekker, Inc., 1997.

Ireson, W. Grant and Clyde F. Coombs Jr., *Handbook of Reliability
Engineering and Management*. New York: McGraw-Hill Book Company,
1988.

Jensen, F. and N. E. Peterson, *Burn-In*. New York: John Wiley and Sons,
1982.

Lloyd, D. K., and M. Lipow, *Reliability Management, Methods and
Management*. 2nd Edition. Milwaukee, WI: American Society for Quality
Control, 1984.

Logothetis, N. and H. P. Wynn, *Quality Through Design*. London, England:
Oxford University Press, 1990.

Mason, R. L., W. G. Hunter, and J. S. Hunter, *Statistical Design and
Analysis of Experiments*. New York: John Wiley & Sons, 1989.

MIL-STD-202, *Test Methods for Electronic and Electrical Component Parts*.
Washington, DC: Department of Defense, 1980.

MIL-STD-750, *Test Methods for Semiconductor Devices*. Washington, DC:
Department of Defense, 1983.

MIL-STD-781, *Reliability Design Qualification and Production Acceptance
Tests: Exponential Distribution*. Washington, DC: Department of Defense,
1977.

MIL-STD-883, *Test Methods and Procedures for Microelectronics.*
Washington, DC: Department of Defense, 1983.

Montgomery, D. C., *Design and Analysis of Experiments.* 2nd Edition. New
York: John Wiley & Sons, 1984.

O'Connor, Patrick D. T., *Practical Reliability Engineering.* 3rd Edition.
Chichester, England: John Wiley & Sons, 1991.

Reliability Analysis Center, *Nonelectronic Parts Reliability Data: 1995.*
Rome, NY: Reliability Analysis Center, 1994.

Ross, P. J., *Taguchi Techniques for Quality Engineering.* New York:
McGraw-Hill, 1988.

Taguchi, Genichi, *Introduction to Quality Engineering.* Unipub/Asian
Productivity Association, 1986.

Taguchi, Genichi, *Systems of Experimental Design.* Unipub/Asian
Productivity Association, 1978.

Chapter 26

Analysis of Test Results

Richard C. Fries, PE, CRE – Datex-Ohmeda, Inc.
Madison, Wisconsin

The heart of reliability is the analysis of data, from which desired reliability parameters can be calculated. These parameters are calculated from testing throughout the product development process. Early calculations are updated as the program progresses and the presence or lack of reliability improvement becomes apparent.

Reliability parameter calculation assumes the product is in the useful life period of the bathtub curve. During this period, the failure rate is constant and the exponential distribution is used for calculations. In standards and handbooks where failure rates and MTBF values are listed, the same assumption is made and the exponential distribution is used.

Calculations of some parameters, such as MTBF, are dependent upon the termination mode of the test. Time terminated tests, where tests are ended after a predetermined time period has elapsed, are calculated different than failure terminated tests, where tests are ended after a predetermined number of units have failed.

The calculations necessary to determine the following parameters will be reviewed:

- Failure rate
- MTBF
- Reliability
- Confidence limits.

In addition, _raphical analysis will be discussed and its application to dealing with reliability data.

26.1   Failure Rate

Failure rate is the number of failures per million hours of operation. For devices in their useful life period, the failure rate is the reciprocal of the MTBF.

$$MTBF = 1/\lambda \qquad\qquad 26.1$$

The failure rate is stated as failures per hour for this equation.

26.1.1   Example 26.1

An EEG machine has a MTBF of 4380 hours. What is the failure rate?

$\lambda = 1/MTBF$
  $= 1/4380$
  $= 0.000228$ failures per hour
  $= 228$ failures per million hours

26.1.2   Example 26.2

Ten power supplies are put on test, to be terminated after each has completed 1000 hours of operation. Two power supplies fail, one at 420 hours and the other at 665 hours. What is the failure rate of the power supplies?

Eight units completed 1000 hours.

$$\text{Total test time} = 8(1000) + 420 + 665$$
$$= 9085 \text{ hours}$$

λ = number of failures/total test time
   = 2/9085
   = 0.000220 failures per hour
   = 220 failures per million hours

26.2   Mean Time Between Failures

Mean Time Between Failures (MTBF) is the time at which 63 % of the operational devices in the field will have failed. MTBF is the reciprocal of the failure rate. It is also calculated from test data dependent upon the type of test run, e.g., time terminated or failure terminated, and upon whether the failed units were replaced or not. Five different methods of MTBF calculation are available:

- Time terminated, failed parts replaced
- Time terminated, no replacement
- Failure terminated, failed parts replaced
- Failure terminated, no replacement
- No failures observed during the test.

26.2.1   Time Terminated, Failed Parts Replaced

$$MTBF = N(td)/r \qquad\qquad 26.2$$

where

N = number of units tested
td = test duration
r = number of failures

26.2.1.1 Example 26.3

The performance of ten pressure monitors is monitored while operating for a period of 1200 hours. The test results are listed below. Every failed unit is replaced immediately. What is the MTBF?

Unit Number	Time of Failure (hours)
1	650
2	420
3	130 and 725
4	585
5	630 and 950
6	390
7	No Failure
8	880
9	No Failure
10	220 and 675

$N = 10$
$r = 11$
$td = 1200$ hours

$$MTBF = N(td)/r$$

$$= 10(1200)/11$$
$$= 1091 \text{ hours}$$

26.2.2   Time Terminated, No Replacement

$$\text{MTBF} = (\Sigma \; T_i) + (N-r)td/r \qquad\qquad 26.3$$

where

N = number of units tested
td = test duration
r = number of failures
T_i = individual failure times

Using the data in Example 26.3,

Unit Number	Time of Failure (hours)
1	650
2	420
3	130
4	585
5	630
6	390
7	No Failure
8	880
9	No Failure
10	220

$$\text{MTBF} = (\Sigma \; T_i) + (N - r)/td/r$$

$$= 650+420+130+585+630+390+880+220) + 2(1200)/8$$
$$= (3905 + 2400)/8$$
$$= 788 \text{ hours}$$

26.2.3   Failure Terminated, Failed Parts Replaced

$$\text{MTBF} = N(td)/r$$

where

N = Number of units tested
td = test duration
r = number of failures

26.2.3.1 Example 26.4

Six TENS units were placed on test until all units failed, the last occurring at 850 hours. The test results are listed below. Every failed unit, except the last one, is replaced immediately. What is the MTBF?

Unit Number	Time of Failure (hours)		
1	130	2	850
3	120 and 655		
4	440		
5	725		
6	580		

$$MTBF = N(td)/r$$
$$= 6(850)/7$$
$$= 729 \text{ hours}$$

26.2.4   Failure Terminated, No Replacement

$$MTBF = (\Sigma\ T_i) + (N-r)td/r$$

Using the data from Example 26.4

Unit Number	Time of Failure (hours)
1	130
2	850
3	120
4	440
5	725
6	580

$$\text{MTBF} = (\Sigma\ T_i\ ) + (\text{N-r})\text{td}/\text{r}$$
$$= (130+850+120+440+725+580) + 0(850)/6$$
$$= 3945 + 0/6$$
$$= 658\ \text{hours}$$

26.2.5 No Failures Observed

For the case where no failures are observed, an MTBF value cannot be calculated. A lower one-sided confidence limit must be calculated and the MTBF stated to be greater than that value.

$$\text{ml} = 2(\text{Ta})/X^2{}_{\alpha;2}$$

where

ml = lower one-sided confidence limit
Ta = total test time
$X^2{}_{\alpha;2}$ = the chi-square value from the table in Appendix
1, where α is the risk level and 2 is the degrees
of freedom

26.2.5.1 Example 26.5

Ten ventilators are tested for 1000 hours without failure. What is the MTBF at a 90% confidence level?

N = 10
td = 1000
r = 0
1 - % = 0.90
% = 0.10
Ta = N(td) = 10(1000) = 10000

$$ml = 2(Ta)/X^2_{\alpha;2}$$
$$= 2(10000)/X^2_{10;2}$$
$$= 20000/4.605$$
$$= 4343 \text{ hours}$$

We can then state that the MTBF > 4343 hours, with 90% confidence.

26.3   Reliability

Reliability has been defined as the probability that an item will perform a required function, under specified conditions, for a specified period of time, at a desired confidence level. Reliability may be calculated from either the failure rate or the MTBF. The resultant number is the percentage of units that will survive the specified time.

Reliability can vary between 0 (no reliability) and 1.0 (perfect reliability). The closer the value is to 1.0, the better the reliability will be. To calculate the parameter "reliability", two parameters are required:

- Either the failure rate or the MTBF
- The mission time or specified period of operation.

$$\text{Reliability} = \exp(-\lambda t)$$
$$= \exp(-t/\text{MTBF})$$

26.3.1   Example 26.6

Using the data in Example 26.2, calculate the reliability of the power supplies for an operating period of 3200 hours.

λ = failure rate = 220 failures per million hours
for the equation, λ must be in failures per hour
thus, 220/1000000 = 0.000220 failures per hour
t = 3200 hours

$$\text{Reliability} = \exp(-\ \lambda t)$$
$$= \exp -(0.000220)(3200)$$
$$= \exp -(0.704)$$
$$= 0.495$$

This states that after 3200 hours of operation, one half the power supplies in operation will not have failed.

26.3.2   Example 26.7

Using the time terminated, no replacement case, calculate the reliability of the pressure monitors for 500 hours of operation.

$$\text{Reliability} = \exp -(\ \lambda\ t)$$
$$= \exp -(t/\text{MTBF})$$
$$= \exp -(500/788)$$
$$= \exp -(0.635)$$
$$= 0.530$$

Thus, 53% of the pressure monitors will not fail during the 500 hours of operation.

26.4   Confidence Level

Confidence level is the probability that a given statement is correct. Thus, when a 90% confidence level is used, the probability that the findings are valid for the device population is 90%.

Confidence level is designated as:

$$\text{Confidence level} = 1 - \alpha$$

where

α = the risk level

26.4.1 Example 26.8

Test sample size is determined using a confidence level of 98%. What is the risk level?

$$\text{Confidence Level} = 1 - \alpha$$
$$\alpha = 1 - \text{confidence level}$$
$$= 1 - 0.98$$
$$= 0.02 \text{ or } 2\%$$

26.5 Confidence Limits

Confidence limits are defined as the extremes of a confidence interval within which the unknown has a designated probability of being included. If the identical test was repeated several times with different samples of a device, it is probable that the MTBF value calculated from each test would not be identical. However, the various values would fall within a range of values about the true MTBF value. The two values which mark the end points of the range are the lower and upper confidence limits. Confidence limits are calculated based on whether the test was time or failure terminated.

26.5.1 Time Terminated Confidence Limits

$$mL = 2(Ta)/X^2_{\alpha;2r+2}$$

where

mL = lower confidence limit
Ta = total test time
$X^2_{\alpha;2r+2}$ = Chi square value from Appendix 1 for α risk level
        and $2r+2$ degrees of freedom

$$mU = 2(Ta)/X^2_{1-\alpha/2;2r}$$

26.5.1.1 Example 26.9

Using the data from the time terminated, no replacement data from Example 26.3, at a 90% confidence limit:

Ta = 6305 hours
α = 1 - confidence level = 0.10
$\alpha/2$ = 0.05
r = 8
2r+2 = 18

$$mL = 2(6305)/X^2{}_{0.05;18}$$
$$= 12610/28.869$$
$$= 437 \text{ hours}$$

$$mU = 2(6305)/X^2{}_{0.95;16}$$
$$= 12610/7.962$$
$$= 1584 \text{ hours}$$

We can thus say:

$$437 < MTBF < 1584 \text{ hours}$$

or the true MTBF lies between 437 and 1584 hours.

26.5.2   Failure Terminated Confidence Limits

$$mL = 2(Ta)/X^2\alpha/2;2r$$

and

$$mU = 2(Ta)/X^2 1-\alpha/2;2r$$

Using the data from the failure terminated, no replacement data from Example 26.4 at a 95% confidence limit:

$Ta = 3945$ hours
$\alpha = 0.05$
$\alpha/2 = 0.025$
$1-\alpha/2 = 0.975$
$r = 6$
$2r = 12$

$mL = 2(3945)/X^2_{0.025;\ 12}$
$= 7890/23.337$
$= 338$ hours

$mU = 2(3945)/X^2_{0.975;12}$
$= 7890/4.404$
$= 1792$ hours

Thus

$$338 < MTBF < 1792$$

26.6   Minimum Life

The minimum life of a device is defined as the time of occurrence of the first failure.

26.7   Graphical Analysis

Graphical analysis is a way of looking at test data or field information. It can show failure trends, determine when a manufacturing learning curve is nearly complete, indicate the severity of field problems or determine the effect of a burn-in program.

Several type of graphical analysis are advantageous in reliability analysis:

- Pareto Analysis
- Graphical Plotting
- Weibull Analysis.

26.7.1   Pareto Analysis

Pareto analysis is a plot of individual failures versus the frequency of the failures. The individual failures are listed on the x-axis and the frequency of occurrence on the y-axis. The result is a histogram of problems and their severity. The problems are usually plotted with the most frequent on the left. Once the results are obtained, appropriate action can be taken. Figure 26-1 is an example of a pareto analysis based on the following data:

Problem	Frequency
Power Supply Problems	10
Leaks	8
Defective Parts	75
Cable Problems	3
Missing Parts	42
Shipping Damage	2

26.7.2   Graphical Plotting

When plotting data, time is usually listed on the x-axis and the parameter to be analyzed on the y-axis.

26.7.2.1 Example 26.10

Nerve stimulators were subjected to 72 hours of burn-in at ambient temperature prior to shipment to customers. Reports of early failures were grouped into 50 hours intervals and showed the following pattern:

Hourly Increment	Number of Failures
0 - 50	12
51 - 100	7
101 - 150	4
151 - 200	1
201 - 250	1

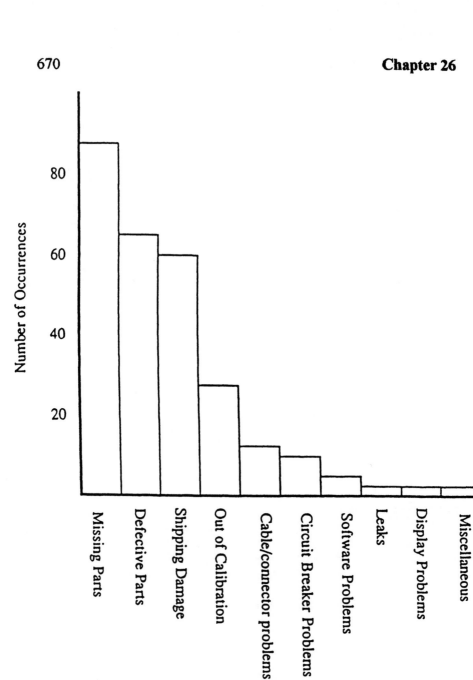

Figure 26-1   Pareto analysis.

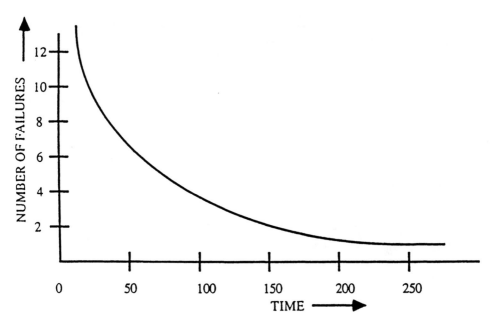

Figure 26-2   Plot of field data.

Figure 26-2 is a plot of the data. The data indicate the number of
failures begins to level off at approximately 200 hours. The burn-in was
changed to an accelerated burn-in, equal to 300 hours of operation.

26.7.3   Weibull Plotting

Weibull paper is a logarithmic probability plotting paper constructed
with the y-axis representing the cumulative probability of failure and the
x-axis representing a time value, in hours or cycles. Data points are
established from failure data, with the failure times arranged in
increasing order or value of occurrence. Corresponding median ranks are
assigned from a percent rank table, based on the sample size. Weibull plotting
was discussed in Chapter 25.

References

Frankel, E. G., *System Reliability and Risk Analysis*. The Hague:
Martinus Nijhoff Publishers, 1984.

Fries, Richard C., *Reliability Assurance for Medical Devices, Equipment and
Software*. Buffalo Grove, IL: Interpharm Press, Inc., 1991.

Fries, Richard C., *Reliable Design of Medical Devices*. New York: Marcel
Dekker, Inc., 1997.

Ireson, W. Grant and Clyde F. Coombs Jr., *Handbook of Reliability
Engineering and Management*. New York: McGraw-Hill Book Company,
1988.

King, J. R., *Probability Charts for Decision Making*. New
Hampshire: Team, 1971.

Lloyd, D. K. and M. Lipow, *Reliability Management, Methods and
Mathematics*. 2nd Edition Milwaukee, WI: The American
Society for Quality Control, 1984.

Mann, N. R. et al., *Methods for Statistical Analysis of Reliability and Life Data*. New York, John Wiley and Sons, 1974.

Nelson, W., *Applied Life Data Analysis*. New York: John Wiley and Sons, 1982.

O'Connor, Patrick D. T., *Practical Reliability Engineering*. 3rd Edition. Chichester, England: John Wiley & Sons, 1991.

Section 5

The Manufacturing/Field Phase

Chapter 27

Quality System Regulations and Manufacturing

Richard C. Fries, PE, CRE – Datex-Ohmeda, Inc.
Madison, Wisconsin

Nearly twenty years ago, the United States Food and Drug Administration established its Good Manufacturing Practices (GMP) for both domestic and foreign manufacturers of medical devices intended for human use. The agency took the position that the failure of manufacturers to follow good manufacturing practices was responsible for a substantial number of device failures and recalls.

The philosophy behind the FDA's requirement that manufacturers adopt GMPs is simple. While the agency's premarket review of devices serves as a check of their safety and effectiveness, it was felt that only compliance with GMPs could ensure that devices were produced in a reliable and consistent manner. At that time, the original GMPs did not in themselves guarantee that a product that was once shown to be safe and effective could be reliably produced.

Recently, spurred by an act of Congress, the FDA has changed its regulations, adding a requirement for design controls and bringing U.S. GMPs into substantive harmony with international requirements. The addition of design controls changes the very nature of the GMP requirements, which now seek to increase the chances that devices will be designed in such a manner as to be safe, effective, and reliable. Further, with the agency embracing the goal of international harmonization, the day may not be far off when manufacturers will be able to establish a single set of manufacturing practices that will satisfy regulatory requirements from New Zealand to Norway. Indeed, the agency has already spoken publicly about the mutual recognition of inspection results among industrialized countries, and has even raised the possibility of third-party audits to replace the need for some FDA inspections.

27.1   History of the Quality System Regulations

Like most U.S. medical device law, the Current Good Manufacturing Practices requirements trace their genesis to the medical device amendments of 1976. Section 520(f) of the Federal Food, Drug, and Cosmetic Act authorized the FDA to establish GMPs. On July 21, 1978, the agency issued its original GMP regulations, which described the facilities and methods to be used in the manufacture, packaging, storage, and installation of medical devices. Aside from some editorial comments, these requirements would remain unchanged for nearly 20 years.

In 1990, Congress passed the Safe Medical Device Act, which gave the FDA authority to add "preproduction design validation controls" to the GMP regulations. The act also encouraged the FDA to work with foreign countries toward mutual recognition of GMP inspections.

The agency went right to work on this and in June, 1990 proposed revised GMPs. Almost seven years of debate and revision followed, but finally, on October 7, 1996, the FDA issued its final rules. The new Quality System Regulations, incorporating the required design controls, went into effect June 1, 1997. The design control provisions, however, were not enforced until June 14, 1998.

The design controls embodied in the new regulations were necessary, the FDA stated, because the lack of such controls had been a major cause of device recalls in the past. A 1990 study suggested that approximately 44% of the quality problems that had led to voluntary recall actions in the previous six years were attributable to errors or deficiencies designed into particular devices, deficiencies that might have been prevented had design controls been in place. With respect to design flaws in software, the data were even more alarming: one study of software related recalls indicated that more than 90% were due to design errors.

Like their predecessors, the new rules are broadly stated. "Because this regulation must apply to so many different types of devices, the regulation does not prescribe in detail how a manufacturer must produce a specific device," explained the FDA. The rules apply to all Class II and Class III devices and to some Class I devices. Failure to comply with the provisions will automatically render any device produced "adulterated" and subject to FDA sanction.

27.2   Scope

On October 7, 1996, FDA published the long-awaited revision of its medical device good manufacturing practices (GMP) regulation in the Federal Register. Manufacturers that have not remained current with the changes in the regulation that the agency has proposed over the past six years are in for a major surprise. And even those that have kept current with the agency's proposals up through the working draft of July 1995 will find a few new twists.

Now renamed as a quality system regulation, FDA's new revision differs significantly from the previous GMP regulation of 1978. It also adds a number of requirements not present in the agency's proposed rule of November 1993, and introduces a number of changes developed since publication of the July 1995 working draft. Specifically, the new quality system regulation contains major additional requirements in the areas of design, management responsibility, purchasing, and servicing.

It is clear that the new regulation has been greatly influenced by the work of the Global Harmonization Task Force. In slightly different wording, the regulation now incorporates all the requirements of the fullest of the quality systems standards compiled by the International Organization for Standardization (ISO). For example, there are now requirements for quality planning, for a quality manual, and for an outline of the general quality procedure. All these new requirements were added in order to bring the regulation into harmony with the quality systems standards currently accepted in the member nations of the European Union (EU), and there is certainly a benefit to their inclusion in the new regulation.

But the regulation also adds documentation requirements that would not have been included if harmonization were not an agency goal, and these requirements must now be met by all U.S. device manufacturers--even if they do not intend to export to the EU. On the up side, the language of the new regulation will allow manufacturers much more flexibility than either the November 1993 proposal or July 1995 working draft would have allowed. Section 22.3 will review the changes that the agency has incorporated into the sections of its newest regulation and will discuss how those changes are likely to affect device manufacturers.

27.3   General Provisions

As mentioned above, FDA has changed the title of its revised regulation from "Good Manufacturing Practice for Medical Devices" to "Quality System Regulation." This change is more than just a matter of nomenclature; it is intended to reflect the expanded scope of the new regulation as well as to bring its terminology into harmony with that of the ISO 9000 family of quality systems standards. While the 1978 GMP regulation focused almost exclusively on production practices, the new regulation encompasses quality system requirements that apply to the entire life cycle of a device. The new rule is therefore properly referred to as a quality system regulation, into which the agency's revised requirements for good manufacturing practices have been incorporated.

The 1978 GMP regulation was a two-tier regulation that included general requirements applicable to all devices and additional requirements that applied only to critical ones. In the new quality system regulation, the notion of a critical device has been removed, and the term is no longer used. However, the new regulation's section on traceability (820.65) makes use of the same general concept, and the definition of traceable device found there is the same as the definition of critical device as presented in the 1978 GMP regulation (820.3(f)). Other critical-device requirements of the 1978 GMP regulation have been melded into appropriate sections of the quality system regulation; for instance, the critical operation requirements are now included in the section on process validation (820.75).

The new regulation's section on scope makes it clear that manufacturers need only comply with those parts of the regulation that apply to them. Thus, for example, only manufacturers who service devices need comply with the servicing requirements. Like the 1978 GMP regulation, the quality system regulation does not apply to component manufacturers, but they are encouraged to use it for guidance.

One important statement in the new regulation's section on scope is the definition of the phrase "where appropriate," which is used in reference to a number of requirements. Contrary to what manufacturers might hope, this phrase doesn't limit application of the regulation's requirements to times when manufacturers believe they are appropriate. Instead, FDA means that a requirement should be considered appropriate "if nonimplementation could reasonably be expected to result in the product not meeting its specified requirements or the manufacturer not being able to carry out any necessary corrective action." In short, a requirement is considered appropriate unless the manufacturer can document justification to the contrary. Unfortunately, industry was not provided an opportunity to comment on the agency's use of this phrase.

Another important issue covered under the scope of the new regulation relates to foreign firms that export devices to the United States. The agency has routinely inspected such firms to determine whether they are complying with GMPs although it has no authority to do so, and must rely on an invitation from the company in question. Some foreign manufacturers have refused to allow FDA to inspect their facilities. The new regulation's section on scope addresses this situation by stating that devices produced by foreign manufacturers that refuse to permit FDA inspections will be considered adulterated and will be detained by U.S. Customs. FDA is basing its authority to impose this penalty on the Federal Food, Drug, and Cosmetic Act (Section 801(a)). It will be interesting to see what occurs if a foreign manufacturer chooses to challenge this position.

27.4   Design for Manufacturability

Design for Manufacturability (DFM) assures that a design can be repeatably manufactured while satisfying the requirements for quality, reliability, performance, availability, and price. One of the fundamental principles of DFM is reducing the number of parts in a product. Existing parts should be simple and add value to the product. All parts should be specified, designed, and manufactured to allow 100% usable parts to be produced. It takes a concerted effort by Design, Manufacturing, and vendors to achieve this goal.

Design for Manufacturability is desirable because it is less costly. The reduction in cost is due to:

- a simpler design with fewer parts
- simple production processes
- higher quality and reliability
- ease of service.

27.4.1   The DFM Process

The theme of DFM is to eliminate nonfunctional parts, such as screws or fasteners, while also reducing the number of functional parts. The remaining parts should each perform as many functions as possible. The following questions help in determining if a part is necessary:

- Must the part move relative to its mating part?

- Must the part be of a different material than its mating part or isolated from all other parts?
- Must the part be separate for disassembly or service purposes?

All fasteners are automatically considered candidates for elimination.

A process that can be expected to have a defect rate of no more that a few parts per million consists of:

- Identification of critical characteristics
- Determination of product elements contributing to critical characteristics
- For each identified product element, determination of the step or process choice that affects or controls required performance
- Determination of a nominal value and maximum allowable tolerance for each product component and process step.
- Determination of the capability for parts and process elements that control required performance
- Assurance that the capability index (Cp) is greater than or equal to 2, where

Cp = (specification width)/process capability.

27.5   Design for Assembly

Design for Assembly is a structured methodology for analyzing product concepts or existing products for simplification of the design and its assembly process. Reduction in parts and assembly operations, and individual part geometry changes to ease assembly are the primary goals. The analysis process exposes many other life cycle cost and customer satisfaction issues which can then be addressed. Design and assembly process quality are significantly improved by this process.

Most textbook approaches to Design for Assembly (DFA) discuss elimination of parts. While this is a very important aspect of DFA, there are also many other factors that affect product assembly. A few rules include:

Overall Design Concept

- the design should be simple with a minimum number of parts
- assure the unit is light weight
- the system should have a unified design approach, rather than look like an accumulation of parts
- components should be arranged and mounted for the most economical assembly and wiring
- components that have a limited shelf life should be avoided
- the use of special tools should be minimized
- the use of wiring and harnesses to connect components should be avoided.

Component Mounting

- the preferred assembly direction is top down
- repositioning of the unit to different orientations during assembly should be avoided
- all functional internal components should mount to one main chassis component
- mating parts should be self aligning
- simple, foolproof operations should be used.

Test Points

- pneumatic test point shall be accessible without removal of any other module
- electrical test points shall include, but not be limited to:

    - reference voltages
    - adjustments

- key control signals
- power supply voltages

- all electronic test points shall be short-circuit protected and easily accessible.

Stress Levels and Tolerances

- the lowest possible stress levels should be used
- the maximum possible operating limits and mechanical tolerances should be maximized
- operations of known capability should be use.

PCBs

- adequate clearance should be provided around circuit board mounting locations to allow for tools
- components should be soldered, not socketed
- PCBs must be mechanically secured and supported
- there must be unobstructed access to test and calibration points
- exposed voltages should be less than 40 volts.

Miscellaneous

- all air intakes should be filtered and an indication that the filter needs to be changed should be given to the user
- the device shall be packed in a recyclable container so as to minimize the system installation time.

27.5.1 Design for Assembly Process

When implementing the Design for Assembly process, the Manufacturer should:

- develop a multi-functional team before the new product architecture is defined. This team should foster a creative climate which will encourage ownership of the new product's design and delivery process.

- establish product goals through a benchmarking process or by creating a model, drawing, or a conception of the product.
- perform a design for assembly analysis of the product. this identifies possible candidates for elimination or redesign, as well as highlighting high cost assembly operations.
- segment the product architecture into manageable modules or levels of assembly.
- apply design for assembly principles to these assembly modules to generate a list of possible cost opportunities.
- apply creative tools, such as brainstorming, to enhance the emerging design and identify further design improvements.
- as a team, evaluate and select the best ideas, thus narrowing and focusing the team's goals.
- make commodity and material selections. Start early supplier involvement to assure economical production.
- with the aid of cost models or competitive benchmarking, establish a target cost for every part in the new design.
- start the detailed design of the emerging product. Model, test, and evaluate the new design for form, fit, and function.
- re-apply the process at the next logical point.
- share the results.

27.6   The Manufacturing Process

The process of producing new product may be said to be a multi-phased process consisting of:

- pre-production activity
- the pilot run build

- the production run
- delivery to the customer.

27.6.1   Pre-Production Activity

Prior to the first manufacturing build, Manufacturing is responsible for completing a myriad of activity.

Manufacturing and Engineering should work together to identify proposed technologies and to assure that the chosen technology is manufacturable.

The selection of suppliers should begin by consulting the current approved suppliers listing to determine if any of the existing suppliers can provide the technology and/or parts. A new supplier evaluation would be necessary if a supplier is being considered as a potential source for a component, subassembly, or device.

A Pilot Run plan must be developed that specifies the quantity of units to be built during the pilot run, the yield expectations and contingency plans, the distribution of those units, the feedback mechanism for problems, the intended production location, staffing requirements, training plan, post production evaluation, and any other key issues specific to the project.

The Manufacturing strategy needs to be developed. The strategy must be documented and communicated to appropriate personnel to ensure it is complete, meets the business objectives, and ultimately is reflected in the design for the product. Developing a strategy for producing the product involves work on five major fronts:

- the production plan
- the quality plan
- the test plan
- the materials plan
- the supplier plan.

The Production Plan details how Manufacturing will produce the product. The first step is defining the requirements of the production process. Some of these requirements will be found in the business proposal and product specification. A Bill of Materials structure is developed for the product which best meets the defined requirements. Based on this Bill of Materials, a process flow diagram can be developed along with specific details of inventory levels and locations, test points, skills, resources, tooling required, and processing times.

The Quality Plan details the control through all phases of manufacture, procurement, packaging, storage, and shipment which collectively assures that the product meets specifications. The plan should cover not only initial production, but also how the plan will be matured over time, using data collected internally and from the field.

The Test Plan specifies the "how" of the Quality Plan. This document must have enough technical detail to assure that the features are incorporated in the product design specification. Care must be taken to ensure that the manufacturer's test strategies are consistent with those of all suppliers.

The Materials Plan consists of defining the operating plan by which the final product, parts, accessories, and service support parts will be managed logistically to meet the launch plans. This involves product structure, lead times, inventory management techniques, inventory phasing/impact estimates, and identification of any special materials considerations that must be addressed. Any production variants which will be in production as well as potentially obsolete product would be detailed.

The Supplier Plan consists of a matrix of potential suppliers versus evaluation criteria. The potential suppliers have been identified using preliminary functional component specifications. The evaluation criteria should include business stability, quality systems, cost, engineering capabilities, and test philosophy.

The DFMA review should be held when a representative model is available. This review should be documented, with action item assigned.

27.6.2 The Pilot Run Build

The objective of this phase is to complete the pilot run and validate the manufacturing process against the objectives set forth in the manufacturing strategy and the product specification.

The Pilot Run build is the first build of devices using the Manufacturing documentation. It is during this phase that training of the assembly force takes place. All training should be documented so no employee is given a task without the appropriate training prior to the task.

The Pilot Run build will validate the manufacturing process against the strategy and the Manufacturing documentation. The validation will determine if Manufacturing has met its objectives, including:

- standard cost
- product quality
- documentation
- tooling
- training
- process control.

The validation will also determine if the production testing is sufficient to ensure that the product meets the specified requirements.

The Pilot Run build also validates the supplier plan and supplier contracts. The validation will determine if the manufacturing plan is sufficient to control the internal processes of the supplier. The method and ground rules for communication between the two companies must be well defined to ensure that both parties keep each other informed of developments which impact the other. It should also confirm that all points have been addressed in the supplier contract and that all the controls and procedures required by the agreement are in place and operating correctly.

Internal failure analysis and corrective action takes place, involving investigating to the root cause all failures during the pilot run. The information should be communicated to the project team in detail and in a timely manner. The project team determines the appropriate corrective action plans.

A Pilot Run review meeting is held to review all aspects of the build, including the Manufacturing documentation. All remaining issues must be resolved and documentation corrected. Sufficient time should be allowed in the project schedule for corrective action to be completed before the production run.

27.6.3   The Production Run

The objective of this phase is to produce high quality product on time, while continuing to fine tune the process using controls which have been put in place. During this phase, the first production order of units and service parts are manufactured. The training effort continues, as new employees are transferred in or minor refinements are made to the process. Line failures at any point in the process should be thoroughly analyzed and the root cause determined. Product cost should be verified at this time.

27.6.4   Customer Delivery

The objective of this phase is to deliver the first production units to the customer, refine the manufacturing process based on lessons learned during the first build, and finally to monitor field unit performance to correct any problems. Following production and shipment of product, continued surveillance of the production process should take place to measure its performance against the manufacturing strategy. The production process should be evaluated for effectiveness as well as unit field performance. Feedback from the field on unit problems should be sent to the project team, where it may be disseminated to the proper area. This subject will be discussed further in Chapter 30.

References

Boothroyd Dewhurst, Inc., *Design for Manufacture and Assembly/Service/Environment and Concurrent Engineering (Workshop Manual)*. Wakefield, RI: Boothroyd Dewhurst, Inc, 1966.

Dash, Glenn, "CGMPs for Medical Device Manufacturers," in *Compliance Engineering.* Volume 14, Number 2, March-April, 1997.

European Committee for Standardization, "Quality Systems--Medical Devices--Particular Requirements for the Application of EN 29001," *European Norm 46001*, Brussels, European Committee for Standardization, 1996.

Food and Drug Administration, "Medical Devices; Current Good Manufacturing Practice (CGMP) Final Rule; Quality System Regulation," *Federal Register.* October 7, 1996.

Food and Drug Administration, *21 CFR Part 820 Medical Devices; Current Good Manufacturing Practice (CGMP) Regulations; Proposed Revisions.* November 23, 1993.

Food and Drug Administration, Code of Federal Regulations, 21 CFR 820, "Good Manufacturing Practice for Medical Devices," *Federal Register.* July 21, 1978.

Food and Drug Administration, "Medical Devices; Current Good Manufacturing Practice (CGMP) Regulations; Proposed Revisions; Request for Comments," *Federal Register.* November 23, 1993.

Food and Drug Administration, "Medical Devices; Working Draft of the Current Good Manufacturing Practice (CGMP) Final Rule; Notice of Availability; Request for Comments; Public Meeting," *Federal Register.* July 24, 1995.

Fries, Richard C., *Reliability Assurance for Medical Devices, Equipment and Software.* Buffalo Grove, IL: Interpharm Press, Inc., 1991.
Fries, Richard C., *Reliable Design of Medical Devices.* New York: Marcel Dekker, Inc., 1997.

Global Harmonization Task Force, "Guidance on Quality Systems for the Design and Manufacture of Medical Devices," Issue 7, August 1994.

Hooten, W. Fred, "A Brief History of FDA Good Manufacturing Practices," in *Medical Device & Diagnostic Industry.* Volume 18, Number 5, May, 1996.

International Organization for Standardization, "Quality Systems--Model for Quality Assurance in Design, Development, Production, Installation, and Servicing," *ISO 9001:1994*, Geneva: International Organization for Standardization (ISO), 1994.

Chapter 28

Configuration Management

Richard C. Fries, PE, CRE – Datex-Ohmeda, Inc.
Madison, Wisconsin

Configuration management is a discipline applying technical and administrative direction and surveillance to:

- identify and document the functional and physical characteristics of configuration items
- audit the configuration items to verify conformance to specifications, interface control documents, and other contract requirements
- control changes to configuration items and their related documentation
- record and report information needed to manage configuration items effectively, including the status of proposed changes and the implementation status of approved changes.

Based on the operations of configuration management, it consists of four major divisions:

- configuration identification
- configuration change control
- configuration status accounting
- configuration audits.

The purpose of configuration management is to maintain the integrity of products as they evolve from specifications through design, development, and production. Configuration management is not an isolated endeavor. It exists to support product development and maintenance.

Applying configuration management techniques to a particular project requires judgements to be exercised. Too little configuration management causes products to be lost, requiring previous work to be redone. Too much configuration management and the organization will never product any products, because everyone will be too busy shuffling paperwork.

Applying configuration management to a project depends on the value of the product, the perceived risks, and the impact on the product in one of the perceived risks actually materializes. The main question to be answered is, what is required to obtain a reasonable degree of assurance that the integrity of the product will be maintained?

28.1   Configuration Identification

The first step in managing a collection of items is to uniquely identify each one. As a process, configuration identification is the selection of the documents to comprise a baseline for the system and the configuration items involve, and the numbers to be affixed to the items and documents.

In the configuration management sense, a baseline is a document, or a set of documents, formally designated and fixed at a specific time during a configuration item's life cycle. By establishing baselines, we can extend the orderly development of the system from specifications into design documentation, and then into hardware and software items themselves. Typically, four baselines are established in each project:

- functional
- allocated
- developmental configuration (software only)
- product.

The four baselines are summarized in Table 28-1.

28.1.1   Functional Baseline

The functional baseline is the initially approved documentation that describes a system's or item's functional characteristics, and the verifications required to demonstrate the achievement of those specified functional characteristics. this is the initial baseline to be established on a project and usually consists of the system specification, a document that establishes the technical characteristics of what the total collection of all the hardware and software is to do. The functional baseline is a part of the formal agreement between a customer and the developer. It is normally established at the time of contract award, although it can be established after contract award at a specified review.

28.1.2   Allocated Baseline

The allocated baseline is the initially approved documentation that describes:

- an item's functional and interface characteristics that are allocated from a higher level configuration item
- interface requirements with interfacing configuration items
- design constraints
- the verification required to demonstrate the achievement of those specified functional and interface characteristics.

The allocated baseline consists of two type of documents:

- specifications for the items themselves
- interface requirements documents.

Baseline	Content	Implementation
Functional	System Specification	Contract award or completion of the peer review
Allocated	Unit Specifications	Not later than the critical design review
	Interface Control Document	Not later than the critical design review
	Software Requirements Specification	Software Requirements Review
	Interface Requirements Specifications	Software Requirements Review
Developmental Configuration	Software Top-Level Design Documents	Preliminary Design Review
	Software Detailed Design Documents	Critical Design Review
	Source, Object, and Executable Code	Unit Test
Product	Hardware Technical Data Package	Physical Configuration Audit
	Software Design Requirements	Physical Configuration Audit
	Source, Object, and Executable Code	
	User and Maintenance Manuals	
	Test Plans, Test Procedures, and Test Reports	

Table 28-1   Summary of Baselines (From Buckley, 1993.)

Specifications for the items themselves are called unit specifications for hardware and the software requirements specification for software. These specifications describe each of the essential requirements of each hardware and software configuration item, including functions, performances, design constraints, and attributes.

Interface requirements documents are of two types: interface control drawings and interface requirements specifications. the interface control drawings identify the hardware interfaces between the hardware configuration items. The interface requirements specifications identify the interfaces between the software configuration items.

28.1.3   Developmental Configuration

The developmental configuration is the software and associated technical documentation, which defines the evolving configuration of a software configuration item under development. It is under the developer's control and describes the software configuration at any stage of the design, coding, and testing effort. Current practice is to implement the developmental configuration in a phased manner as the individual components achieve specific values.

The developmental configuration is established incrementally. Items of the developmental configuration are baselined when they are reviewed with peers. Substantial efforts have been made as part of these reviews and the results reflect agreements reached with others. Although the documents remain under the control of the originating organization, some means of identifying the reviewed documents and tracking their changes is required.

28.1.4   Product Baseline

The product baseline is the initially approved documentation that describes all the necessary functional and physical characteristics of the configuration item, any required interoperability characteristics of a configuration item, and the selected functional and physical characteristics designated for production acceptance testing. Typically, for hardware, the product baseline consists of the technical data package, including engineering drawings and associated lists, and all the rest of the items necessary to ensure that the hardware products can be fabricated by a third party. For software, the product baseline includes the software code on electronic media and the other items required to assure the code can be reproduced and maintained.

The product baseline is established on completion of formal acceptance testing of the system and the completion of a physical configuration audit.

28.2   Configuration Audits

An audit is an independent evaluation of a product to ascertain compliance to specifications, standards, contractual agreements, or other criteria. In the area of configuration management, there are three types of audits:

- functional configuration audits
- physical configuration audits
- in-process audits.

Each audit has a different purpose.

28.2.1   Functional Configuration Audits

The purpose of a functional configuration audit is to validate that the development of a configuration item has been completed satisfactorily, and that the configuration item has achieved the performance and functional characteristics specified in the functional or allocated configuration. The audits are held at the end of the development cycle, following completion of all the testing on items that have been developed. The goal of the audits is to obtain a reasonable degree of confidence that the items have met all their requirements.

There are a number of cautions that should be observed at this point. First, the functional configuration audit is not the time to review the test program itself for adequacy. The judgement that the test program was adequate for the intended purposes should have already been made.

Second, there is sometimes a viewpoint expressed that if anything changed, the entire test program should be reinitiated. There are judgements to be made, and extreme calls on either end of the spectrum should be avoided. Regression or check tests should be used in doubtful cases.

Third, there are cases in which there has been only one test made, with one test report and a series of actions. In such circumstances, convening a functional configuration audit to review that one test may not be warranted. For this reason, in software, functional configuration audits are not usually held.

28.2.2 Physical Configuration Audits

The physical configuration audit is a technical examination of a designated configuration item to verify that the configuration item, as built, conforms to the technical documentation that defines it. On the hardware side, a physical configuration audit is an audit of the actual product itself against its technical data package. The reason for this audit for hardware is straightforward. It has been previously verified, at the functional configuration audit, that the item constructed as part of the development cycle met all the requirements in the specification. Now, if the technical data package provides accurate instructions on how to build identical items, them many of the items that meet those specifications can be produced without the exhaustive testing required for the initial item. Confirmatory and first-item testing will take place during production, but these can be done on a sampling basis, rather than on 100% of the production items.

28.2.3 In-Process Audits

In-process audits are performed to determine whether the configuration management process, established in an organization, is being followed and to ascertain what needs to be improved. The task of conducting an in-process audit is usually relegated to the Quality Assurance function.

28.3 Configuration Management Metrics

Configuration management metrics can be obtained from the configuration management library, which holds the source files, both documents and source code. By examining the documentation in the source file, the following can be obtained:

- documentation sizes
- documentation changes
- size of documentation changes.

Documentation sizes can be easily measured in words, using any standard word-counting program. Metrics can then be provided for individual documents, indicidual types of documents, and documents grouped by configuration item.

Documentation changes are the actual number of changes for each document identified above, where one change is defined s one formal issue of a set of page changes to an original document. The size of document changes consists of the acutal size, in words, for the changes for each document identified above.

In a similar manner to documentation metrics, the following source code metics are also easily obtained:

- the number of source files of code
- the number of revisions to source file code
- actual number of source line of code.

28.4   FDA's View of Configuration Management

In the March, 1996 draft of their design control guidance document, the FDA states that the procedures for controlling change include methods for:

- controlling the identification of development status
- requesting and approving changes
- ensuring that changes are properly integrated through formal change control procedures
- obtaining approval to implement a change
- version identification, issue, and control.

Change control procedures require the complete documentation of approved changes and the communication of configuration changes to all who are effected. Design changes are reviewed to determine whether they influence previously approved design verification or validation results. In general, for any approved document, subsequent changes to that document should be approved by the same authority that approved the original design. In addition, the request for a change should be accompanied by an assessment of the total impact of the change.

The FDA believes configuration management refers to the documentation to be controlled, the procedures for controlling it, and the responsibilities of those managing the documentation. It includes a system of traceability including traceability of components, service manuals, and procedures that could be affected by a change. The controlled documents are configuration items and collectively form the device configuration.

Typically the device configuration includes specifications, design documents, test documents, and all other deliverables including those documents required for regulatory records.

The draft document has been issued for review and comment by medical device manufacturers.

28.5   Status Accounting

Status accounting is the recording activity. It follows up on the results of configuration management activities. It keeps track of the current configuration identification documents, the current configuration of the delivered software, the status of changes being reviewed, and the status of implementation of approved changes.

Status accounting refers to the record-keeping functions inherent in the other configuration management activities and to the specialized management information system that must exist to rovide all the technical information. Thus, for each document authored, reviewed, approved, and distributed, recordings are made of all the current data for a document, specification, or change in order to communicate this information to the project/users/support activities as fast as it becomes available. The data must be in a form to allow traceability from top to bottom and bottom to top.

The first step in establishing a configuration status accounting capability is to identify the overall reporting requirements. Then these reporting requirements are used to determine the detailed requirements for the supporting facility. Acquisition of the resources, including hardware, software,

communications, space, and people, can then be initiated. The database can
then be initialized and the initial reports produced. Establishing this capability
requires substantial efforts and should be initiated as early as possible in the
development process. Updating the database will be a continuing activity, and
the reports themselves will change as the user's needs evolve.

References

Berlack, H. Ronald, *Software Configuration Management*. New York: John
Wiley & Sons, Inc., 1992.

Buckley, Fletcher J., *Implementing Configuration Management: Hardware,
Software, and Firmware*. New York: The Institute of Electrical and Electronic
Engineers, Inc., 1993.

Evans, Michael W. and John J. Marciniak, *Software Quality Assurance and
Management*. New York: John Wiley & Sons, Inc., 1987.

Food and Drug Administration, *Draft of Design Control Guidance for
Medical Device Manufacturers*. March, 1996.

IEEE Std 828, *IEEE Standard for Software Configuration Management
Plans*. New York: The Institute of Electrical and Electronic Engineers, Inc.,
1990.

IEEE Std 1042, *IEEE Guide to Software Configuration Management*. New
York: The Institute of Electrical and Electronic Engineers, Inc., 1986.

MIL-STD-483, *Configuration Management Practices for Systems,
Equipment, Munitions, and Computer Programs*. Washington, DC:
Department of Defense, 1979.

MIL-STD-973, *Configuration Management*. Washington, DC: Department
of Defense, 1992.

O'Connor, Patrick D. T., *Practical Reliability Engineering*. 3rd Edition. Chichester, England: John Wiley & Sons, 1991.

Chapter 29

The Quality System Audit

Tina Juneau – Lunar Inc.
Madison, Wisconsin

There are two important areas to focus time and energy when discussing a Quality Systems Audit: Preparation and Audit Day. Each has its own importance and potential outcome on the audit, but each area should be approached separately. While the organization can never know the path that any auditor will take, the time spent in preparation can help ensure that audit day goes smoothly.

29.1   Preparation

There are three main areas that the organization should focus efforts when preparing for a Quality Systems Audit: Documentation, Employees and Escorts. Much of this preparation will occur as the company establishes the quality system. However, these areas should always be reviewed prior to any outside audit.

29.1.1   Documentation

Perhaps the most important part of the preparation for the Quality System Audit is writing the documentation that is required. This may be the reason that many people view the ISO 9001 standard as strictly a documentation activity. While there are certain elements which require procedures or other documentation to be available the organization has a great deal of flexibility not only in how many procedures it writes, but in how the documentation is stored and controlled. Any documentation that is established should serve a purpose to your organization. If it does not, determine if it is truly required in the first place.

It is important to remember that documents can be in either hard copy or electronic media thus completely avoiding the dreaded procedure binder that plagues most companies. Of course either method of distributing documentation must ensure proper controls are in place for the auditors to objectively evaluate the system.

The organization should avoid any major procedural or process changes immediately prior to any audit. Each process will need time to develop and the auditors will need ample evidence that the system has been implemented and is effective. If many documentation changes occur immediately prior to the audit there many not be enough supporting evidence in place.

Once the quality manual, procedures, work instructions and records are established the company must ensure that employees know the location of all documentation and how to access it. Employees should have been involved in the preparation so that they take ownership of their procedures and the documentation accurately reflects the processes used in all areas. If electronic methods are used, employees must know how to use the system to retrieve documentation. All persons must have access, understand the system and be able to demonstrate its use to an auditor.

If documentation is maintained in hard copy only strategic distribution locations can be established to ensure that all employees can get to required procedures. Electronic documentation needs to have similar control over the access to the master copies. Who will have the ability to update the system and who will remove old or obsolete copies? The organization also needs to consider how it will control documents which may be printed off the system.

29.1.2 Employees

Employees throughout the organization must be prepared for the upcoming audit to be sure that they are ready as well. Since employees have been made a part of the ongoing efforts to gain certification they will be somewhat familiar with the general system. They will have experienced the audit process with your internal audit program and will be familiar with how to respond to questions about their position and the quality system.

There are several questions that auditors will likely ask employees if they are interviewed during the visit. The organization should make employees aware of these questions and prepare them for how to answer them. Common questions are listed below:

- What do you do?
- How do you know how to perform this activity?
- How do you know you have the latest/most current
  procedure or documentation?
- What kind of training have you had about ISO 9001?
- How does your position affect quality?
- What is your quality policy?
- Who is your Management Representative?

The organization's internal audit team can help with this training by asking these questions during internal audits prior to a third party audit team coming to the facility.

During the audit process employees should always be comfortable asking either the auditor or one of the escorts to further explain a question. If the employee does not understand the terms used by the auditor they should be told to ask for clarification or have the question repeated. Employees should not try to answer questions outside of their realm of responsibility and should direct the auditors to a supervisor or the person in charge when necessary. Many organizations will instruct employees to only answer the auditor's questions and not offer additional information. If the quality system has been well implemented employees should not feel that they have anything to hide and should be able to freely discuss the system during the audit. It is important that employees know to treat auditors with respect, to be polite, and to be honest. Any information that the organization attempts to hide will most likely be brought to light during the investigation and will cause greater harm than if the issue was dealt with in an outright manner.

It is sometimes helpful to have the quality policy printed on business size cards and distributed to the employee so that it can be easily referenced if needed. Some companies also post the quality policy in various locations around the facility so that it is easy seen by many people. Employees do not need to have the quality policy memorized, but they should know its intent.

Employees must be able to trace their documentation through the system by identifying work instructions or procedures as needed. Employees must know where documentation is located, how to ensure it is the current or most recent revision and what process to follow if the document needs to be changed.

Employees must also be aware of where training records are located and the organization should ensure that all records are up to date. Training records should include quality system as well as job specific training. It may help to have records of training received at outside classes or seminars in addition to the training provided on site. Annual updates and refresher training should be recorded as necessary to show ongoing efforts to raise awareness of the quality system.

29.1.3   Escorts

Although the preparation of the documentation and employees is a vital part of the pre-audit activity, it is the preparation of the escorts that may be most important to a successful audit. The escorts will accompany the auditors at all times during their visit and be the main interface between them and the organization.

Generally the Management Representative is an escort during all outside audits. They may be accompanied by other individuals who are well versed in the requirements of the quality system and with all of the process areas. Escorts should be aware of any open issues such as internal audit findings, corrective actions, or problems regarding the quality system. This will allow them to explain the area better to the auditors if it is brought to light during the audit or help steer auditors away from the area if needed. They should be familiar with ongoing improvement efforts and prepared to discuss the changes that are in process.

Prior to the audit a schedule will be sent. It is important for the escorts to inform the various areas about when they will be involved and escorts should know key employees throughout the organization and their roles in the quality system. During the audit the escorts will then be able to call upon these individuals as further resources. Escorts should speak to these key people prior to the audit to ensure that they understand the audit process and are prepared to deal with the auditors.

During the audit the escorts will explain the quality system in great detail. If they are able to answer the questions in adequate detail the auditors may not need to further their investigation in the specific area. Because of this it is very important to consider who will act as an escort during the audits.

29.2   What To Expect On Audit Day

29.2.1   Open to Close

Prior to the first day of the audit your organization should be well informed regarding the schedule of the audit. Generally you will be sent a timeline that details each area to be audited and the departments which will be involved. Occasionally there are conflicts or discrepancies in the audit plan that can be worked out in advance. These may include altering the schedule to accommodate certain departments needs or changing the location of an area that will be covered. For example, most auditors assume that training will be handled in the Human Resource department but if your organization handled all training within the individual departments you will need to inform the auditors. These details can usually be worked out in advance. In preparation for the upcoming audit many auditors will also ask for copies of the organization's quality manual and a few key procedures to be sent to them for early review. This allows for less time to be spent reading material while onsite and gives the auditors time to prepare for the way your system has been implemented.

The organization should ensure that the auditors have a few comforts available to them. If possible have a conference room available as the central audit room. Ensure that the auditors belongings will be secure there. Auditors may need access to a copier and a phone during the course of the audit and the location and use (if necessary) of these items should be discussed.

On the first day of the audit there will be an Opening meeting. Members of the organization's executive staff may wish to attend this meeting which will cover the plan and scope of the audit. Managers from the areas being audited may wish to attend in case there are any last minute changes to the audit plan, however the organization should limit the number of people in attendance so that it is not overwhelming.

To help orientate the auditors to your facility it may help to have a brief tour and overview of the organization. After the opening meeting and tour the auditors will begin to execute their audit plan. Every audit will cover a few main areas of the quality system and these will certainly be a major focus of the certification audit. Management Responsibility, Quality System, Corrective and Preventive Action and Internal Audits. Most audits will cover the first two areas after the opening meeting. During this time they will ensure management's commitment to the system and look for any major changes since the last audit. Many auditors will reserve the final area to be audited for Internal Audits. This ensures that the focus of the audit is not turned by findings identified in internal audits and focuses the investigation to the internal audit program rather than the issues it has brought up. If internal audits are on the schedule earlier in the audit, the organization may ask to have it moved.

Once the general areas of management are finished the auditors will move into other areas of the quality system. Depending on the scope of the audit and number of auditors present they may elect to split up and cover various aspects of the system. Because of this ensure that escorts with greatest knowledge of the areas are paired with the auditors visiting those areas. Most auditors will speak with the manager or supervisor of the area and may talk directly to some employees. The escorts should always introduce the auditor to the relevant people in each department and help ensure that each element is presented correctly.

During the audit any issues should be presented immediately by the audit team. If the organization is able to correct the issue immediately they should do so, and present the evidence to the audit team. While it may not avoid the finding from being written in a report it will ensure that the report also states that the issue was corrected while the team was onsite. Escorts must ensure that they take good notes during the audit. They should identify each area the auditors go to, who they interview and what information they review. They should note any areas that the auditors do not investigate as well as those that were covered. This helps ensure that if there are open issues the organization can correct them.

At the end of the day auditors will likely wish to have some time to discuss and document their activities. They will then hold an informal wrap-up meeting where they will discuss any issues they have found with the escorts. At this time the organization may clear up any misunderstandings and present additional evidence to the audit team regarding any of the areas that were visited. Once any issues are discussed, the auditors may discuss any changes in the schedule review the plan for the following day and stop for the evening.

29.2.2   Possible Outcomes

During the course of the day the escorts will be aware of how the audit is going. They will be able to tell if there are many issues that have been identified or if there are only a few discrepancies that were found. Most auditors have four categories or levels of deviations that they record.

The least severe will be called a recommendation. These items are usually considered an auditor's preference for how something is done. The organization should not feel obligated to change their system based on an auditor's recommendation. In fact you may receive conflicting recommendations from auditors over the course of time.

A second level issue will be listed as an observation. This is more severe than a recommendation, but is usually not written as a formal discrepancy. Auditors may make note in the audit report of their observations and review the areas involved at the following audit to see if the issue has been corrected. If the organization is unsure if the auditors expect the issue to be corrected, they should ask them at the closing meeting. Observations are usually a very minor observance of a discrepancy in the system. Although it identifies a problem the issue was not found to be widespread or it may involve a less critical element of the quality system. The organization will want to address this issue prior to the next audit.

If the auditors identify any minor deviations in the quality system they will almost certainly be written as a formal request for correction. A minor deviation identifies a breakdown in the system and must be corrected. The auditors will write the deviation and identify the evidence they have gathered to illustrate the problem. The organization will be asked to sign the formal request and eventually to submit their corrective actions to the audit team to show that the issue was handled in a timely manner. Any minor deviations will be listed in the audit report and certification may be held until the corrective action has been received.

The most severe discrepancies only occur where an entire element of the system has either been eliminated or was never properly implemented. This is considered a major discrepancy or a systematic problem in the quality system. Issues of this magnitude may result in the organization being denied certification. The auditors will always require the organization to be re-audited for a major discrepancy once the issue has been addressed.

29.3   Surveillance

Once the organization has received certification, they can expect to be re-audited on a yearly basis to ensure they maintain the quality system. The time period for surveillance audits may vary between registrars. Some will conduct the certification audit and two annual surveillance audits, rotating on a three year schedule. Others maintain a five year schedule and conduct four surveillance audits with a full certification audit every sixth year.

Surveillance audits are conducted in the same manner as a certification audit except that the audit will cover fewer elements. The elements to be audited will rotate for each visit with the exception of the four elements mentioned earlier; Management Review, Quality System, Corrective Action and Internal Audits. These areas are core monitors of the system and will be on each audit schedule. Because of the limited scope, a surveillance audit will usually be conducted in half the time that was spend on the certification audit.

As the organization builds its reputation with the registrar, it can expect the audits to go more smoothly. Each subsequent auditor will review the organizations audit file prior to his/her visit. If the organization has built a reputation for limited problems identified, the auditors will come in with a different attitude. This does not mean that they will not conduct a full and detailed audit, but they will expect that the organization will perform well. It will change the way they approach the audit, and should help ease the tension that can sometimes develop. The organization can expect smooth audits as long as they maintain their system as promised.

References

Fries, Richard C., *Reliable Design of Medical Devices*. New York: Marcel Dekker, Inc., 1997.

ISO 9001, *Quality systems - Model for quality assurance in design, development, production, installation and servicing*. Switzerland: International Organization for Standardization, 1994.

Steudel, H.J & Associates, Inc,. *What Every Employee Needs to Know About ISO 9000*. Madison, WI: 1995.

Chapter 30

Analysis of Field Data

Richard C. Fries, PE, CRE – Datex-Ohmeda, Inc.
Madison, Wisconsin

The goal of the Product Development process is to put a safe, effective and reliable medical device in the hands of a physician or other medical personnel where it may be used to improve health care. The device was designed and manufactured to be safe, effective and reliable. The manufacturer warranties the device for a certain period of time, usually one year. Is this the end of the manufacturer's concern about the device? It should'nt be. There is too much valuable information to be obtained.

When a product is subjected to reliability activities during design and development, testing is performed to determine the degree of reliability present and the confidence in that determination. There is, however, no guarantee that the product, as manufactured and shipped, has that same degree of reliability. The most meaningful way to determine the degree of reliablity within each device is to monitor its activity in the field.

Analysis of field data is the means of determining how a product is performing in actual use. It is a means of determining the reliability growth over time. It is a measure of how well the product was specified, designed and manufactured. It is a source of information on the effectiveness of the shipping configuration. It is also a source for information for product enhancements or new designs.

Field information may be obtained in any of several ways, including:

- Analysis of Field Service Reports
- Failure Analysis of Failed Units
- Warranty Analysis.

30.1   Analysis of Field Service Reports

The type of data necessary for a meaningful analysis of product reliability is gathered from Field Service Reports. The reports contains such vital information as:

- Type of product
- Serial number
- Date of service activity
- Symptom of the problem
- Diagnosis
- List of parts replaced
- Labor hours required
- Service representative.

The type of product allows classification by individual model. The serial number allows a history of each individual unit to be established and traceability to the manufacturing date. The date of service activity helps to indicate the length of time until the problem occurred.

The symptom is the problem, as recognized by the user. The diagnosis is the description of the cause of the problem from analysis by the service representative. The two may be mutually exclusive, as the cause of the problem may be remote from the user's original complaint. The list of parts replaced is an adjunct to the diagnosis and can serve to trend parts usage and possible vendor problems. The diagnosis is then coded, where it may be sorted later.

The required labor hours help in evaluating the complexity of a problem, as represented by the time involved in repair. It, along with the name of the Service Representative, acts as a check on the efficiency of the individual representative, as average labor hours for the same failure code may be compared on a representative to representative basis. The labor hours per problem may be calculated to assist in determining warranty cost as well as determining the efficiency of service methods.

The only additional data, which is not included in the Field Service Report is the date of manufacture of each unit and the length of time since manufacture that the problem occurred. The manufacturing date is kept on file in the Device History Record. The length of time since manufacture is calculated by subtracting the manufacturing date from the date of service.

30.1.1   The Database

Field Service Reports are sorted by product upon receipt. The report is scanned for completeness. Service representatives may be contacted where clarification of an entry or lack of information would lead to an incomplete database record. The diagnoses are coded, according to a list of failures, as developed by Reliability Assurance, Design Engineering and Manufacturing Engineering (Table 30-1). Manufacturing date and the length of time since manufacture are obtained. The data is then ready to be entered into the computer.

The data is entered into a computer data base, where it may be manipulated to determine the necessary parameters. Each Field Service Report is input to a single database record, unless the service report contains multiple failure codes. Table 30-2 shows a sample database record.

The data is first sorted by service date, so trending can be accomplished by a predetermined time period, such as a fiscal quarter. Data within that time frame is then sorted by problem code, indicating the frequency of problems during the particular reporting period. A pareto analysis of the problems can then be developed. Data is finally sorted by serial number, which

Failure Code	Failure
Base Machine	
101	Missing parts
102	Shipping Damage
103	Circuit Breaker Wiring Damage
104	Regulator Defect
105	Shelf Latch Broken
Monitor	
201	Display Problems
202	Control Cable Defect
203	Power Board Problem
204	Control Board Problem
205	Unstable Reference Voltage

Table 30-1   List of Failure Codes

gives an indication of which devices experienced multiple service calls and/or experienced continuing problems.

Percentages of total problems are helpful in determining primary failures. Spread sheets are developed listing the problems versus manufacturing dates and the problems versus time since manufacturing. The spread sheet data can then be plotted and analyzed.

Field	Field Content
1	Service date
2	Device serial number
3	Manufacturing date
4	Time in use (hours)
5	Failure code
6	Failed parts 1
7	Failed parts 2
8	Failed parts 3
9	Failed parts 4
10	Failed parts 5
11	Time to repair (hours)
12	Service representative ID

Table 30-2   Sample Database Record

30.1.2 Data Analysis

The most important reason for collecting the field data is to extract the most significant problem information and put it in such a form that the cause of product problems may be highlighted, trended and focused upon. The cause of the problem must be determined and the most appropriate solution implemented. A "band-aid" solution is unacceptable.

Pareto analysis is used to determine what the major problems are. The individual problems are plotted along the x-axis and the frequency on the y-axis. The result is a histogram of problems, where the severity of the problem is indicated, leading to the establishment of priorities in addressing solutions.

Several graphical plots are helpful in analyzing problems. One is the plot of particular problems versus length of time since manufacturing. This plot is used to determine the area of the life cycle in which the problem occurs. Peaks of problem activity indicate infant mortality, useful life or wearout, depending on the length of time since manufacture.

A second plot of interest is that of a particular problem versus the date of manufacture. This plot is a good indication of the efficiency of the manufacturing process. It shows times where problems occur, e.g., the rush to ship product at the end of a fiscal quarter, lot problems on components, or vendor problems The extent of the problem is an indication of the correct or incorrect solution.

Another useful plot is that of the total number of problems versus the date of manufacture. The learning curve for the product is visible at the peaks of the curve. It can also be shown how the problems for subsequent builds decrease as manufacturing personnel become more familiar and efficient with the process.

Trending of problems, set against the time of reporting is an indicator of the extent of a problem and how effective the correction is. Decreasing numbers indicate the solution is effective. Reappearing high counts indicate the initial solution did not address the cause of the problem.

The database is also useful for analyzing warranty costs. The data can be used to calculate warranty expenses, problems per manufactured unit and warranty costs as a percentage of sales. A similar table can be established for installation of devices.

30.2   Failure Analysis of Field Units

Most failure analysis performed in the field is done at the board level. Service Representative usually solve problems by board swapping, since they are not equipped to troubleshoot at the component level. Boards should be returned to be analyzed to the component level. This not only yields data for trending purposes, but highlights the real cause of the problem. It also gives data on problem parts or problem vendors.

Product Code	Parameters	Cost 1/95	Cost 2/95	Cost Year to Date
4425	Normal Warranty	$	$	$
	Recall Warranty	$	$	$
	Total Warranty	$	$	$
	Setup Cost	$	$	$
	Total Cost	$	$	$
	Sales	$	$	$
	Warranty/Sales			
	Setup/Sales			
	Total/Sales			
	Number of Units Shipped			
	Number of Units Setup			
	Number Warranty Units			
	Number of Recall Units			
	Warranty/Unit	$	$	$
	Recall/Unit	$	$	$
	Setup/Unit	$	$	$
	Total/Unit	$	$	$

Table 30-3   Warranty Analysis

The most important process in performing field failure analysis is focusing on the cause of the problem, based on the symptom. It does no good to develop a fix for a symptom, if the cause is not known. To do so only creates additional problems. Analysis techniques, such as fault tree analysis of FMEA may help to focus on the cause.

Once the component level analysis is completed, pareto charts may be made, highlighting problem areas and prioritizing problem solutions. The major problems can be placed in a spread sheet and monitored over time. Graphical plots can also be constructed to monitor various parameters over time.

30.3   Warranty Analysis

Warranty analysis is an indication of the reliability of a device in its early life, usually the first year. Warranty analysis (Table 30-3) is a valuable source of information on such parameters as warranty cost as a percentage of sales, warranty cost per unit, installation cost per unit and percentage of shipped units experiencing problems. By plotting this data, a trend can be established over time.

References

AAMI, *Guideline for Establishing and Administering Medical Instrumentation.* Arlington, VA: Association for the Advancement of Medical Instrumentation, 1984.

Fries, R. C. et. al., "A Reliability Assurance Database for Analysis of Medical Product Performance," in *Proceedings of the Symposium on e Engineering of Computer-Based Medical Systems.* New York: The Institute of Electrical and Electronic Engineers, 1988.

MIL-HDBK-472, *Maintainability Prediction*. Washington, DC: Department of Defense, 1966.

Section 6

Appendices

Appendix 1

Chi Square Table

$\upsilon\backslash\gamma$	0.975	0.950	0.900	0.050	0.100	0.050	0.025
1	0.001	0.004	0.016	0.455	2.706	3.841	5.024
2	0.051	0.103	0.211	1.386	4.605	5.991	7.378
3	0.216	0.352	0.584	2.366	6.251	7.815	9.348
4	0.484	0.711	1.064	3.357	7.779	9.488	11.143
5	0.831	1.145	1.610	4.351	9.236	11.070	12.832
6	1.237	1.635	2.204	5..348	10.645	12.592	14.449
7	1.690	2.167	2.833	6.346	12.017	14.067	16.013
8	2.180	2.733	3.490	7.344	13.362	15.507	17.535
9	2.700	3.325	4.168	8.343	14.684	16.919	19.023
10	3.247	3.940	4.865	9.342	15.987	18.307	20.483
11	3.816	4.575	5.578	10.341	17.275	19.675	21.920
12	4.404	5.226	6.304	11.340	18.549	21.026	23.337
13	5.009	5.892	7.042	12.340	19.812	22.362	24.736
14	5.629	6.571	7.790	13.339	21.064	23.685	26.119
15	6.262	7.261	8.547	14.339	22.307	24.996	27.488
16	6.908	7.962	9.312	15.338	23.542	26.296	28.845
17	7.564	8.672	10.085	16.338	24.769	27.587	30.191
18	8.231	9.390	10.865	17.338	25.989	28.869	31.526

υ\γ	0.975	0.950	0.900	0.050	0.100	0.050	0.025
19	8.907	10.117	11.651	18.338	27.204	30.144	32.852
20	9.591	10.851	12.443	19.337	28.412	31.410	34.170
21	10.283	11.591	13.240	20.337	29.615	32.671	35.479
22	10.982	12.338	14.041	21.337	30.813	33.924	36.781
23	11.688	13.091	14.848	22.337	32.007	35.172	38.076
24	12.401	13.848	15.659	23.337	33.196	36.415	39.364
25	13.120	14.611	16.473	24.337	34.382	37.652	40.646
26	13.844	15.379	17.292	25.336	35.563	38.885	41.923
27	14.573	16.151	18.114	26.336	36.741	40.113	43.194
28	15.308	16.928	18.939	27.336	37.916	41.337	44.461
29	16.047	17.708	19.768	28.336	39.087	42.557	45.722
30	16.791	18.493	20.599	29.336	40.256	43.773	46.979

Appendix 2

Percent Rank Tables

Sample Size = 1

Order Number	2.5	5.0	10.0	50.0	90.0	95.0	97.5
1	2.50	5.00	10.00	50.00	90.00	95.00	97.50

Sample Size = 2

Order Number	2.5	5.0	10.0	50.0	90.0	95.0	97.5
1	1.258	2.532	5.132	29.289	68.377	77.639	84.189
2	15.811	22.361	31.623	71.711	94.868	97.468	98.742

Sample Size = 3

Order Number	2.5	5.0	10.0	50.0	90.0	95.0	97.5
1	0.840	1.695	3.451	20.630	53.584	63.160	70.760
2	9.430	13.535	19.580	50.000	80.420	86.465	90.570
3	29.240	36.840	46.416	79.370	96.549	98.305	99.160

Sample Size = 4

Order Number	2.5	5.0	10.0	50.0	90.0	95.0	97.5
1	0.631	1.274	2.600	15.910	43.766	52.713	60.236
2	6.759	9.761	14.256	38.573	67.954	75.140	80.588
3	19.412	24.860	32.046	61.427	85.744	90.239	93.241
4	39.764	47.287	56.234	84.090	97.400	98.726	99.369

Sample Size = 5

Order Number	2.5	5.0	10.0	50.0	90.0	95.0	97.5
1	0.505	1.021	2.085	12.945	36.904	45.072	52.182
2	5.274	7.644	11.223	31.381	58.389	65.741	71.642
3	14.663	18.926	24.644	50.000	75.336	81.074	85.337
4	28.358	34.259	41.611	68.619	88.777	92.356	94.726
5	47.818	54.928	63.096	87.055	97.915	98.979	99.495

Sample Size = 6

Order Number	2.5	5.0	10.0	50.0	90.0	95.0	97.5
1	0.421	0.851	1.741	19.910	31.871	39.304	45.926
2	4.327	6.285	9.260	26.445	51.032	58.180	64.123
3	11.812	15.316	20.091	42.141	66.681	72.866	77.722
4	22.278	27.134	33.319	57.859	79.909	84.684	88.188
5	35.877	41.820	48.968	73.555	90.740	93.715	95.673
6	54.074	60.696	68.129	89.090	98.259	99.149	99.579

Sample Size = 7

Order Number	2.5	5.0	10.0	50.0	90.0	95.0	97.5
1	0.361	0.730	1.494	9.428	28.031	34.816	40.962
2	3.669	5.338	7.882	22.489	45.256	52.070	57.872
3	9.899	12.876	16.964	36.412	59.618	65.874	70.958
4	18.405	22.532	27.860	50.000	72.140	77.468	81.595
5	29.042	34.126	40.382	63.588	83.036	87.124	90.101
6	42.128	47.930	54.744	77.151	92.118	94.662	96.331
7	59.038	65.184	71.969	90.752	98.506	99.270	99.639

Sample Size = 8

Order Number	2.5	5.0	10.0	50.0	90.0	95.0	97.5
1	0.316	0.639	1.308	8.300	25.011	31.234	36.942
2	3.185	4.639	6.863	20.113	40.625	47.068	52.651
3	8.523	11.111	14.685	32.052	53.822	59.969	65.086
4	15.701	19.290	23.966	44.016	65.538	71.076	75.514
5	24.486	28.924	43.462	55.984	76.034	80.710	84.299
6	34.914	40.031	46.178	67.948	85.315	88.889	91.477
7	47.349	52.932	59.375	79.887	93.137	95.361	96.815
8	63.058	68.766	74.989	91.700	98.692	99.361	99.684

Sample Size = 9

Order Number	2.5	5.0	10.0	50.0	90.0	95.0	97.5
1	0.281	0.568	1.164	7.413	22.574	28.313	33.627
2	2.814	4.102	6.077	17.962	36.836	42.914	48.250
3	7.485	9.775	12.950	28.624	49.008	54.964	60.009
4	13.700	16.875	21.040	39.308	59.942	65.506	70.070
5	21.201	25.137	30.097	50.000	69.903	74.863	78.799
6	29.930	34.494	40.058	60.692	78.960	83.125	86.300
7	39.991	45.036	50.992	71.376	87.050	90.225	92.515
8	51.750	57.086	63.164	82.038	93.923	95.898	97.186
9	66.373	71.687	77.426	92.587	98.836	99.432	99.719

Sample Size = 10

Order Number	2.5	5.0	10.0	50.0	90.0	95.0	97.5
1	0.253	0.512	1.048	6.697	20.567	25.887	30.850
2	2.521	3.677	5.453	16.226	33.685	39.416	44.502
3	6.674	8.726	11.583	25.857	44.960	50.690	55.610
4	12.155	15.003	18.756	35.510	55.173	60.662	65.245
5	18.709	22.244	26.732	45.169	64.578	69.646	73.762
6	26.238	30.354	35.422	54.831	73.268	77.756	81.291
7	34.755	39.338	44.827	64.490	81.244	84.997	87.845
8	44.390	49.310	55.040	74.143	88.417	91.274	93.326
9	55.498	60.584	66.315	83.774	94.547	96.323	97.479
10	69.150	74.113	79.433	93.303	98.952	99.488	99.747

Sample Size = 11

Order Number	2.5	5.0	10.0	50.0	90.0	95.0	97.5
1	0.230	0.465	0.953	6.107	18.887	23.840	28.491
2	2.283	3.332	4.945	14.796	31.024	36.436	41.278
3	6.022	7.882	10.477	23.579	41.516	47.009	41.776
4	10.926	13.508	16.923	32.380	51.076	56.437	60.974
5	16.749	19.958	24.053	41.189	59.947	65.019	69.210
6	23.379	27.125	31.772	50.000	68.228	72.875	76.621
7	30.790	34.981	40.053	58.811	75.947	80.042	83.251
8	39.026	43.563	48.924	67.620	83.077	86.492	89.074
9	48.224	52.991	58.484	76.421	89.523	92.118	93.978
10	58.722	63.564	68.976	85.204	95.055	96.668	97.717
11	71.509	76.160	81.113	93.893	99.047	99.535	99.770

Sample Size = 12

Order Number	2.5	5.0	10.0	50.0	90.0	95.0	97.5
1	0.211	0.427	0.874	5.613	17.460	22.092	26.465
2	2.086	3.046	4.524	13.598	28.750	33.868	38.480
3	5.486	7.187	9.565	21.669	38.552	43.811	48.414
4	9.925	12.285	15.419	29.758	47.527	52.733	57.186
5	15.165	18.102	21.868	37.583	55.900	60.914	65.112
6	21.094	24.530	28.817	45.951	63.772	68.476	72.333
7	27.667	31.524	36.228	54.049	71.183	75.470	78.906
8	34.888	39.086	44.100	62.147	78.132	81.898	84.835
9	42.814	47.267	52.473	70.242	84.581	87.715	90.075
10	51.586	56.189	61.448	78.331	90.435	92.813	94.514
11	61.520	66.132	71.250	86.402	95.476	96.954	97.914
12	73.535	77.908	82.540	94.387	99.126	99.573	99.789

Sample Size = 13

Order Number	2.5	5.0	10.0	50.0	90.0	95.0	97.5
1	0.195	0.394	0.807	5.192	16.232	20.582	24.705
2	1.921	2.805	4.169	12.579	26.784	31.634	36.030
3	5.038	6.605	8.800	20.045	35.978	41.010	45.447
4	9.092	11.267	14.161	27.528	44.426	49.465	53.813
5	13.858	16.566	20.050	35.016	52.343	57.262	61.426
6	19.223	22.396	26.373	52.508	59.824	64.520	68.422
7	25.135	28.705	33.086	50.000	66.914	71.295	74.865
8	31.578	35.480	40.176	57.492	73.627	77.604	80.777
9	38.574	42.738	47.657	64.984	79.950	83.434	86.142
10	46.187	50.535	55.574	72.472	85.839	88.733	90.908
11	54.553	58.990	64.022	79.955	91.200	93.395	94.962

| 12 | 63.970 | 68.366 | 73.216 | 87.421 | 95.831 | 97.195 | 98.079 |
| 13 | 75.295 | 79.418 | 83.768 | 94.808 | 99.193 | 99.606 | 99.805 |

Sample Size = 14

Order Number	2.5	5.0	10.0	50.0	90.0	95.0	97.5
1	0.181	0.366	0.750	4.830	15.166	19.264	23.164
2	1.779	2.600	3.866	11.702	25.067	29.673	33.868
3	4.658	6.110	8.148	18.647	33.721	38.539	42.813
4	8.389	10.405	13.094	25.608	41.698	46.566	50.798
5	12.760	15.272	18.513	32.575	49.197	54.001	58.104
6	17.661	20.607	24.316	39.544	56.311	60.959	64.862
7	23.036	26.358	30.455	46.515	63.087	67.497	71.139
8	28.861	32.503	36.913	53.485	69.545	73.642	76.964
9	35.138	39.041	43.689	60.456	75.684	79.393	82.339
10	41.896	45.999	50.803	67.425	81.487	84.728	87.240
11	49.202	53.434	58.302	74.392	86.906	89.595	91.611
12	57.187	61.461	66.279	81.353	91.852	93.890	95.342
13	66.132	70.327	74.933	88.298	96.134	97.400	98.221
14	76.836	80.736	84.834	95.170	99.250	99.634	99.819

Sample Size = 15

Order Number	2.5	5.0	10.0	50.0	90.0	95.0	97.5
1	0.169	0.341	0.700	4.516	14.230	18.104	21.802
2	1.658	2.423	3.604	10.940	23.557	27.940	31.948
3	4.331	5.685	7.586	17.432	31.279	36.344	40.460
4	7.787	9.666	12.177	23.939	39.279	43.978	48.089
5	11.824	14.166	17.197	30.452	46.397	51.075	55.100
6	16.336	19.086	22.559	36.967	53.171	57.744	61.620
7	21.627	24.373	28.218	43.483	59.647	64.043	67.713
8	26.586	29.999	34.152	50.000	65.848	70.001	73.414
9	32.287	35.957	40.353	56.517	71.782	75.627	78.733
10	38.380	42.256	46.829	63.033	77.441	80.914	83.664
11	44.900	48.925	53.603	69.548	82.803	85.834	88.176
12	51.911	56.022	60.721	76.061	87.823	90.334	92.213
13	59.540	63.656	68.271	82.568	92.414	94.315	95.669
14	68.052	72.060	76.443	89.060	96.396	97.577	98.342
15	78.198	81.896	85.770	95.484	99.300	99.659	99.831

Sample Size = 16

Order Number	2.5	5.0	10.0	50.0	90.0	95.0	97.5
1	0.158	0.320	0.656	4.240	13.404	17.075	20.591
2	1.551	2.268	3.375	10.270	22.217	26.396	30.232
3	4.047	5.315	7.097	16.365	29.956	34.383	38.348
4	7.266	9.025	11.380	22.474	37.122	41.657	45.646
5	11.017	13.211	16.056	28.589	43.892	48.440	52.377
6	15.198	17.777	21.041	34.705	50.351	54.835	58.662
7	19.753	22.669	26.292	40.823	56.544	60.899	64.565
8	24.651	27.860	31.783	46.941	62.496	66.663	70.122
9	29.878	33.337	37.504	53.059	68.217	72.140	75.349
10	35.435	39.101	43.456	59.177	73.708	77.331	80.247
11	41.338	45.165	49.649	65.295	78.959	82.223	84.802
12	47.623	51.560	56.108	71.411	83.944	86.789	88.983
13	54.354	58.343	62.878	77.526	88.620	90.975	92.734
14	61.652	65.617	70.044	83.635	92.903	94.685	95.953
15	69.768	73.604	77.783	89.730	96.625	97.732	98.449
16	79.409	82.925	86.596	95.760	99.344	99.680	99.842

Sample Size = 17

Order Number	2.5	5.0	10.0	50.0	90.0	95.0	97.5
1	0.149	0.301	0.618	3.995	12.667	16.157	19.506
2	1.458	2.132	3.173	9.678	21.021	25.012	28.689
3	3.779	4.990	6.667	15.422	28.370	32.619	36.441
4	6.811	8.465	10.682	21.178	35.187	39.564	43.432
5	10.314	12.377	15.058	26.940	41.639	46.055	49.899
6	14.210	16.636	19.716	32.704	47.807	52.192	55.958
7	18.444	21.191	24.614	38.469	53.735	58.029	61.672
8	22.983	26.011	29.726	44.234	59.449	63.599	67.075
9	27.812	31.083	35.039	50.000	64.961	68.917	72.188
10	32.925	36.401	40.551	55.766	70.274	73.989	77.017
11	38.328	41.971	46.265	61.531	75.386	78.809	81.556
12	44.042	47.808	52.193	67.296	80.284	83.364	85.790
13	50.101	53.945	58.361	73.060	84.942	87.623	89.686
14	56.568	60.436	64.813	78.821	89.318	91.535	93.189
15	63.559	67.381	71.630	84.578	93.333	95.010	96.201
16	71.311	74.988	78.979	90.322	96.827	97.868	98.542
17	80.494	83.843	87.333	96.005	99.382	99.699	99.851

Sample Size = 18

Order Number	2.5	5.0	10.0	50.0	90.0	95.0	97.5
1	0.141	0.285	0.584	3.778	12.008	15.332	18.530
2	1.375	2.011	2.995	9.151	19.947	23.766	27.294
3	3.579	4.702	6.286	14.58`	26.942	31.026	34.712
4	6.409	7.970	10.064	20.024	33.441	37.668	41.418
5	9.695	11.643	14.177	25.471	39.602	43.888	47.637
6	13.343	15.634	18.549	30.921	45.502	49.783	53.480
7	17.299	19.895	23.139	36.371	51.184	55.405	59.007
8	21.530	24.396	27.922	41.823	56.672	60.784	64.255
9	26.019	29.120	32.885	47.274	61.980	65.940	69.243
10	30.757	34.060	38.020	52.726	67.115	70.880	73.981
11	35.745	39.216	43.328	58.177	72.078	75.604	78.470
12	40.993	44.595	48.618	63.629	76.861	80.105	82.701
13	46.520	50.217	54.498	69.079	81.451	84.336	86.657
14	52.363	56.112	60.398	74.529	85.823	88.357	90.305
15	58.582	62.332	66.559	79.976	89.936	92.030	93.591
16	65.288	68.974	73.058	85.419	93.714	95.298	96.421
17	72.706	76.234	80.053	90.849	97.005	97.989	98.625
18	81.470	84.668	87.992	96.222	99.416	99.715	99.859

Sample Size = 19

Order Number	2.5	5.0	10.0	50.0	90.0	95.0	97.5
1	0.133	0.270	0.553	3.582	11.413	14.587	17.647
2	1.301	1.903	2.835	8.678	18.977	22.637	26.028
3	3.383	4.446	5.946	13.827	25.651	29.580	33.138
4	6.052	7.529	9.514	18.989	31.859	35.943	39.578
5	9.147	10.991	13.394	24.154	37.753	41.912	45.565
6	12.576	14.747	17.513	29.322	43.405	47.580	51.203
7	16.289	18.750	21.832	34.491	48.856	52.997	56.550
8	20.252	22.972	26.327	39.660	54.132	58.194	61.642
9	24.447	27.395	30.983	44.830	59.246	63.188	66.500
10	28.864	32.009	35.793	50.000	64.207	67.991	71.136
11	33.500	36.812	40.754	55.170	69.017	72.605	75.553
12	38.358	41.806	45.868	60.340	73.673	77.028	79.748
13	43.450	47.003	51.144	65.509	78.168	81.250	83.711
14	48.797	54.420	56.595	70.678	82.487	85.253	87.424
15	54.435	58.088	62.247	75.846	86.606	89.009	90.853
16	60.422	64.057	68.141	81.011	90.486	92.471	93.948
17	66.682	70.420	74.349	86.173	94.054	95.554	96.617
18	73.972	77.363	81.023	91.322	97.165	98.097	98.699
19	82.353	85.413	88.587	96.418	99.447	99.730	99.867

Sample Size = 20

Order Number	2.5	5.0	10.0	50.0	90.0	95.0	97.5
1	0.127	0.256	0.525	3.406	10.875	13.911	16.843
2	1.235	1.807	2.691	8.251	18.096	21.611	24.873
3	3.207	4.217	5.642	13.147	24.477	28.262	31.698
4	5.733	7.135	9.021	18.055	30.419	34.366	37.893
5	8.657	10.408	12.693	22.967	36.066	40.103	43.661
6	11.893	13.955	16.587	27.880	41.489	45.558	49.105
7	15.391	17.731	20.666	32.795	46.727	50.782	54.279
8	19.119	21.707	24.906	37.711	51.803	55.803	59.219
9	23.058	25.865	29.293	42.626	56.733	60.642	63.946
10	27.196	30.195	33.817	47.542	61.525	65.307	68.472
11	31.528	34.693	38.475	52.458	66.183	69.805	72.804
12	36.054	39.358	43.267	57.374	70.707	74.135	76.942
13	40.781	44.197	48.197	62.289	75.094	78.293	80.881
14	45.721	49.218	53.273	67.205	79.334	82.269	84.609
15	50.895	54.442	58.511	72.120	83.413	86.045	88.107
16	56.339	59.897	63.934	77.033	87.307	89.592	91.343
17	62.107	65.634	69.581	81.945	90.979	92.865	94.267
18	68.302	71.738	75.523	86.853	94.358	95.783	96.793
19	75.127	78.389	81.904	91.749	97.309	98.193	98.765
20	83.157	86.089	89.125	96.594	99.475	99.744	99.873

Sample Size = 21

Order Number	2.5	5.0	10.0	50.0	90.0	95.0	97.5
1	0.120	0.244	0.500	3.247	10.385	13.295	16.110
2	1.175	1.719	2.562	7.864	17.294	20.673	23.816
3	3.049	4.010	5.367	12.531	23.405	27.055	30.377
4	5.446	6.781	8.577	17.209	29.102	32.921	36.342
5	8.218	9.884	12.062	21.891	34.522	38.441	41.907
6	11.281	13.245	15.755	26.574	39.733	43.698	47.166
7	14.588	16.818	19.619	31.258	44.771	48.739	52.175
8	18.107	20.575	23.632	35.943	49.661	53.594	56.968
9	21.820	24.499	27.779	40.629	54.416	58.280	61.565
10	25.713	28.580	32.051	45.314	59.046	62.810	65.979
11	29.781	32.811	36.443	50.000	63.557	67.189	70.219
12	34.021	37.190	40.954	54.686	67.949	71.420	74.287
13	38.435	41.720	45.584	59.371	72.221	75.501	78.180
14	43.032	46.406	50.339	64.057	76.368	79.425	81.893
15	47.825	51.261	55.229	68.742	80.381	83.182	85.412
16	52.834	56.302	60.267	73.426	84.245	86.755	88.719
17	58.093	61.559	65.478	78.109	87.938	90.116	91.782
18	63.658	67.079	70.898	82.791	91.423	93.219	94.554
19	69.623	72.945	76.595	87.469	94.633	95.990	96.951
20	76.184	79.327	82.706	92.136	97.438	98.281	98.825
21	83.890	86.705	89.615	96.753	99.500	99.756	99.880

Sample Size = 22

Order Number	2.5	5.0	10.0	50.0	90.0	95.0	97.5
1	0.115	0.233	0.478	3.102	9.937	12.731	15.437
2	1.121	1.640	2.444	7.512	16.559	19.812	22.844
3	2.906	3.822	5.117	11.970	22.422	25.947	29.161
4	5.187	6.460	8.175	16.439	27.894	31.591	34.912
5	7.821	9.411	11.490	20.911	33.104	36.909	40.285
6	10.729	12.603	15.002	25.384	38.117	41.980	45.370
7	13.865	15.994	18.674	29.859	42.970	46.849	50.222
8	17.198	19.556	22.483	34.334	47.684	51.546	54.872
9	29.709	23.272	26.416	38.810	52.275	56.087	59.342
10	24.386	27.131	30.463	43.286	56.752	60.484	63.645
11	28.221	31.126	34.619	47.762	61.119	64.746	67.790
12	32.210	35.254	38.881	52.238	65.381	68.874	71.779
13	36.355	39.516	43.248	56.714	69.537	72.869	75.614
14	40.658	43.913	47.725	61.190	73.584	76.728	79.291
15	45.128	48.454	52.316	65.666	77.517	80.444	82.802
16	49.778	53.151	57.030	70.141	81.326	84.006	86.135
17	54.630	58.020	61.883	74.616	84.998	87.397	89.271
18	59.715	63.091	66.896	79.089	88.510	90.589	92.179
19	65.088	68.409	72.106	83.561	91.825	93.540	94.813
20	70.839	74.053	77.578	88.030	94.883	96.178	97.094
21	77.156	80.188	83.441	92.488	97.556	98.360	98.879
22	84.563	87.269	90.063	96.898	99.522	99.767	99.885

Sample Size = 23

Order Number	2.5	5.0	10.0	50.0	90.0	95.0	97.5
1	0.110	0.223	0.457	2.969	9.526	12.212	14.819
2	1.071	1.567	2.337	7.191	15.884	19.020	21.949
3	2.775	3.652	4.890	11.458	21.519	24.925	28.038
4	4.951	6.168	7.808	15.734	26.781	30.364	33.589
5	7.460	8.981	10.971	20.015	31.797	35.493	38.781
6	10.229	12.021	14.318	24.297	36.626	40.390	43.703
7	13.210	15.248	17.816	28.580	41.305	45.098	48.405
8	16.376	18.634	21.442	32.863	45.856	49.644	52.919
9	19.708	22.164	25.182	37.147	50.291	54.046	57.226
10	23.191	25.824	29.027	41.431	54.622	58.315	61.458
11	26.820	29.609	32.971	45.716	58.853	62.461	65.505
12	30.588	33.515	37.012	50.000	62.988	66.485	69.412
13	34.495	37.539	41.147	54.284	67.029	70.391	73.180
14	38.542	41.685	45.378	58.569	70.973	74.176	76.809
15	42.734	45.954	49.709	62.853	74.818	77.836	80.292
16	47.081	50.356	54.144	67.137	78.558	81.366	83.624
17	51.595	54.902	58.695	71.420	82.184	84.752	86.790
18	56.297	59.610	63.374	75.703	85.682	87.979	89.771
19	61.219	64.507	68.203	79.985	89.029	91.019	92.540
20	66.411	69.636	73.219	84.266	92.192	93.832	95.049
21	71.962	75.075	78.481	88.542	95.110	96.348	97.225
22	78.051	80.980	84.116	92.809	97.663	98.433	98.929
23	85.151	87.788	90.474	97.031	99.543	99.777	99.890

Sample Size = 24

Order Number	2.5	5.0	10.0	50.0	90.0	95.0	97.5
1	0.105	0.213	0.438	2.847	9.148	11.735	14.247
2	1.026	1.501	2.238	6.895	15.262	18.289	21.120
3	2.656	3.495	4.682	10.987	20.685	23.980	26.997
4	4.735	5.901	7.473	15.088	25.754	29.227	32.361
5	7.132	8.589	10.497	19.192	30.588	34.181	37.384
6	9.773	11.491	13.694	23.299	35.246	38.914	42.151
7	12.615	14.569	17.033	27.406	39.763	43.469	46.711
8	16.630	17.796	20.493	31.513	44.160	47.873	51.095
9	18.799	21.157	24.058	35.621	48.449	52.142	55.322
10	22.110	24.639	27.721	39.729	52.461	56.289	59.406
11	25.553	28.236	31.476	43.837	56.742	60.321	63.357
12	29.124	31.942	35.317	47.946	60.755	64.244	67.179
13	32.821	35.756	39.245	52.054	64.683	68.058	70.876
14	36.643	39.679	43.258	56.163	68.524	71.764	74.447
15	40.594	43.711	47.359	60.271	72.279	75.361	77.890
16	44.678	47.858	51.551	64.379	75.942	78.843	81.201
17	48.905	52.127	55.840	68.487	79.507	82.204	84.370
18	53.289	56.531	60.237	72.594	82.967	85.431	87.385
19	57.849	60.086	64.754	76.701	86.306	88.509	90.227
20	62.616	65.819	69.412	80.808	89.503	91.411	92.868
21	67.639	70.773	74.246	84.912	92.527	94.099	95.265
22	73.003	76.020	79.315	89.013	95.318	96.505	97.344
23	78.880	81.711	84.738	93.105	97.762	98.499	98.974
24	85.753	88.265	90.852	97.153	99.562	99.787	99.895

Sample Size = 25

Order Number	2.5	5.0	10.0	50.0	90.0	95.0	97.5
1	0.101	0.205	0.421	2.735	8.799	11.293	13.719
2	0.984	1.440	2.148	6.623	14.687	17.612	20.352
3	2.547	3.352	4.491	10.553	19.914	23.104	26.031
4	4.538	5.656	7.166	14.492	24.802	28.172	31.219
5	6.831	8.229	10.062	18.435	29.467	32.961	36.083
6	9.356	11.006	13.123	22.379	33.966	37.541	40.704
7	12.072	13.948	16.317	26.324	38.331	41.952	45.129
8	14.950	17.030	19.624	30.270	42.582	46.221	49.388
9	17.972	20.238	23.032	34.215	46.734	50.364	53.500
10	21.125	23.559	26.529	38.161	50.795	54.393	57.479
11	24.402	26.985	30.111	42.108	54.722	58.316	61.335
12	27.797	30.513	33.774	46.054	58.668	62.138	65.072
13	31.306	34.139	37.514	50.000	62.486	65.861	68.694
14	34.928	37.862	41.332	53.946	66.226	69.487	72.203
15	38.665	41.684	45.228	57.892	69.889	73.015	75.598
16	42.521	45.607	49.205	61.839	73.471	76.441	78.875
17	46.500	49.636	53.266	65.785	76.968	79.762	82.028
18	50.612	53.779	57.418	69.730	80.736	82.970	85.050
19	54.871	58.048	61.669	73.676	83.683	86.052	87.928
20	59.296	62.459	66.034	77.621	86.877	88.994	90.644
21	63.917	67.039	70.533	81.565	89.938	91.771	93.169
22	68.781	71.828	75.198	85.508	92.834	94.344	95.462
23	73.969	76.896	80.086	89.447	95.509	96.648	97.453

| 24 | 79.648 | 82.388 | 85.313 | 93.377 | 97.852 | 98.560 | 99.016 |
| 25 | 86.281 | 88.707 | 92.201 | 97.265 | 99.579 | 99.795 | 99.899 |

Appendix 3

Glossary

ACCELERATED TESTING

> Testing at higher than normal stress levels to increase the failure rate and shorten the time to wearout.

ACCEPTABLE QUALITY LEVEL (AQL)

> The maximum percent defective that, for the purpose of sampling inspection, can be considered satisfactory for a process average.

ACCEPTANCE

> Sign-off by the purchaser.

ACTIVE REDUNDANCY

> That redundancy wherein all redundant items are operating simultaneously.

AMBIENT

> Used to denote surrounding, encompassing, or local conditions and is usually applied to environments.

ARCHIVING

> The process of establishing and maintaining copies of controlled items such that previous items, baselines and configurations can be re-established should there be a loss or corruption.

ASSESSMENT

> The review and auditing of an organization's Quality Management System to determine that it meets the requirements of the standards, that it is implemented, and that it is effective.

AUDITEE

> An organization to be audited.

AUDITOR

> A person who has the qualifications to perform quality audits.

BASELINE

> A definition of configuration status declared at a point in the project life cycle.

BURN-IN

> The operation of items prior to their end application to stabilize their characteristics and identify early failures.

CALIBRATION

> The comparison of a measurement system or device of unverified accuracy to a measurement system or device of known and greater

accuracy, to detect and correct any variation from required
performance specifications of the measurement system or device.

CERTIFICATION

The process which seeks to confirm that the appropriate minimum best
practice requirements are included and that the quality management
system is put into effect.

CERTIFICATION BODY

An organization which sets itself up as a supplier of product or process
certification against established specifications or standards.

CHANGE NOTICE
A document approved by the design activity that describes and
authorizes the implementation of an engineering change to the product
and its approved configuration documentation.

CHECKLIST

An aid for the auditor listing areas and topics to be covered by the
auditors.

CHECKSUM

The sum of every byte contained in an input/output record used for
assuring the integrity of the programmed entry.

CLIENT

A person or organization requesting an audit.

COMPLIANCE AUDIT

An audit where the auditor must investigate the Quality System, as put
into practice, and the organization's results.

CONDITIONING

> The exposure of sample units or specimens to a specific environment for a specified period of time to prepare them for subsequent inspection.

CONFIDENCE

> The probability that may be attached to conclusions reached as a result of application of statistical techniques.

CONFIDENCE INTERVAL

> The numerical range within which an unknown is estimated to be.

CONFIDENCE LEVEL

> The probability that a given statement is correct.

CONFIDENCE LIMITS

> The extremes of a confidence interval within which the unknown has a designated probability of being included.

CONFIGURATION

> A collection of items at specified versions for the fulfillment of a particular purpose.

CONTROLLED DOCUMENT

> Documents with a defined distribution such that all registered holders of control documents systematically receive any updates to those documents.

CORRECTIVE ACTION

All action taken to improve the overall Quality Management System as a result of identifying deficiencies, inefficiencies, and non-compliances.

CREEP

Continuous increase in deformation under constant or decreasing stress.

CRITICAL ITEM

An item within a configuration item which, because of special engineering or logistic considerations, requires an approved specification to establish technical or inventory control.

CYCLE

An ON/OFF application of power.

DEBUGGING

A process to detect and remedy inadequacies.

DEFECT

Any nonconformance of a characteristic with specified requirements.

DEGRADATION

A gradual deterioration in performance.

DELIVERY

Transfer of a product from the supplier to the purchaser.

DERATING

> The use of an item in such a way that applied stresses are below rated values.

DESIGN ENTITY

> An element of a design that is structurally and functionally distinct from other elements and that is separately named and referenced.

DESIGN REVIEW

> A formal, documented, comprehensive and systematic examination of a design to evaluate the design requirements and the capability of the design to meet these requirements and to identify problems and propose solutions.

DESIGN VIEW

> A subset of design entity attribute information that is specifically suited to the needs of a software project activity.

DEVIATION

> A specific written authorization, granted prior to manufacture of an item, to depart from a particular requirement(s) of an item's current approved configuration documentation for a specific number of units or a specified period of time.

DEVICE

> Any functional system, whether hardware, software, or a combination of the two.

DISCRETE VARIABLE

> A variable which can take only a finite number of values.

DOCUMENT

Contains information which is subject to change.

DOWN TIME

The total time during which the system is not in condition to perform
its intended function.

EARLY FAILURE PERIOD

An interval immediately following final assembly, during which the
failure rate of certain items is relatively high.

ENTITY ATTRIBUTE

A named characteristic or property of a design entity that provides a
statement of fact about the entity.

ENVIRONMENT

The aggregate of all conditions which externally influence the
performance of an item.

EXTERNAL AUDIT

An audit performed by a customer or his representative at the facility
of the supplier to assess the degree of compliance of the quality system
with documented requirements.

EXTRINSIC AUDIT

An audit carried out in a company by a third party organization or a
regulatory authority, to assess its activities against specific
requirements.

FAIL-SAFE

The stated condition that the equipment will contain self-checking features which will cause a function to cease in case of failure, malfunction, or drifting out of tolerance.

FAILURE

The state of inability of an item to perform its required function.

FAILURE ANALYSIS

Subsequent to a failure, the logical, systematic examination of any item, its construction, application, and documentation to identify the failure mode and determine the failure mechanism.

FAILURE MODE

The consequence of the mechanism through which the failure occurs.

FAILURE RATE

The probability of failure per unit of time of the items still operating.

FATIGUE

A weakening or deterioration of metal or other material, or of a member, occurring under load, specifically under repeated, cyclic or continuous loading.

FAULT

The immediate cause of a failure.

FAULT ISOLATION

The process of determining the location of a fault to the extent necessary to effect repair.

FEASIBILITY STUDY

The study of a proposed item or technique to determine the degree to which it is practicable, advisable, and adaptable for the intended

FIRMWARE

The combination of a hardware device and computer instructions or computer data that reside as read-only software on the hardware device.

FORM

The shape, size, dimensions, mass, weight, and other visual parameters which uniquely characterize an item.

GRADE

An indicator or category or rank relating to features or characteristics that cover different sets of needs for products or services intended for the same functional use.

INHERENT FAILURE

A failure basically caused by a physical condition or phenomenon internal to the failed item.

INHERENT RELIABILITY

Reliability potential present in the design.

INSPECTION

The examination and testing of supplies and services to determine whether they conform to specified requirements.

INSTALLATION

Introduction of the product to the purchaser's organization.

INTERNAL AUDIT

> An audit carried out within an organization by its own personnel to assess compliance of the quality system to documented requirements.

ITEM

> Any entity whose development is to be tracked.

MAINTAINABILITY

> The measure of the ability of an item to be retained in or restored to a specified condition when maintenance is performed by personnel having specified skill levels, using prescribed procedures and resources, at each prescribed level of maintenance and repair.

MAINTENANCE

> The servicing, repair, and care of material or equipment to sustain or restore acceptable operating conditions.

MAJOR NON-COMPLIANCE

> Either the non-implementation, within the quality system of a requirement of ISO 9001, or a breakdown of a key aspect of the system.

MALFUNCTION

> Any occurrence of unsatisfactory performance.

MANUFACTURABILITY

> The measure of the design's ability to consistently satisfy product goals, while being profitable.

MEAN TIME BETWEEN FAILURE (MTBF)

A basic measure of reliability for repairable items.

MEAN TIME TO FAILURE (MTTF)

A basic measure of maintainability.

MEAN TIME TO REPAIR (MTTR)

The sum of repair times divided by the total number of failures, during a particular interval of time, under stated conditions.

METHOD

A prescribed way of doing things.

METRIC

A value obtained by theoretical or empirical means in order to determine the norm for a particular operation.

MINIMUM LIFE

The time of occurrence of the first failure of a device.

MINOR NON-COMPLIANCE

A single and occasional instance of a failure to comply with the quality system.

MODULE

A replaceable combination of assemblies, subassemblies, and parts common to one mounting.

NON-COMPLIANCE

The non-fulfillment of specified requirements.

OBJECTIVE EVIDENCE

Qualitative or quantitative information, records, or statements of fact pertaining to the quality of an item or service or to the existence and the implementation of a quality system element, which is based on observation, measurement, or test, and which can be verified.

OBSERVATION

A record of an observed fact which may or may not be regarded as a non-compliance.

PARAMETER

A quantity to which the operator may assign arbitrary values, as distinguished from a variable, which can assume only those values that the form of the function makes possible.

PARSING

The technique of marking system or subsystem requirements with specified attributes in order to sort the requirements according to one or more of the attributes.

PERFORMANCE STANDARDS

Published instructions and requirements setting forth the procedures, methods, and techniques for measuring the designed performance of equipments or systems in terms of the main number of essential technical measurements required for a specified operational capacity.

PHASE

A defined segment of work.

POPULATION

The total collection of units being considered.

PRECISION

The degree to which repeated observations of a class of measurements conform to themselves.

PREDICTED

That which is expected at some future time, postulated on analysis of past experience and tests.

PREVENTIVE MAINTENANCE

All actions performed in an attempt to retain an item in specified condition by providing systematic inspection, detection, and prevention of incipient failures.

PROBABILITY

A measure of the likelihood of any particular event occurring.

PROBABILITY DISTRIBUTION

A mathematical model which represents the probabilities for all of the possible values a given discrete random variable may take.

PROCEDURES

Documents that explain the responsibilities and authorities related to particular tasks, indicate the methods and tools to be used, and may include copies of, or reference to, software facilities or paper forms.

PRODUCT

Operating system or application software including associated documentation, specifications, user guides, etc.

PROGRAM

The program of events during an audit.

PROTOTYPE

A model suitable for use in complete evaluation of form, design, and performance.

PURCHASER

The recipient of products or services delivered by the supplier.

QUALIFICATION

The entire process by which products are obtained from manufacturers or distributors, examined and tested, and then identified on a qualified products list.

QUALITY

The totality of features or characteristics of a product or service that bear on its ability to satisfy stated or implied needs.

QUALITY ASSURANCE

All those planned and systematic actions necessary to provide adequate confidence that a product or service will satisfy given requirements for quality.

QUALITY AUDIT

A systematic and independent examination to determine whether quality activities and related results comply with planned arrangements and whether these arrangements are implemented effectively and are suitable to achieve objectives.

QUALITY CONTROL

The operational techniques and activities that are used to fulfill requirements for quality.

QUALITY MANAGEMENT

That aspect of the overall management function that determines and implements quality policy.

A technique covering Quality Assurance and Quality Control aimed at ensuring defect free products.

QUALITY POLICY

The overall intention and direction of an organization regarding quality as formally expressed by top management.

Management's declared targets and approach to the achievement of quality.

QUALITY SYSTEM

The organizational structure, responsibilities, procedures, processes, and resources for implementing quality management.

RECORD

Provides objective evidence that the Quality System has been effectively implemented.

A piece of evidence that is *not* subject to change.

REDUNDANCY

Duplication, or the use of more than one means of performing a function in order to prevent an overall failure in the event that all but one of the means fails.

REGRESSION ANALYSIS

> The fitting of a curve or equation to data in order to define the functional relationship between two or more correlated variables.

RELIABILITY

> The probability that a device will perform a required function, under specified conditions, for a specified period of time.

RELIABILITY GOAL

> The desired reliability for the device.

RELIABILITY GROWTH

> The improvement a reliability parameter caused by the successful correction of deficiencies in item design or manufacture.

REPAIR

> All actions performed as a result of failure, to restore an item to a specified condition.

REVIEW

> An evaluation of software elements or project status to ascertain discrepancies from planned results and to recommend improvement.

REVIEW MEETING

> A meeting at which a work product or a set of work products are presented to project personnel, managers, users, customers, or other interested parties for comment or approval.

REVISION

> Any change to an original document which requires the revision level to be advanced.

RISK

The probability of making an incorrect decision.

SAFETY FACTOR

The margin of safety designed into the application of an item to insure that it will function properly.

SCHEDULE

The dates on which the audit is planned to happen.

SCREENING

A process of inspecting items to remove those that are unsatisfactory or those likely to exhibit early failure.

SERVICE LEVEL AGREEMENT

Defines the service to be provided and the parameters within which the service provider is contracted to service.

SHELF LIFE

The length of time an item can be stored under specified conditions and still meet specified requirements.

SIMULATION

A set of test conditions designed to duplicate field operating and usage environments as closely as possible.

SINGLE POINT FAILURE

The failure of an item which would result in failure of the system and is not compensated for by redundancy or alternative operational procedures.

SOFTWARE

> A combination of associated computer instructions and computer data definitions required to enable the computer hardware to perform computational or control functions.

SOFTWARE DESIGN DESCRIPTION

> A representation of a software system created to facilitate analysis, planning, implementation, and decision making.

> A blueprint or model of the software system.

SOURCE CODE

> The code in which a software program is prepared.

SPECIFICATION

> A document which describes the essential technical requirements for items, material, or services.

STANDARDS

> Documents that state very specific requirements in terms of appearance, formal and exact methods to be followed in all relevant cases.

STANDARD DEVIATION

> A statistical measure of dispersion in a distribution.

STANDBY REDUNDANCY

> That redundancy wherein the alternative means of performing the function is not operating until it is activated upon failure of the primary means of performing the function.

SUB-CONTRACTOR

The organization which provides products or services to the supplier.

SUPPLIER

The organization responsible for replication and issue of product.

The organization to which the requirements of the relevant parts of an ISO 9000 standard apply.

SYSTEM

A group of subsystems, including any required operator functions, which are integrated to perform a related operation.

SYSTEM COMPATIBILITY

The ability of the subsystems within a system to work together to perform the intended mission of the system.

TESTING

The process of executing hardware or software to find errors.

A procedure or action taken to determine, under real or simulated conditions, the capabilities, limitations, characteristics, effectiveness, reliability, and suitability of a material, device, or method.

TOLERANCE

The total permissible deviation of a measurement from a designated value.

TOOL

The mechanization of the method or procedure.

TOTAL QUALITY

A business philosophy involving everyone for continuously improving an organization's performance.

TRACEABILITY

The ability to track requirements from the original specification to code and test.

TRADE-OFF

The lessening of some desirable factor(s) in exchange for an increase in one or more other factors to maximize a system's effectiveness.

USEFUL LIFE PERIOD

The period of equipment life following the infant mortality period, during which the equipment failure rate remains constant.

VALIDATION

The process of evaluating a product to ensure compliance with specified and implied requirements.

VARIABLE

A quantity that may assume a number of values.

VARIANCE

A statistical measure of the dispersion in a distribution.

VARIANT

An instance of an item created to satisfy a particular requirement.

VERIFICATION

The process of evaluating the products of a given phase to ensure correctness and consistency with respect to the products and standards provided as input to that phase.

VERSION

An instance of an item or variant created at a particular time.

WEAROUT

The process which results in an increase in the failure rate or probability of failure with increasing number of life units.

WEAROUT FAILURE PERIOD

The period of equipment life following the normal failure period, during which the equipment failure rate increases above the normal rate.

WORK INSTRUCTIONS

Documents that describe how to perform specific tasks and are generally only required for complex tasks which cannot be adequately described by a single sentence or paragraph with a procedure.

WORST CASE ANALYSIS

A type of circuit analysis that determines the worst possible effect on the output parameters by changes in the values of circuit elements. The circuit elements are set at the values within their anticipated ranges which produce the maximum detrimental output changes.

Index

Accelerated testing, 638
Alarms, 380
Anthropometry, 376
Australian regulations, 150
Australian standards, 150

Biocompatibility, 395
Block diagram, 306
Breach of warranty, 518
Business proposal, 219

Canadian market, 133
CE mark, 103
Chinese regulations, 163
Chinese standards, 163
Coding, 346
Component derating, 314

Component selection, 310
Configuration audits, 698
Configuration metrics, 699
Configuration management, 348,
    693
Confidence level, 665
Confidence limits, 666
Conformity assessment, 60, 94
Copyrights, 536

Declaration of conformity, 102
    to recognized standards, 38
Defects, 520
Design
    changes, 320
    control, 11
    process, 139
    reviews, 322

[Design]
    specification, 234
Design for assembly, 683
Design for manufacturability, 682
Design for variation, 319, 448
Design history file (DHF), 250
Design of experiments, 319
Device classification. 5,22,91,137
Device history record (DHR), 253
Device master record (DMR), 252
Device regulation, 4
Dynamic testing, 610

Effectiveness, 134
Environmental protection, 317
Environmental testing, 631
Essential requirements, 78
European directives, 52
European Organization for Testing
    and Certification, 62
European regulations, 50
European standardization bodies,
    53
European standards development
    process, 55
Extracts, 406

Failure rate, 658
Failure to warn, 522
Field data, 715
Field service reports, 716
510(k)
    abbreviated, 36
    special, 34
    traditional, 26
Food and Drug Administration
    (FDA), 3
    inspection, 14

[Food and Drug Administration
    (FDA)]
    listing, 9
    registration, 9
    software standards, 171

Global Harmonization Task Force,
    69
Good Laboratory Practices (GLP),
    10
Good Manufacturing Practices
    (GMP), 10
Graphical analysis, 668

Hardware design, 305
Harmonized standards, 81
Hazards, 262
Hazard analysis, 266
Human factors, 11, 353
    process, 361

Implant registration, 141
Intellectual property, 527
Investigational device exemption,
    40
In vitro diagnostic devices (IVDD),
    142
ISO/IEC 12207, 174
ISO 9001, 107
    requirements, 110

Japanese regulations, 158
Japanese standards, 158

Labeling, 137, 383

Liability, 515
Load protection, 317

Manufacturing process, 686
Manuals, 456
Mean time between failures
    (MTBF), 659
Medical Device Directives, 75
    process, 77
Medical informatics, 67
Minimum life, 668
Mitigations, 262
Modeling techniques, 609

Negligence, 516
Notified body, 98

Patents, 528
Plumbing features, 146
Product definition process, 207
PMA, 38
Product misuse, 318
Product specification, 232
Programming language, 337

Quality, 420
Quality function deployment
    (QFD), 210
Quality system
    audit, 705
    regulation, 677
Redundancy, 306
Reliability, 419, 664
    prediction, 433
Risk analysis, 279
    matrix, 291

Risks, 262
Russian regulations, 162
Russian standards, 162

Safety, 134
    margin, 316
Safety requirements specification,
    301
Software
    architectural design, 343
    classification, 43
    configuration management, 348
    design, 327
    design method, 335
    design specification (SDS), 243
    development planning, 328
    development process model,
        330, 340
    engineering management, 328
    estimating, 338
    hazard analysis, 294, 341
    human factors, 385
    integration, 347
    quality assurance plan (SQAP),
        236
    regulations, 12
    requirements specification
        (SRS), 240, 340
    scheduling, 338
    standards history, 169
    standards organizations, 171
    validation, 601, 624
    verification, 601, 621
Specification review, 234
Status accounting, 701
Static verification, 604
Strict liability, 517
Sudden death testing, 642

Technical documentation file
    (TDF), 253
Test development, 588
Test execution, 597
Testing, 555
Test reporting, 597
Trademarks, 542
Trade secrets, 547
Translations, 495
Translator, 508
Type testing, 97

Unreliability, 420
User documentation, 451
User interface, 371

Validation, 579, 601, 624
Verification, 579, 601, 621

Warranty analysis, 721